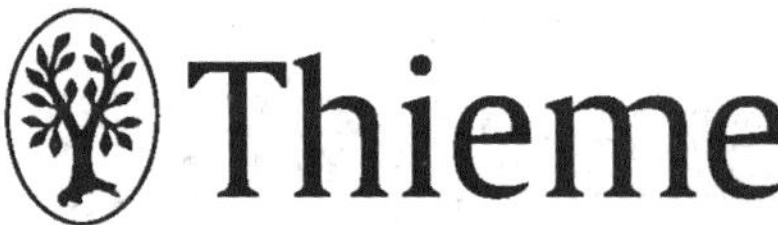
Thieme

Spinal Deformity Surgery

Tips from the Masters

Salman Sharif, FRCS (SN), FRCS (England)
President, World Spinal Column Society;
Chief of Neurosurgery
Liaquat National Hospital
Karachi, Pakistan

Nikolay Peev, MD, PhD (Neurosurgery), FRCS (England)
Consultant Neurosurgeon and Spinal Surgeon
Belfast Health and Social Care Trust
Belfast, UK

Michael Steinmetz, MD, FAANS
Prof & Chair, William P & Amanda C Madar Endowed
Cleveland Clinic Learner College of Medicine
Ohio, USA

Thieme
Delhi • Stuttgart • New York • Rio de Janeiro

Publishing Director: Ritu Sharma
Development Editor: Dr Ambika Kapoor
Director-Editorial Services: Rachna Sinha
Project Manager: Sumbul Jafri
Vice President Sales and Marketing: Arun Kumar Majji
Managing Director & CEO: Ajit Kohli

Thieme Medical and Scientific Publishers Private Limited.
A - 12, Second Floor, Sector - 2, Noida - 201 301, Uttar Pradesh, India, +911204556600
Email: customerservice@thieme.in
www.thieme.in

Cover design: © Thieme
Cover image source: © Thieme

Page make-up by RECTO Graphics, India

Printed in India by Nutech Print Services

5 4 3 2 1

ISBN: 978-93-90553-33-4
eISBN: 978-93-90553-41-9

Contents

Foreword

The specialty of "spinal surgery" is evolving into its surgical discipline stemming from orthopaedic surgery and neurosurgery contributions over the past several decades. However, traditionally, the subspecialty of spinal deformity surgery has been under the domain primarily of orthopaedic spinal surgeons both in the United States and around the world. But as further evidence of the disappearing delineation of pathways that spinal surgeons care for and surgically treat various patients, we have now a seminal textbook *Spinal Deformity Surgery: Tips from the Masters* edited by three prominent neurosurgical spinal surgeons from across the globe: Dr. Salman Sharif from Pakistan, Dr. Nikolay Peev from the United Kingdom, and Dr. Michael Steinmetz from the United States. This just further illustrates the cross-pollination of spinal surgery among the two specialties. In addition, this textbook is sponsored by the World Spinal Column Society, demonstrating the true international nature and participation of educational efforts of this global spine organization. So, it is truly inspiring how spinal surgery, and specifically the subspecialty of spinal deformity surgery, has progressed over the last 30 years that I have been in practice both from a collaboration of orthopaedic and neurosurgical spinal surgeons and the global cooperation of this society and all for the betterment of the patients that we treat.

In this comprehensive review of the current state-of-the-art of spinal deformity surgical care, the editors have assembled a global faculty to focus on conventional topics such as radiographic measurements and biomechanics as pertaining to spinal deformity patients, along with varying diagnostic groupings of deformity conditions such as adolescent idiopathic, congenital, neuromuscular, and degenerative scoliosis, and the not too uncommon problem of iatrogenic spinal deformity that occurs following previous degenerative and deformity operations. Lastly, specialty-specific chapters focusing on topics such as the role of limited surgery for these patients, use of spinal osteotomies, minimally invasive surgery, and controversial topics such as dynamic instrumentation for deformity conditions are expertly presented.

All of the chapters in the book are very well written, with "pearls" highlighted when appropriate throughout the text to help emphasize the salient points of the topics presented. I personally found three chapters especially detailed and educational (Chapters 9, 14, and 18).

I would like to congratulate Dr. Salman Sharif, Dr. Nikolay Peev, Dr. Michael Steinmetz, and all the contributing surgeon authors for their outstanding effort for this textbook. *Spinal Deformity Surgery: Tips from the Masters* will be an important reference and educational tool for both orthopaedic and neurosurgical trainees and practitioners of spinal deformity surgery in the coming years, and further elevates this highly specialized and challenging subspecialty of spinal surgery into a class of its own. I hope that this contribution will continue to optimize the care of patients suffering from various spinal deformities worldwide. For this, we owe a debt of gratitude to all who helped make this textbook a reality!

Lawrence G. Lenke, MD
Professor of Orthopaedic Surgery (In Neurological Surgery)
Chief of Spinal and Spinal Deformity Surgery
Columbia University Vagelos College of Physicians and Surgeons;
Surgeon-in-Chief
Och Spine Hospital at New York-Presbyterian/Allen
New York, USA

Preface

Spinal Deformity Surgery: Tips from the Masters covers all the essential topics, making it very appealing for both young and seasoned spine surgeons. This book epitomizes the mission of the World Spine, which is to advance spine care worldwide by connecting spine surgeons from across the globe, through high-quality education, training, and collaborative activities. It is funded by the World Spinal Column Society (WSCS) and written by 52 authors who hail from countries spanning four continents.

Over the past few decades, surgeons have gained a better understanding of the spine and learned a variety of treatment options, among which are different fixation procedures and devices. With these advancements come the need to understand the consequences of the different types of fixations. To date, a considerable amount of clinical and experimental data exists suggesting that fixation of a spinal section can provoke compensatory movements in the adjacent segments, thus changing the local and global biomechanics. Nowadays, applying the principles of spinal biomechanics in the treatment of spinal problems is believed to be a condition sine qua non, or essential, for immediate and long-lasting good outcomes of applied surgical procedures.

At a time when more and more surgeons are taking on deformity surgeries, this distinctive book, with its easy-to-read format and superb illustrations, provides an excellent insight into the various procedures performed by spine masters around the globe. Other than writing the tips and tricks of different procedures in every chapter, the authors have also included scientific evidence from recent landmark papers with a brief conclusion.

This book takes us through the history of spinal deformity and explains the techniques of radiographic measurements of the deformity, with examples of commonly seen deformities. It also has a chapter on biomechanics and the deformities associated with it. Harmony of curves in sagittal balance is a very important topic which is essential in ensuring patients have a better quality of life. Other than these exceptional topics, new and innovative chapters include the role of limited surgery in adult deformity, correction of the deformity using minimally invasive surgical techniques, lateral interbody fusion for degenerative scoliosis, cranial femoral traction in severe scoliosis, and dynamic instrumentation for deformity and osteotomies.

We would like to acknowledge Dr. Areeba Tariq, Dr. Muhammad Rafay, and Mr. Imad Ullah from the Department of Neurosurgery at Liaquat National Hospital & Medical College, Karachi, Pakistan for helping us in publishing this book.

We sincerely hope that this amazing book will help surgeons all over the world in providing the best possible treatment to patients with spinal problems.

Happy reading!

Salman Sharif, FRCS (SN), FRCS (England)
Nikolay Peev, MD, PhD (Neurosurgery), FRCS (England)
Michael Steinmetz, MD, FAANS

World Spinal Column Society

The World Spinal Column Society (WSCS) is a fast-growing society. Its mission is to advance spine care worldwide by connecting spine surgeons in advanced and emerging nations through high-quality education, training, and collaborative activities.

The WSCS is also an educational and scientific forum for the advancement of knowledge in the field of spine surgery and for the education of the patients, the clinicians, and the researchers. Our aim is to advance the science, art, and practice of spine surgery and promulgate the maintenance of professional standards in order to provide the best professional care to patients with spinal problems.

The WSCS holds meetings, conferences, live surgeries, and cadaver courses to provide sharing platforms for clinical and research members. We are proud of growing the number of members and participants to our meetings and invite you to work together with us to achieve the best in spine health care.

For more information about the WSCS, please visit www.worldspinalcolumn.org or email at info@worldspinalcolumn.org.

Presidents

Edward Benzel (2000–2005)
Luis Pimenta (2000–2005)
Mehmet Zileli (2007–2014)
Abdelfattah Saoud (2014–2016)
Sait Naderi (2016–2018)
Ioannis Polythodorakis (2018–2020)

Executive Committee (2020–2022)

President	Salman Sharif (Pakistan)
Vice President	Lilyana Angelov (USA)
Treasurer	Sandeep Vaishya (India)
Secretary	Paulo Pereira (Portugal)
Joint Secretary	Joachim Oertel (Germany)

Contributors

Abdelfattah Saoud, MD, PhD, FAANS/CNS
Professor of Orthopaedic & Spine Surgery;
Vice President for Education & Students' Affairs
Ain Shams University
Cairo, Egypt

Abhishek Mannem, MD
Clinical Fellow
VERTEBRA Unit European Back Institute-Polyclinic
Bordeaux Nord Aquitaine
Bordeaux, France

Adrian Kelly, FC Neurosurgery
Head of the Neurospine Department
Department of Neurosurgery
Dr George Mukhari Hospital, Sefako Makgatho
Health Sciences University
Pretoria, South Africa

Aftab Younus, FC Orthopaedics
Head of Orthopedic and Spine Surgery Department
Helen Joseph Hospital, University of the
Witwatersrand
Johannesburg, South Africa

Alexandra J. White, BA
Student
Cleveland Clinic Lerner College of Medicine of Case
Western Reserve University
Cleveland, Ohio, USA

Ali Fahir Ozer, MD
Professor of Neurosurgery
KOC University School of Medicine, Spine Center
Istanbul, Turkey

Amjad Shad, MBBS, FCPS, FRCS (SN)
Professor & Consultant Neurosurgeon
University Hospital Coventry
Coventry, UK

Areeba Tariq, MBBS
Resident
Department of Neurosurgery
Liaquat National Hospital & Medical College
Karachi, Pakistan

Arvind G. Kulkarni, MS, FCPS
Consultant Spine Surgeon
Mumbai Spine Scoliosis and Disc
Mumbai, Maharashtra, India

Assem Sultan, MD
Resident
Orthopaedic Surgery Department
Cleveland Clinic
Cleveland, Ohio, USA

Brian T. David, PhD
Assistant Professor
Department of Neurosurgery, Rush University
Medical Center
Chicago, Illinois, USA

Çağrı Canbolat, MD
Neurosurgery Specialist
Memorial Hizmet Hospital
Istanbul, Turkey

Davor Dasic, MD, MRCS Eng, FRCS (SN)
Registrar
Department of Neurosurgery
University Hospital Coventry and Warwickshire
Coventry, UK

Edward C. Benzel, MD
Chairman, Emeritus
Neurological Surgery
Cleveland Clinic Foundation
Cleveland, Ohio, USA

Emanuele Quarto, MD
Clinical Fellow
VERTEBRA Unit European Back Institute-Polyclinic
Bordeaux Nord Aquitaine
Bordeaux, France

Eric Momin, MD
Resident
Department of Neurosurgery
University of Wisconsin School of Medicine
Madison, Wisconsin, USA

Eric Schmidt, MD
Resident
Department of Neurosurgery
Cleveland Clinic of Case Western Reserve School of
Medicine
Cleveland, Ohio, USA

Fardad T. Afshari, MB BChir, MRCS, PhD
Registrar
Department of Neurosurgery
University Hospital Coventry and Warwickshire
Coventry, UK

Inyang Udo-Inyang, Jr., MD
Orthopedic Spine Surgeon
Orthopaedic Institute of Ohio
Lima, Ohio, USA

Jacob Hoffmann, MD
Attending consultant
Department of Orthopedic Surgery
Cleveland Clinic Akron General Hospital
Akron, Ohio, USA

Jason W. Savage, MD
Director, Spine Surgery Fellowship Program
Director, Adult Spinal Deformity Program
Cleveland Clinic;
Associate Professor of Surgery
Case Western Reserve University and Cleveland Clinic Lerner College of Medicine
Cleveland, Ohio, USA

Jean Charles Le Huec, MD, PhD
Professor and Spine Surgeon;
Chief of Spine Unit and Chairman of Department of Orthopaedic
VERTEBRA Unit European Back Institute-Polyclinic Bordeaux Nord Aquitaine
Bordeaux University Hospital
Bordeaux, France

Kemal Paksoy, MD
Neurosurgery Specialist
Department of Neurosurgery
Memorial Bahcelievler Hospital
Istanbul, Turkey

Kyle McGrath, BS
Student
Ohio University Heritage College of Osteopathic Medicine
Dublin, Ohio, USA

Laurent Balabaud, MD
Spine Surgeon
VERTEBRA Unit European Back Institute-Polyclinic
Bordeaux Nord Aquitaine
Bordeaux, France

Matthew H. Trawczynski, BA
Medical Student
Department of Neurosurgery
Rush University Medical Center
Chicago, Illinois, USA

Mehmet Zileli, MD
Professor
Department of Neurosurgery
Ege University Faculty of Medicine
Bornova, Izmir, Turkey

Michael McLarnon, MSc (Dist)
Medical Student (5th year)
Queen's University Belfast, School of Medicine
Belfast, UK

Michael Steinmetz, MD, FAANS
Prof & Chair, William P & Amanda C Madar Endowed
Cleveland Clinic Learner College of Medicine
Ohio, USA

Muhammad Tariq Imtiaz, MD
Consultant Physician
National Neurosciences Institute
King Fahad Medical City
Riyadh, Saudi Arabia

Muhammad Yassar Jazaib Ali, MBBS
Resident
Department of Neurosurgery
Liaquat National Hospital & Medical College
Karachi, Pakistan

Murat Korkmaz, MD
Assistant Professor of Orthopedics,
KOC University School of Medicine, Spine Center
Istanbul,Turkey

Nathaniel P. Brooks, MD
Associate Professor of Neurological Surgery
University of Wisconsin School of Medicine and Public Health
Madison, Wisconsin, USA

Nikolay Peev, MD, PhD (Neurosurgery), FRCS (England)
Consultant Neurosurgeon and Spinal Surgeon
Belfast Health and Social Care Trust
Belfast, UK

Noorulain Iqbal, MBBS
Resident
Department of Neurosurgery
The Walton Centre NHS Foundation Trust
Liverpool, UK

Onur Yaman, MD
Professor
Department of Neurosurgery
Memorial Bahcelievler Hospital
Istanbul, Turkey

Parmod Kumar Bithal, MD
Former Subspecialty Consultant
Neuroanesthesia, King Fahad Medical City
Riyadh, Saudi Arabia

Paul Page, MD
Resident
Department of Neurosurgery
University of Wisconsin School of Medicine
Madison, Wisconsin, USA

R. Douglas Orr, MD, FRCSC
Staff Physician
Center for Spine Health & Orthopedic Spine Surgeon
Lutheran Hospital, Cleveland Clinic
Cleveland, Ohio, USA

Richard G. Fessler, MD, PhD
Professor
Department of Neurosurgery
Rush University Medical Center
Chicago, Illinois, USA

Salman Sharif, FRCS (SN), FRCS (England)
President, World Spinal Column Society;
Chief of Neurosurgery
Liaquat National Hospital
Karachi, Pakistan

Sameer Ruparel, MS, DNB
Consultant Spine Surgeon
Gleneagles Global Hospital
Mumbai, Maharashtra, India

Stacey Darwish, MD
Consultant Orthopaedic Spine Surgeon
Mater Misericordiae University Hospital
Dublin, Ireland

Tansu Gürsoy, MD
Neurosurgery Specialist
Memorial Hizmet Hospital
Istanbul, Turkey

Taofiq D. Sanusi, BSc, MBBS, MSc, DIC, Pg Cert, MRCS, FRCS(SN), FEBNS
Post CCT Clinical Fellow
Neurosurgery Department
Royal Victoria Hospital
Belfast, UK

Thibault Cloché, MD
Spine Surgeon
VERTEBRA Unit European Back Institute-Polyclinic
Bordeaux Nord Aquitaine
Bordeaux, France

Tyler J. Calton, MD
Resident
Department of Orthopaedic surgery Cleveland Clinic Akron general
Ohio, USA

Vikram Chakravarthy, MD
Resident Physician
Neurological Surgery
Cleveland Clinic Foundation
Cleveland, Ohio, USA

Wendy Thompson, MD
Spine Surgeon
VERTEBRA Unit European Back Institute-Polyclinic
Bordeaux Nord Aquitaine
Bordeaux, France

William J. Kemp, MD
Resident Physician
Neurological Surgery
Cleveland Clinic Foundation
Cleveland, Ohio, USA

Yousuf Shaikh, FCPS
Sr. Registrar
Department of Neurosurgery
Liaquat National Hospital & Medical College
Karachi, Pakistan

Ziev B. Moses, MD
Clinical Fellow
Department of Neurosurgery
Rush University Medical Center
Chicago, Illinois, USA

1 History of Spinal Deformity Correction

Areeba Tariq, Yousuf Shaikh, and Salman Sharif

Introduction

Spinal deformity is one of the oldest diseases known to mankind. Throughout history of mankind, different methods to treat deformity have been found and new techniques are always emerging.

Presurgical Techniques

In earlier times, spinal deformity was considered a punishment from God and patients were left to die from deformity and its complications. The oldest record of deformity correction comes from Shrimad Bhagwat Mahapuranam, an Indian religious mythological book written somewhere between 3500 BC and 1800 BC, where Lord Krishna (a Hindu deity) treated a female devotee suffering from scoliosis by exerting pressure on her back with traction upward on her chin.[1] Earlier attempts to correct spinal deformity were mostly nonsurgical with use of external braces, traction, and casts.[2,3]

The first detailed description of anatomy and treatment of spine deformities comes from Hippocrates (460–370 BC),[4] who advocated the use of scamnum and succussion (shaking) methodologies for patients with such deformities. Both techniques involved traction and were not very successful (**Fig. 1.1**). Till the 16th century, most of the work done for deformity correction involved traction of some type. In the 15th and 16th centuries, Francis Glisson (1597–1677), Giovanni Alfonso Borelli (1608–1679), Nicholas Andry (1658–1759), and many others started using braces of different kinds for deformed spine.

Pearl

Traction and manipulation were the first and most commonly employed primitive techniques for deformity correction. These were not very successful. Different kinds of braces for deformed spine were in use in the 15th and 16th centuries.

Surgical Techniques

Initial surgical attempts to treat scoliosis were reported in the mid- to late 19th century. Prior to the 20th century, it was believed that scoliosis, regardless of origin, was caused by poor posture. Thus, most attempts to resolve this deformity were aimed at correcting posture by one way or another.

Prefusion to Fusion Era

Jules Rene Guerin (1801–1886), a French orthopaedic, performed percutaneous myotomies of the vertebral musculature accompanied by postoperative bracing for scoliosis.[5] This was the first step in direction of surgical management of deformity. In 1891, Hadra attempted wiring of the spinous processes in a patient with Pott disease (having progressive deformity) and successfully stabilized the spinal fracture.[6] In 1902, Fritz Lange, attempted internal fixation on a spondylitis patient with a hunch-back deformity.[7] He used 4-mm-thick steel rods under the muscles on either side of the spine and tied them on the upper and the lower ends with silver wires. Although the steel rods remained intact, abscess formation routinely occurred at the ends where the silver wires were

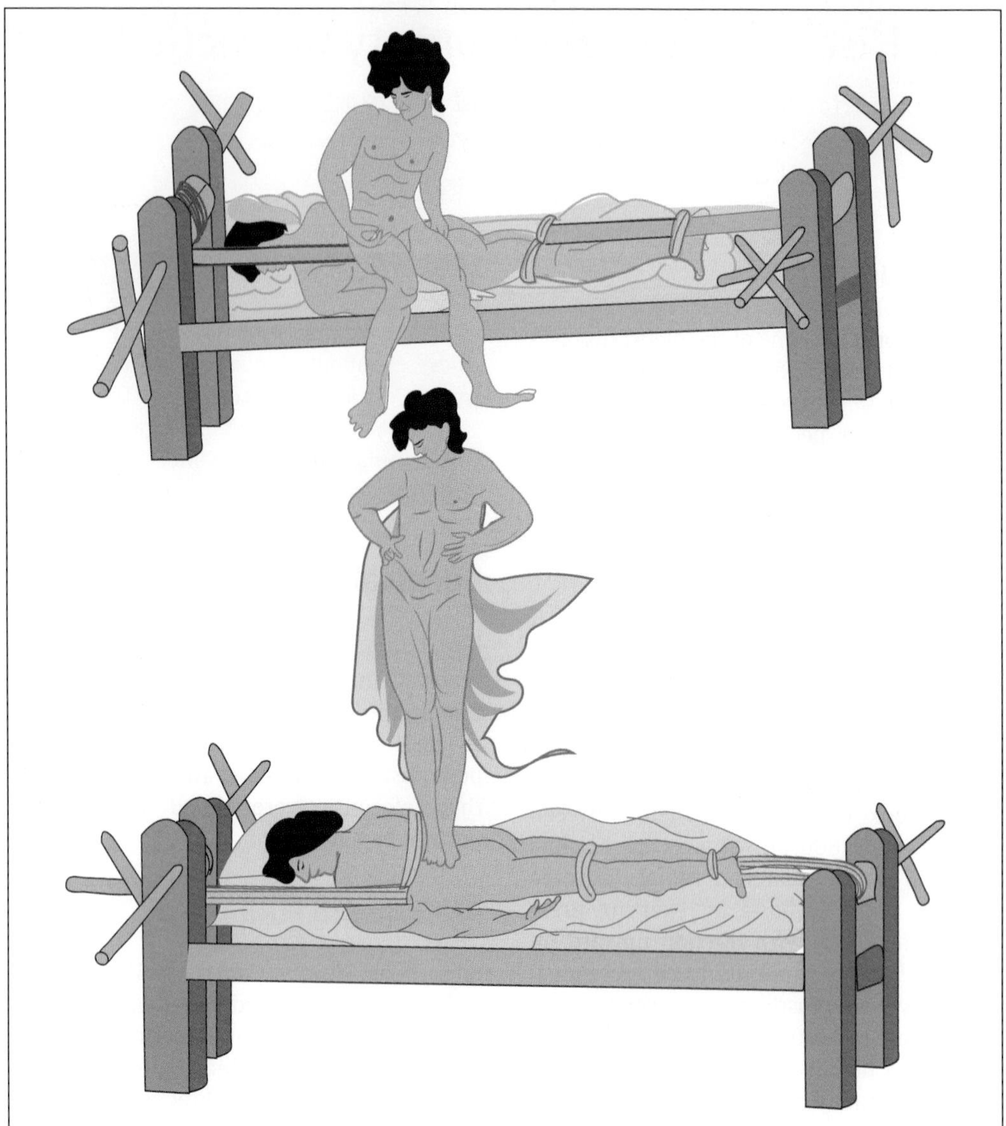

Fig. 1.1 Hippocrates advised the use of pressure and traction to correct deformities.

secured. After 6 years, in 1908, he performed the same procedure using 5-mm-diameter and 10-cm-length rods. At this time, he used wires with tin knobs at the ends to attempt to reduce the irritation. This made other surgeons use internal fixation for deformed spine due to polio and tuberculosis.

Russel Hibbs (1869–1933) is credited with performing the first true spinal fusion, in 1911. He was the first person who described the concept of promoting fusion in spine and routinely used spinous process and other autologous bone grafts on a tuberculous spine.[3,8] He would fracture the lamina and spinous process and bring them close together. Patients were postoperatively kept in a brace until fusion was achieved. Based on his results, he concluded that fusion was the only logical means to arrest spinal deformity. This landmark claim to achieve fusion was widely accepted among the surgeons and many different types of bone autografts were explored in this regard. Fred Albee used Tibia whereas de Quervain used scapular spine for autograft.[9] Many modifications followed, and the application of such techniques further extended to patients with trauma or degenerative pathologies. Gallie, in 1915, used boiled human allograft bone to achieve fusion, and Forbes recommended multisectioning of the spinous processes of the lumbar spine. Rib grafting was also favored by many surgeons, thus adding to pool of different surgical fusion procedures available for deformity correction.[10]

Pearl

Russel Hibbs first introduced the concept of spinal fusion by using bone graft and concluded that the fusion was the only logical means to arrest spinal deformity.

Up to this point, all these fusion surgeries were performed through a posterior approach. The first ever anterior approach was attempted by William von Lackum in 1924. However, due to poor results and postoperative kyphosis, the procedure was subsequently abandoned.[5]

Joseph Risser (in 1920), along with Hibbs, introduced a body jacket that provided more effective correction for lumbar curves than surgery alone.[11] In 1952, a localizer cast was introduced, which allowed early ambulation of the patient, later referred to as the Risser cast.[12] Risser also developed the Risser sign; according to which the excursion of ossification of the iliac epiphysis occurred sequentially from the anterolateral margin of each ilium. By the time the ossification reached the ilium at the iliosacral junction, vertebral growth was presumed to have terminated. This radiological feature was appreciated in anteroposterior X-rays of spine and was used as a marker of skeletal growth arrest. This subsequently helped in timing the surgical intervention as it is often dictated by whether further longitudinal skeletal growth is anticipated or not.[13]

Vertebral resection operations came into existence in 1932. Compere[14] was the first to report having performed hemivertebral resection in two patients. But due to unfavorable results, the procedure was not recommended by Compere. Another attempt with dorsal wedge resection of vertebra was performed by Philip Wiles in 1941. His approach was the first ever to address kyphotic deformity and not just coronal. However, yet again the results were poor and only two procedures were done by him.[15]

Paul Harrington is well known for his internal fixation treatment of scoliosis. He initially attempted to put screws in facet joints to arrest deformity progression, but the results were short lived. He subsequently used a distraction rod which was made of steel and was secured with hooks on the vertebra. Since this fixation technique was not supplemented by fusion, yet again the results were disappointing. But, with the addition of fusion techniques, the results improved[16,17] (**Fig. 1.2**).

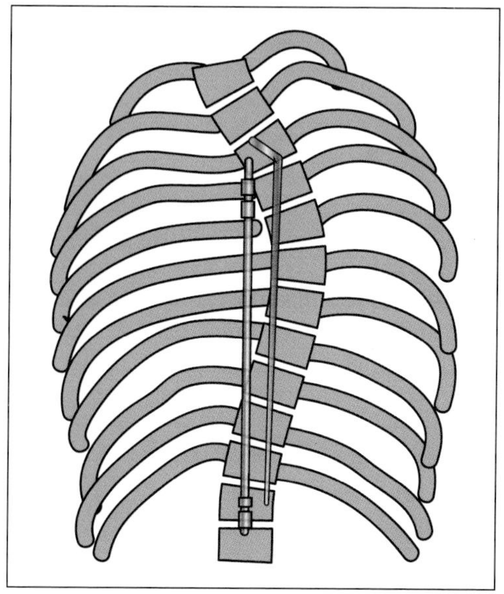

Fig. 1.2 Harrington rod held in place by wires.

Pearl

Paul Harrington first used Harrington rods in an attempt to correct deformity, which were later improved by adding fusion techniques.[16,17]

In 1964, Allen Dwyer became the first successful surgeon to have used an anterolateral approach to treat scoliosis by using internal fixation.[18] He performed staged surgeries consisting of a posterior release, followed by an instrumented anterior curve correction. He inserted titanium screws into the vertebral body on the convex side and with the aid of plates over these screws, a titanium cable was threaded through the screw heads, and the distance shortened between the screws by a tensioning device. By continuing this process down each level of the spine, a bent column would become straighter. His patients wore a jacket to restrict movement for up to 3 months postoperatively. Most of the patients had deformity corrected this way but had atelectasis and pneumothorax as common complications.

Pearl

Allen Dwyer first performed successful anterior approach to spinal deformity, by stage posterior release followed by anterior curve correction.[17]

Zielke instrumentation (ventral derotation spondylodesis [VDS]) was introduced in 1976 as a modification for Dwyer's procedure and served as a foundation for further developments.[19,20] The results of deformity correction were much better with Zielke instrumentation as compared to Dwyer instrumentation for similar curves. In VDS, the screws were placed more posteriorly through the vertebral bodies. This not only helped in correction of scoliosis, but also derotated the spine[20] (**Fig. 1.3**).

Yves Cotrel and Jean Dubousset described the Cotrel-Dubousset (CD) instrumentation in 1988.[21] It was a segmental instrumentation of the spine designed to facilitate selective and three-dimensional correction of spinal deformities. The goal of this system was to combine the rigidity of segmental fixation with curve derotation to obtain correction. The system comprised of pedicular screws and laminar hooks which were secured on to rods. This also marked the first use of pedicle screws, described in vertebral fusion operations, for scoliosis. In addition, the rods were fixed to each other using the device for transverse traction. This formed a frame of construct and was thought to diminish rotational and torsional forces. The results of this technique were very promising.

Since the Zielke instrumentation was successful in addressing both coronal and sagittal deformity, multiple modifications were made to the basic approach. The Texas Scottish Rite Hospital system of anterior instrumentation was introduced which used two rods.[22] This made the construct much more rigid, which was less prone to fracture. The instruments consisted of the vertebral body screws with adjunctive staples and a rod with a hexagonal end. The hexagonal end eliminated the use of an outrigger device application and facilitated better visualization of the surgical field.

As placement of lumbar pedicle screws became increasingly common, it was time to utilize them for thoracic spine. For a

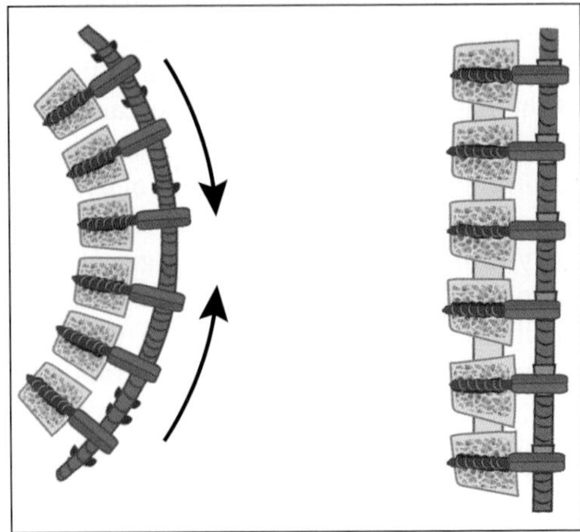

Fig. 1.3 Zielke instrumentation technique to correct scoliosis.

very long time, transpedicular approach to thoracic spine was considered difficult or impractical due to risk of spinal cord injury or small pedicles. But with time, smaller screws and utilization of rib head were done. Connecting two to three screws with rod was an easy task. But problems arose when long constructs with monoaxial screws were attached to the rod. This was not only difficult but time consuming as well. Development of polyaxial head screws significantly improved the ease of connection of screws to the rods. Most recently, uniaxial, pedicle screws have been developed to attempt to improve three-dimensional balance, allowing motion in the sagittal plane but not in the coronal plane. This design allows for improved coronal plane correction while preserving sagittal plane alignment.

Table 1.1 and **Fig. 1.4** depict milestones in the history of deformity correction.

Pearl

Polyaxial pedicle screws now represent the backbone for majority of spinal deformity correction.

The Future

As further work is done on internal fixation, new techniques of spinal fusion have been developed. Thoracoscopic releases, performed anteriorly, can allow for a less invasive method to effect curve correction.[24] Additional minimally invasive surgical procedures have been recently introduced for spinal deformity. The use of percutaneous pedicle screw instrumentation in deformity surgery is now being performed by increasing the number of surgeons. Minimally invasive techniques are known to reduce intraoperative blood loss, postoperative pain, as well as shorten hospital stay. These methods were long ignored by surgeons owing to technical difficulties, larger learning curve, and longer operating times. However, as experience has increased, operating times are now comparable between the open and minimally invasive groups. Since the advent of minimally invasive techniques, tubular approaches are used to achieve lumbar interbody fusion. Complete facetectomies are performed with distraction of intervertebral disc space for placement of larger grafts or cages. This also

Table 1.1 Landmarks in deformity surgery[22]

Surgical era		
1902	Fritz Lange	Internal fixation using 4 mm steel rods under muscles and tied them with silver wires
1911	Russel Hibbs	First describes the concept of fusion using spinous process and lamina
1924	William von Lackum	Describes two-stage surgery with first ever anterior approach
1941	Philip Wiles	First ever dorsal wedge resection of vertebra to address kyphotic deformity
1955	F.G. Allen	Devised a “Jack,” surgically implanted expandable rod
1962	Paul Harrington	Used threaded compression rod and distraction bar that used hooks
1964	Allen Dwyer	First to perform staged posterior followed by anterior approach
1976	Klaus Zielke	Optimized Dwyer approach with ventral derotation spondylodesis rod
1988	Yves Cotrel	First ever use of pedicle screws and hooks to hold rods for fixation
2001	L. Pimenta	Extreme Lateral Interbody Fusion (XLIF) technique which was true lateral retroperitoneal approach

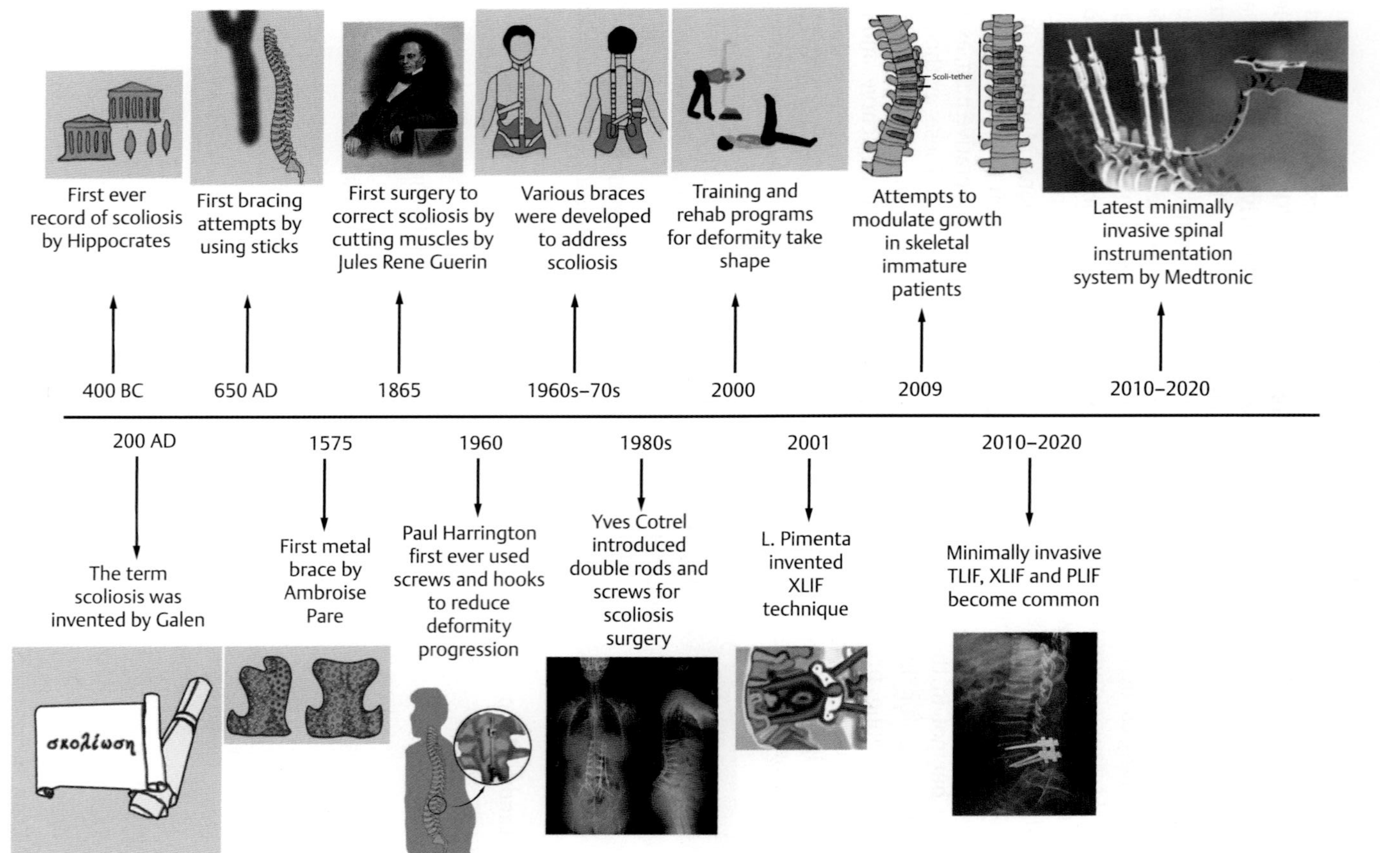

Fig. 1.4 Milestones in the history of deformity correction.

significantly improved neurological outcome attributed to no dural traction while placement of cages. Fusion is then subsequently achieved by adding bone graft over the entire construct.

The first ever percutaneous lumbar pedicle screw was placed by Matthews and Long in 1995.[25] He used plates to connect the screws which were placed over dorsolumbar fascia. This form of instrumentation was slightly modified by Lowery et al in 2000 when he used rods instead of plates to connect the adjacent screws.[26] But because the construct was kept above the fascia, it led to significant postoperative pain which necessitated its removal. A major breakthrough came in 2002 when Foley and Gupta introduced Sextant manufactured by Medtronic.[26] This was a complete instrumentation set that allowed percutaneous pedicle screw fixation, end-plate curettage, distraction, compression, and rod placement. Since then, many such systems have been introduced with the latest offering of CDH Longitude by Medtronic that allows placement of contoured rods up to six spinal segments. There have been numerous studies where the adequacy of neural decompression was compared between minimally invasive and open techniques. This led to innovation of hybrid procedures where screws are placed minimally invasive but a midline incision is given to perform complete laminectomy and facetectomy. Irrespective of the technique used, the basic idea remained same which was to achieve fusion rather than just fixation. Another newer potentially promising innovation for spinal deformity is the Extreme Lateral Interbody Fusion (XLIF) technique, initially described by Pimenta in 2001.[28] The XLIF procedure is a true lateral approach, through the retroperitoneal space, to access the lumbar intervertebral disc space. Recently hybrid procedures are also becoming common. These include open and minimally invasive techniques, such as lateral transpsoas fusions and/or mini-open transforaminal lumbar interbody fusion (TLIF), followed by posterior laminectomy and/or osteotomies.

No matter what technique is used, all constructs are bound to eventually fail if a solid bony arthrodesis cannot be achieved.[5] The use of autologous bone grafting has been considered the gold standard in the deformity surgeries; however, it comes with price of donor site morbidity. Consequently, alternative graft preparations that do not have this adverse effect are being continually sought, and demineralized bone matrix, ceramics composed of tricalcium phosphate, hydroxyapatite, and bone morphogenic proteins (BMP) among many other compounds have been used for this purpose.

Another development in deformity correction is the use of intraoperative monitoring to prevent neurological injury. Previously, somatosensory-evoked potentials (SSEPs) were used,[29] but, recently, use of motor-evoked potential (MEP) have improved monitoring. The type of MEP monitoring most often used in the present-day clinical setting is transcranial magnetic cortical stimulation MEP monitoring.[30]

Conclusion

The history of spinal deformity correction is interesting and reflects the quest for development of newer techniques to treat a disorder. Today's surgeon is equipped with better techniques and instruments for correction of deformity and further advancements welcome new techniques that can shorten intraoperative timing and recovery time, increase early mobility, and decrease complications.

References

1. Kumar K. Spinal deformity and axial traction. Spine 1996;21(5):653–655
2. Byrd JA III. Current theories on the etiology of idiopathic scoliosis. Clin Orthop Relat Res 1988; (229):114–119

3. Cho SK, Kim YJ. History of spinal deformity surgery part I: The Pre-modern Era. Korean J Spine 2011;8(8):1–8
4. Marketos SG, Skiadas P. Hippocrates. The father of spine surgery. Spine 1999;24(13): 1381–1387
5. Hall JE. Spinal surgery before and after Paul Harrington. Spine 1998;23(12):1356–1361
6. Hadra BE. The classic: Wiring of the vertebrae as a means of immobilization in fracture and Potts' disease. Berthold E. Hadra. Med Times and Register, Vol 22, May 23, 1891. Clin Orthop Relat Res 1975; (112):4–8
7. The classic. Support for the spondylitic spine by means of buried steel bars, attached to the vertebrae. By Fritz Lange. 1910. Clin Orthop Relat Res 1986; (203):3–6
8. Howorth MB. Evolution of spinal fusion. Ann Surg 1943;117(2):278–289
9. de Quervain FJ, Hoessly H. Operative immobilization of the spine; 1917
10. Tarpada SP, Morris MT, Burton DA. Spinal fusion surgery: a historical perspective. J Orthop 2016;14(1):134–136
11. Risser JC. The application of body casts for the correction of scoliosis. Instr Course Lect 1955;12:255–259
12. Risser JC. Scoliosis: past and present. J Bone Joint Surg Am 1964;46(1):167–199
13. Risser JC. Treatment of scoliosis during the past 50 years. Clin Orthop Relat Res 1966; 44(44):109–113
14. Compere EL. Excision of hemivertebrae for correction of congenital scoliosis. J Bone Joint Surg 1932; 14:555 -562
15. Wiles P. Resection of dorsal vertebrae in congenital scoliosis. J Bone Joint Surg Am 1951;33 A(1):151–154
16. Dickson JH, Harrington PR. The evolution of the Harrington instrumentation technique in scoliosis. J Bone Joint Surg Am 1973; 55(5):993–1002
17. Harrington PR. Treatment of scoliosis. Correction and internal fixation by spine instrumentation. J Bone Joint Surg Am 1962; 44-A(4):591–610
18. Dwyer AF, Newton NC, Sherwood AA. An anterior approach to scoliosis. A preliminary report. Clin Orthop Relat Res 1969;62(62): 192–202
19. Halm HF, Liljenqvist U, Niemeyer T, Chan DP, Zielke K, Winkelmann W. Halm-Zielke instrumentation for primary stable anterior scoliosis surgery: operative technique and 2-year results in ten consecutive adolescent idiopathic scoliosis patients within a prospective clinical trial. Eur Spine J 1998;7(5): 429–434
20. Moe JH, Purcell GA, Bradford DS. Zielke instrumentation (VDS) for the correction of spinal curvature. Analysis of results in 66 patients. Clin Orthop Relat Res 1983; (180):133–153
21. Cotrel Y, Dubousset J, Guillaumat M. New universal instrumentation in spinal surgery. Clin Orthop Relat Res 1988;227(227):10–23
22. Bischoff R, Bennett JT, Stuecker R, Davis JM, Whitecloud TS III. The use of Texas Scottish-Rite instrumentation in idiopathic scoliosis. A preliminary report. Spine 1993;18(16): 2452–2456
23. Heary RF, Madhavan K. The history of spinal deformity. Neurosurgery 2008; 63(3, Suppl): 5–15
24. McAfee PC, Regan JR, Zdeblick T, et al. The incidence of complications in endoscopic anterior thoracolumbar spinal reconstructive surgery. A prospective multicenter study comprising the first 100 consecutive cases. Spine 1995;20(14):1624–1632
25. Matthews HH, Long BH. Endoscopy assisted percutaneous anterior interbody fusion with subcutaneous suprafascial internal fixation: evolution of technique and surgical considerations. Orthop Int. 1995;3:496–500
26. Lowery GL, Kulkarni SS. Posterior percutaneous spine instrumentation. Eur Spine J 2000; 9(1, Suppl 1):S126–S130
27. Foley KT, Gupta SK. Percutaneous pedicle screw fixation of the lumbar spine: preliminary clinical results. J Neurosurg 2002; 97(1, Suppl):7–12
28. Pimenta L. Lateral endoscopic transpsoas retroperitoneal approach for lumbar spine surgery. 2001; In: Paper Presented at: VIII Brazilian Spine Society Meeting .
29. Nash CL Jr, Lorig RA, Schatzinger LA, Brown RH. Spinal cord monitoring during operative treatment of the spine. Clin Orthop Relat Res 1977; (126):100–105
30. Edmonds HL Jr, Paloheimo MP, Backman MH, Johnson JR, Holt RT, Shields CB. Transcranial magnetic motor evoked potentials (tcMMEP) for functional monitoring of motor pathways during scoliosis surgery. Spine 1989; 14(7):683–686

2 Radiographic Measurements of Spinal Deformity

Noorulain Iqbal, Salman Sharif, and Onur Yaman

Introduction

The spine is composed of parts with different alignment and biomechanical properties, which collectively contribute to global alignment. Although the regional spinal curves may vary occiput to the pelvis in different individuals, global spinal alignment is maintained in a narrower range. This is mandatory for maintaining the spine's horizontal gaze and balance over the pelvis and femoral heads.

Spinal deformities are deviations from the normal alignment of the spine. Spinal alignment is evaluated clinically and radiographically. The chapter discusses the different radiological measurements of spinal alignment.

Vertebral Labeling

The key to vertebral labeling is following a consistent numbering of the vertebras. It is essential to differentiate between normal and abnormal spinal alignment. O'Brien et al[1] described how a clear understanding of deformity's normal and altered anatomy has significant implications. This is crucial for the effective interpretation of radiographic images and formulation of surgical plans.[1] Although numbering vertebras can look reasonably straightforward, the challenge is labeling the vertebras on a spine with a deformity. The steps of labeling the vertebras are explained in **Box 2.1**.

Box 2.1 The steps for labeling the vertebras are as follows

- Start at the first vertebra with ribs and label that T1
- Continue labeling vertebra until the last one with ribs is identified (T11, T12, T13)
- If there are 11 definite ribs with 6 vertebras below and it is not clear if the 12th vertebra has a rib, call it T12, and label the 5 lumbar vertebras below
- The first vertebra below the last vertebra with ribs is considered L1, in all other cases
- L5 junctions are reviewed for lumbarization or sacralization
- A sacralized L5 requires measurement of coronal and sagittal Cobbs to S1, as well as a sagittal balance from C7 to S1

Pearl

When classifying the curve type, choosing the surgical approach and instrumentation system, and defining the ideal level of fusion, the apex of the curve and significant vertebrae must be known.[2]

Identification of Types of Curves and Significant Vertebras

Major and minor structural curves characterize deformities of the spine. Their location, magnitude, and flexibility define structural curves. The first step to assess any deformity is to classify the structure as scoliotic, kyphotic, lordotic, scoliokyphotic, or scoliolordotic. The major and minor structural curves form a pattern further defining the spinal deformity. The curve's location can be identified by where the apex of the curve is located (**Table 2.1**).

Pearl

Using a two-dimensional radiographic image of a three-dimensional deformity for measuring the Cobb angle has limitations because it does not take vertebral rotation into account. However, it is still the gold standard for diagnosis, monitoring, therapeutic planning, and epidemiologic analysis of scoliosis.

The *apex* of the curve is defined as the vertebra or intervertebral disc that is maximally laterally displaced and minimally angulated, as shown in **Fig. 2.1a**. *End vertebrae* are the most rostral and caudal vertebrae that tilt the most into the concavity of the curve, which is used to measure the Cobb angle (**Fig. 2.1b**). *Neutral vertebrae*'s pedicles are symmetric and do not show rotation on standing frontal. Neutral vertebrae may be at the same level as end vertebrae, either above or below the curve, but are never nearer to the apex than the end vertebrae. Stable vertebrae are those who have a central sacral vertical line (CSVL) that cuts through or nearly cuts through them at a level below the end vertebra of the distal curve.[3]

Coronal Parameters

The concept of coronal balance is essential to the multidimensional approach to deformity surgery. The most important coronal balance interpretation measurements are the proximal thoracic, the main thoracic, and the thoracolumbar (TL) Cobb angles and C7–CSVL distance.

Coronal Cobb Measurements: Proximal Thoracic, Main Thoracic, Thoracolumbar

To quantify spinal deformity, Cobb angle is the most commonly used measurement. It is formed by the intersection between a line parallel to the superior end vertebra's end plate and a parallel line to the inferior end vertebra's end plate.

As shown in **Fig. 2.2**, a line is drawn perpendicular from the goniometer aligned with the proximal vertebra's upper end plate and then from the distal end vertebra's lower end plate. We measure the Cobb angle between two perpendiculars and label the end vertebrae accordingly.

Table 2.1 Location of apex of the curve

Curve	Apex
Occipitocervical	Occiput to C2
Cervical coronal	C2–C3 disc to C6–C7 disc
Cervicothoracic junction	C7–T1
Proximal thoracic	T1–T2 disc to T5 disc
Main thoracic	T5–T6 disc to T11–T12 disc
Thoracolumbar	T12–L1
Lumbar	L1–L2 disc through L4–L5 disc
Lumbosacral	L5–S1

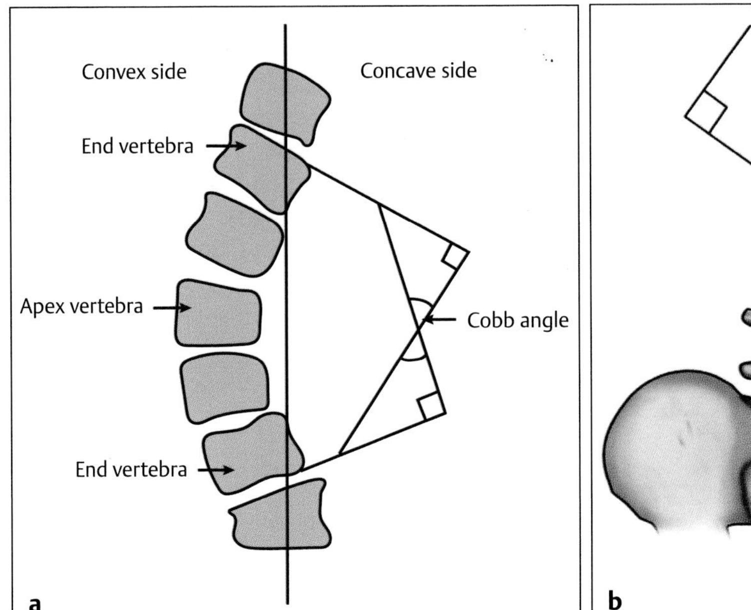

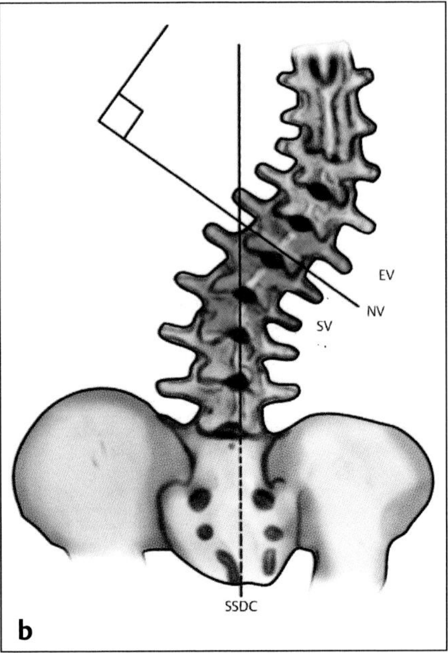

Fig. 2.1 (a, b) Apex vertebra, end vertebra (EV), neutral vertebra (NV) and stable vertebra (SV). The apex of the curve is the vertebra or intervertebral disc that is maximally laterally displaced and minimally angulated. EV, the most rostral and caudal vertebra that maximally tilt into the concavity of the curve, are used to measure the Cobb angle. The NV show no rotation; their pedicles are in normal symmetric positions. SV are the most cephalad vertebrae that are bisected by the central sacral vertical line (CSVL).

Pitfalls in Cobb Angle Measurements

The following should be kept in mind when measuring the Cobb angle:

- Over the course of a day, the Cobb angle of a curve can change by 5 degrees, particularly in the afternoon.[4]
- Scoliosis can make it difficult to position the patient accurately for a frontal view due to the vertebral rotation it causes. Cobb angles may be greater than those plotted on radiographs. Thus, follow-up imaging must be taken with the patient in the same position as at initial imaging.[5]
- During surgery, it has been reported that Cobb angle decreases in prone position under anesthesia. A loss of correction can occur as a postoperative rebound effect when the patient stands postoperatively.[6]
- It has been reported that radiographic acquisitions can cause errors of 2 to 7 degrees when measuring Cobb angles.[7] It is suggested to use a consistently defined end vertebra in the initial curve assessment and follow-ups.[7–9]
- There is a variation of 5 to 10 degrees in intraobserver Cobb angle measurement, whereas the interobserver variation is even more significant.[8,10] According to Carman et al, when radiographs obtained at two different time points were compared to assess curve progression, a measured difference of 10 degrees in the Cobb angle had a 95% chance of representing a true difference.[9]

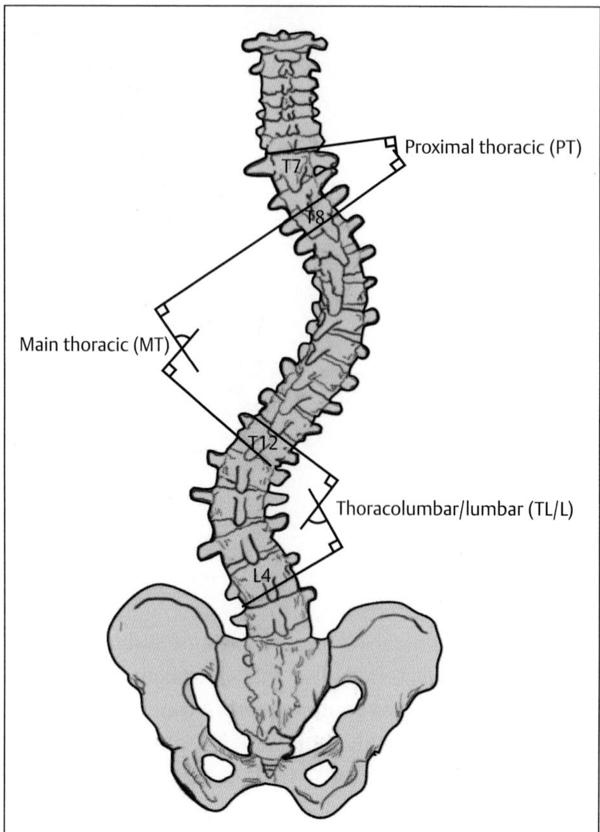

Fig. 2.2 Coronal Cobb angle: The goniometer is aligned with the proximal end vertebra's upper end plate and marked, and then a perpendicular line is drawn. Then the lower end plate of the distal end vertebra is marked and its perpendicular line is drawn. The Cobb angle is measured between the two perpendicular lines.

Pearl

A lack of accurate knowledge of vertebral rotation can lead to unnecessary surgery, or the misplacement of pedicle screws can result in spinal cord injuries.

Nash-Moe Classification

According to the Scoliosis Research Society, the Nash-Moe classification is the standardized method of quantifying the scoliotic spine's vertebral rotation.[11,12] Clinically, it can be used to assess preoperatively and postoperatively curve progression.[11,13]

The apical vertebral body is divided into six equal segments using the Nash-Moe classification and helps to identify the segment that contains the pedicles. The axial vertebral rotation has five grades according to the position of the pedicle, as shown in **Fig. 2.3**. Pedicle outline on the convex side moves on the vertebral outline as the vertebral body rotates in an evolving curve. Similarly, concave counterparts become less apparent, eventually disappearing.

Pearl

A spinal deformity causing coronal malalignment causes pelvic obliquity which results in abnormal gait in patients who can walk and asymmetric ischial compression in a sitting posture in patients who cannot walk. In addition, pelvic obliquity can cause costal pain.

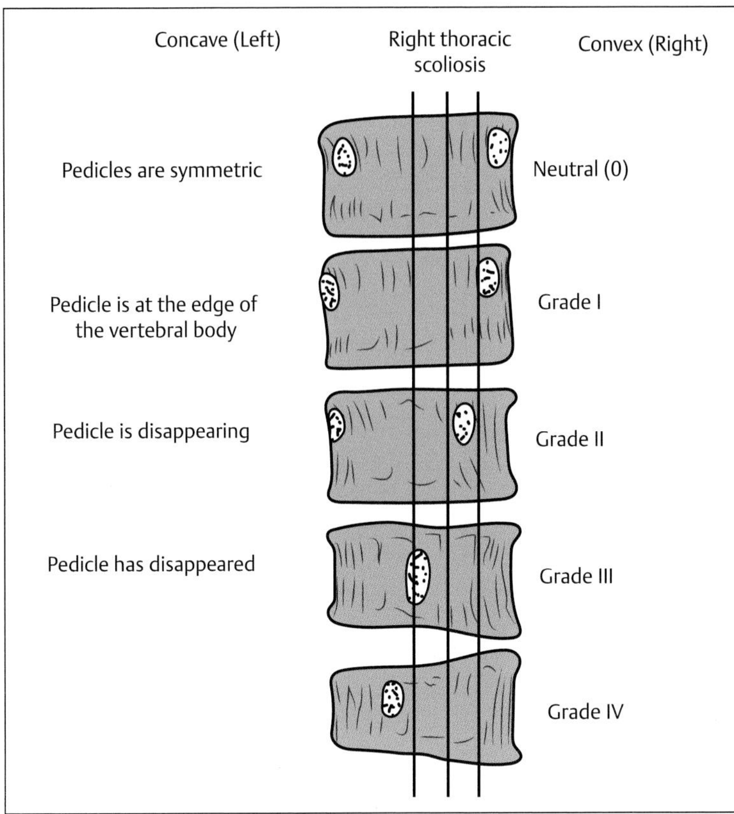

Fig. 2.3 Nash-Moe classification quantifies the scoliotic spine's vertebral rotation into five grades (0–IV). This classification divides the vertebrae into six equal segments, and helps to identify the segment that contains the pedicles.

Apical Vertebral Translation and Coronal Balance

An apical vertebral translation (AVT) depicts the distance in millimeters from the central sacral line (CSVL) to the midpoint of the apical body/disc (apex) horizontally.

The technique of measuring the AVT is as follows:

- C7 plumb line (C7PL) represents the head's position in space by showing a vertical line perpendicular to the floor starting from the C7 centroid.
- A CSVL indicates an individual's coronal position in their pelvis when a vertical line is drawn perpendicularly to the floor from the geometric center of the first sacral vertebrae.
- An AVT measurement is made when C7PL and CSVL coincide, as shown **Fig. 2.4**.
- When C7PL and CSVL do not overlap, AVT of the proximal and main thoracic curves is determined from C7PL, and the thoracolumbar and lumbar curves are determined from CSVL (**Fig. 2.4b**).

Pearl

Decompensated patients have the apical translation measured from the central sacral line (CSVL), while for the thoracic spine it is measured from the C7 plumb line (C7PL).

Coronal malalignment refers to the deviation for more than 20 millimeters of the C7PL from the pelvic midline.[14] To assess coronal balance, a long-standing full-length radiograph is required. From the centroid of the C7 vertebral body, a vertical line is drawn downward (perpendicular to the floor), and

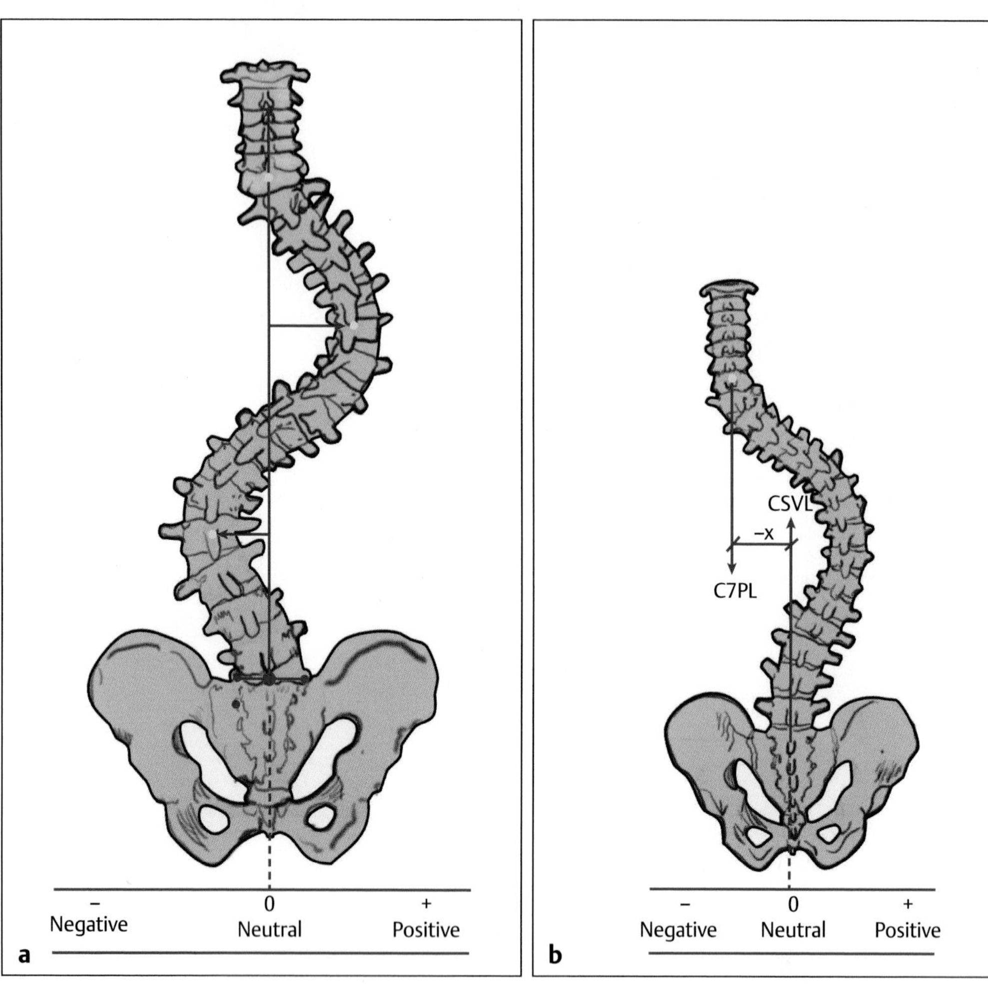

Fig. 2.4 (a, b) Coronal balance and apical vertebral translation. The C7 plumb line (C7PL) is drawn perpendicular to the floor from the C7 centroid. The central sacral vertical line (CSVL) is a vertical line drawn up perpendicular to the floor from the center of S1. **(a)** When the C7PL and CSVL coincide, the apical vertebral translation (AVT). **(b)** When the C7PL and CSVL do not coincide, the AVT of the proximal and main thoracic curve is measured from the C7PL, and that of the thoracolumbar and lumbar curve is measured from CSVL. To assess coronal balance, the horizontal distance between the C7PL and the CSVL is measured. A positive balance implies that the plumb line passes to the right of the midline by more than 2 cm, and a negative balance means displacement to the left by more than 2 cm as shown in **(b)**. Neutral balance is when C7PL equals the CSVL or is within 2 cm as shown in **(a)**.

a horizontal distance is measured between this vertical line and the CSVL. A positive balance implies that the PL passes more than 2 cm to the right of the midline, and a negative balance means displacement to the left by 2 cm or more[15] (**Fig. 2.4b**). Neutral balance is when C7PL equals the CSVL or is within 2 centimeters (**Fig. 2.4a**). A patient's coronal balance is evaluated in a standing or sitting position when they are ambulatory or disabled, and it has been studied in cerebral palsy patients with good results.[16,17]

Thoracic Trunk Shift

Pearl

- In patients with scoliosis, trunk imbalance negatively affects pelvic obliquity, function, and self-image.[18]
- There is a greater likelihood of trunk imbalance in cases involving thoracolumbar/lumbar (TL/L) curves than thoracic curves due to pain and/or its magnitude.[19]

Floman et al initially described trunk imbalance in 1982,[20] defined as the trunk's frontal plane shift. A thoracic shift is measured by first identifying the apical thoracic vertebra in standing posteroanterior (PA) or anteroposterior (AP) scoliosis X-rays. A horizontal line AB is drawn through the center of that vertebra, touching the ribs' boundary on either side. At point (c) along line segment AB, a line is dropped perpendicularly, known as the vertical trunk reference line (VTRL). Then from the midpoint of the S1 upward, a vertical line is drawn parallel to the sides of the radiograph known as the center sacral vertical line (CSVL). The term "trunk shift" refers to a difference of at least 2 cm between the VTRL and CSVL[21] **(Fig. 2.5)**. When the trunk shift is right of the CSVL, the value is positive; when it is left of the CSVL, it is negative.

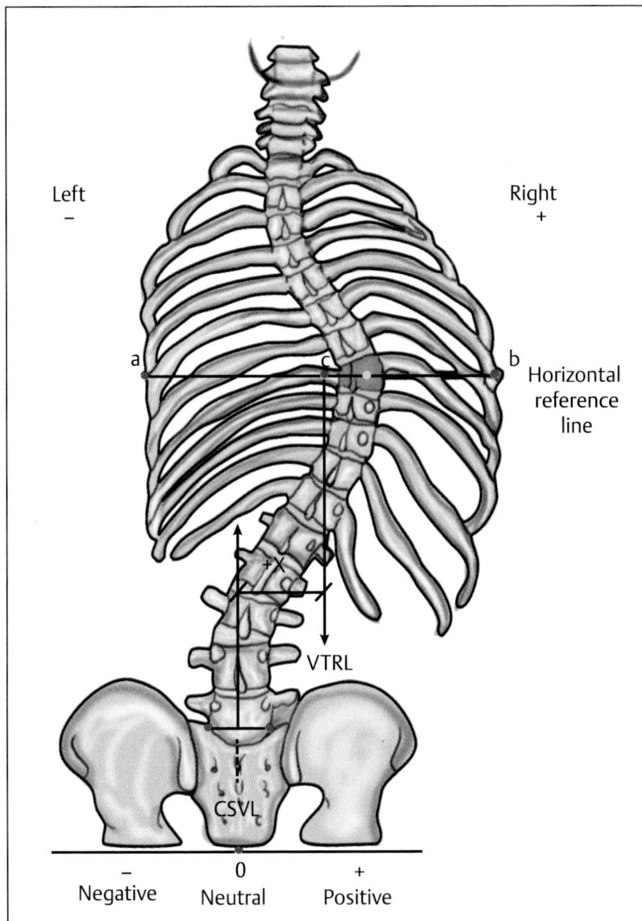

Fig. 2.5 Trunk shift is measured by first identifying the apical thoracic vertebra in standing posteroanterior (PA) or anteroposterior (AP) scoliosis X-rays. A horizontal line AB is drawn through the center of that vertebra, touching the ribs' boundary on either side. At the midpoint of line segment AB, point (c) is identified, and a perpendicular line is dropped as a reference line, known as the vertical trunk reference line (VTRL). Then, the center sacral vertical line (CSVL) is drawn from the midpoint of the S1 upward and parallel to the sides of the radiograph. Now, the distance between the VTRL and CSVL is measured in millimeters. This measurement refers to the thoracic trunk shift. A trunk shift to the right of the CSVL is a positive value, and to the left of the CSVL, a negative value.

Pearls

- As determined by self-assessment surveys such as the Scoliosis Research Society (SRS)-22 questionnaire, Short Form 12-item survey, and Oswestry Disability Index profiles, Glassman et al and others found the sagittal balance to be the most important and reliable radiologic predictor of clinical outcome.[22]
- The normal sagittal vertical axis (SVA) is less than 5 cm and is age dependent.23

Sagittal Parameters

Sagittal Balance and Sagittal Vertical Axis

Sagittal balance describes how the head and pelvis relate in sagittal space. Spinopelvic harmony is disrupted by pathological processes, resulting in deformities that lead to adaptive changes in the pelvis and lower limbs. Leg alignment can greatly affect spinal posture. We now also know that pelvic posture changes also affect spinal alignment, which is described later in the chapter. In sagittal malalignment, there is an exaggerated or reduced degree of lordosis or kyphosis. Persistent pain and disability are more likely to be associated with sagittal malalignment, in contrast to the size and location of the curve, or coronal plane decompensation.[5]

The sagittal vertical axis (SVA) is the simplest and most frequently used measurement for evaluating global spinal balance. The SVA is calculated by measuring the distance from the posterior–superior S1 corner to the C7PL. The C7PL is considered a crucial point of the global spinal balance.[24] Kuntz et al, in his literature review, states that the worldwide parameter of the spine over the pelvis and femoral head is a constant, reliable index of sagittal balance, and it is maintained within narrow ranges.[25]

Technique

Using a lateral standing full-length film, a line is drawn vertically from the midpoint of the C7 vertebral body perpendicular to the floor (**Fig. 2.6a**). The sagittal balance is considered neutral if C7PL passes through the superior end plate or is within 2 cm of the posterosuperior aspect of the S1 vertebral body. The sagittal balance is considered positive when the plumb line is more than 2 cm in front, and it is negative when it passes behind the posterior corner of the S1 vertebral body[15,26] (**Fig. 2.6b**).

Spinosacral Angle

The SVA measures distance; therefore, it requires calibrated images instead of indicators based on angles. The spinosacral angle (SSA) is a fundamental parameter of balance and is formed by the sacral end plate surface and the line joining C7 to the sacral end plate center **(Fig. 2.7)**. The normal value of this parameter is 135 ± 8 degrees, and it is a fixed angle as it integrates the C7 position with the sacral slope (SS).

C7 Plumb Line/Sacrofemoral Distance Ratio (C7/SFD Ratio)

Using the C7/SFD ratio (Barrey index) as a replacement for a distance metric like SVA, Barrey et al proposed a ratio that is applicable to all radiographs.[27,28] The SFD is calculated using the distance between the vertical bicoxofemoral axis and the vertical line that passes through the sacrum corner posteriorly. In addition, the distance from C7PL to the sacrum's posterior corner (that is, SC7 D) was measured. Based on the SC7-SF distance ratio, they calculated the C7/SFD ratio **(Fig. 2.8)**. The C7/SFD ratio is 0 if the C7PL is directed at the posterosuperior corner of the sacrum, and if directed on the bicoxofemoral axis, it is 1.

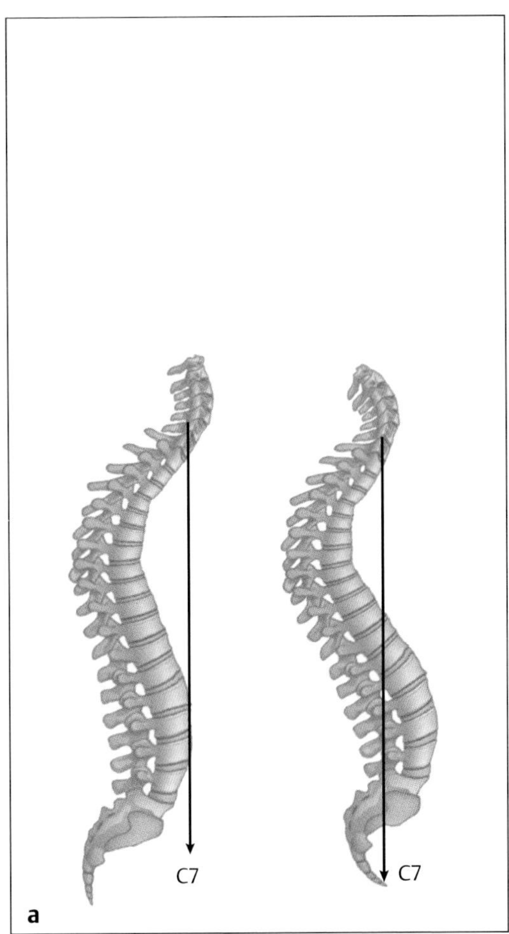

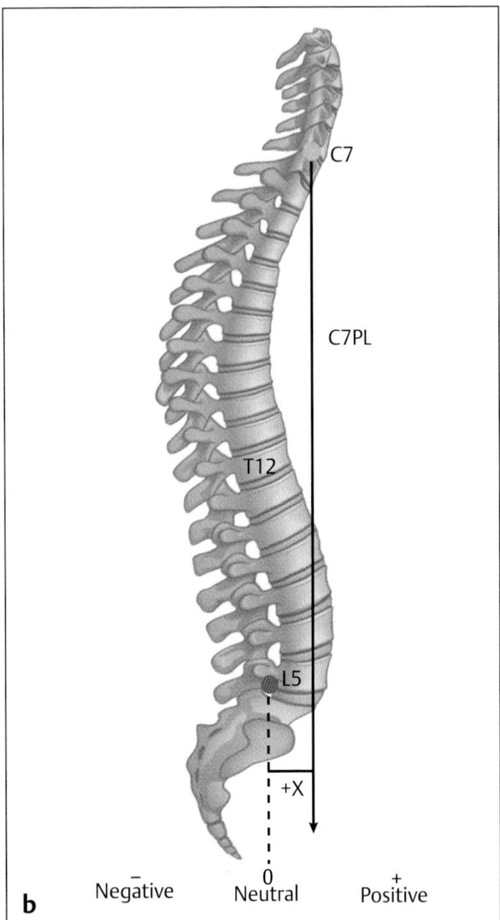

Fig. 2.6 (a, b) The sagittal vertical axis (SVA) is the distance between the C7 plumb line (C7PL) and the posterior superior S1 corner. On a lateral full-length radiograph, a C7PL is drawn, normally the C7PL should pass through or be within 2 cm of the posterosuperior corner of the S1 (neutral balance). The sagittal balance is positive, if the C7PL passes more than 2 cm in front of the posterosuperior corner of the S1. And the sagittal balance is considered negative, if the plumb line passes more than 2 cm behind the posterosuperior corner of the S1 vertebral body.

Pearl

The global sagittal balance can be estimated using the spinosacral angle and the C7/sacrofemoral distance (SFD) ratio.

T9-Tilt Angle

Duval-Beaupère et al describe the T9 tilt as an indicator of the spine balance at the level of the body mass center.[29,30] The T9 tilt is the angle between the line connecting the midpoint of the femoral head's axis with the center of the T9 vertebral body and the vertical line crossing the midpoint of the femoral head's axis[31] (**Fig. 2.9**). When the axis of the femoral head is projected posterior to the center of the T9 vertebral body, the tilt is positive; when anterior, it is negative.[32]

T1 Pelvic Angle

The T1 pelvic angle (TPA) involves both sagittal balance and pelvic retroversion.[33,34]

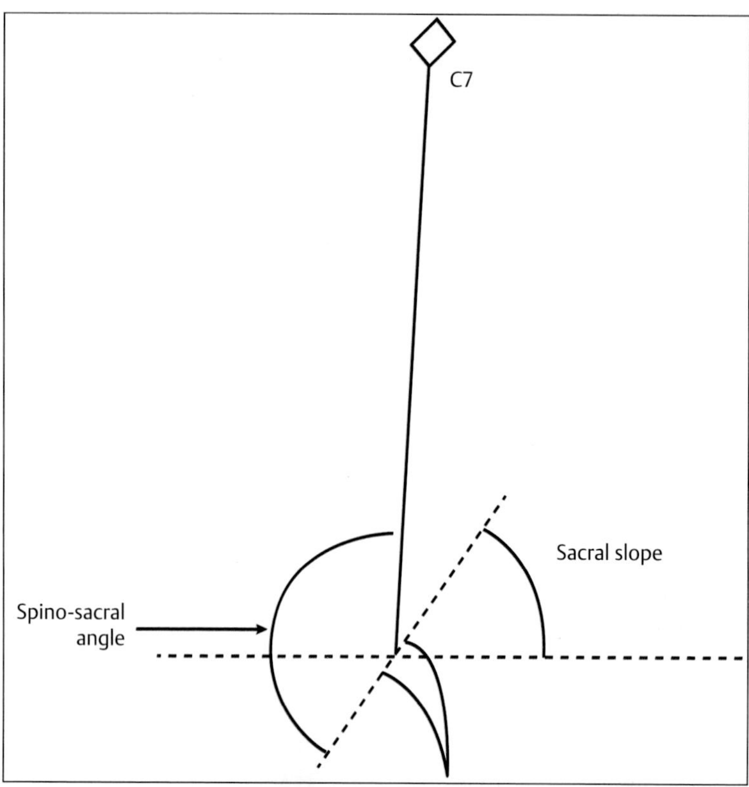

Fig. 2.7 Spinosacral angle is the angle between a line from the center of C7 to the center of the sacral end plate and the surface of the sacral end plate.

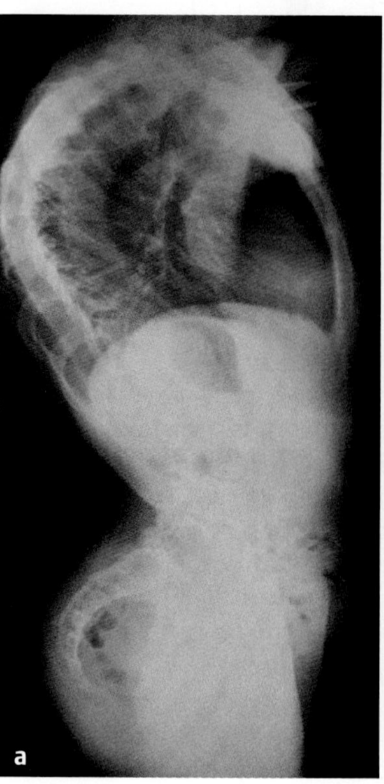

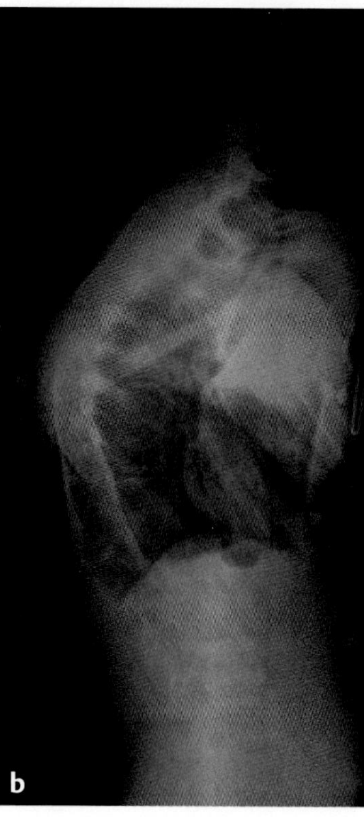

Fig. 2.8 (a, b) Barry's Index is the C7/SFD ratio. The sacrofemoral distance (SFD) is the horizontal distance between the vertical bicoxofemoral axis and the vertical line passing through the sacrum's posterior corner. The sacral C7 distance (S-C7 D) is the horizontal distance between the C7PL and the sacrum's posterior corner. The C7/SFD ratio is calculated using the ratio between SC7 D and SFD.

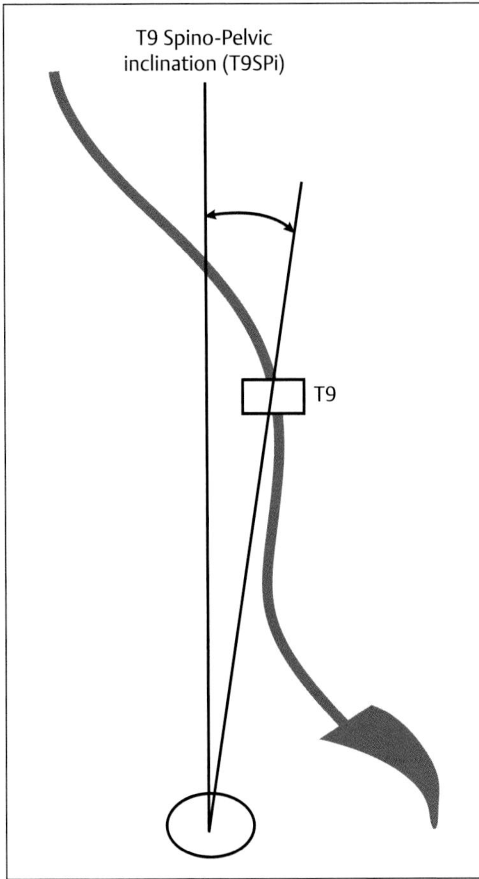

Fig. 2.9 T9 tilt angle is the angle between the line linking the midpoint of the femoral head's axis with the center of the T9 vertebra body and the vertical line crossing the midpoint of the femoral head's axis.

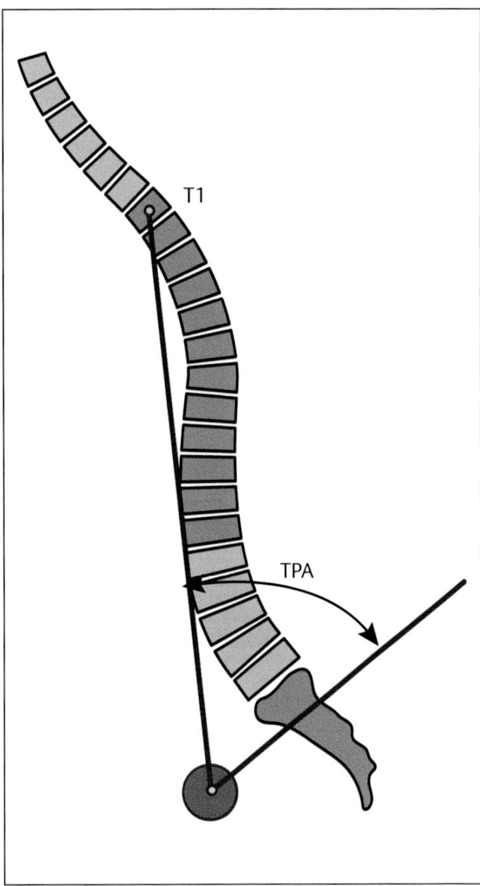

Fig. 2.10 T1 pelvic angle (TPA): the angle between the line from the femoral head axis to the centroid of T1 and the line from the femoral head axis to the middle of the S1 end plate.

This angle is formed between a line connecting the center of T1 with the center of femoral heads and a line connecting the center of the S1 end plate **(Fig. 2.10)**. TPA includes both measurements of spinal vertical alignment and pelvic tilt (PT).[33,34]

Pearl

According to Ryan et al, the goal of surgery should be a T1 pelvic angle of around 10 degrees. Patients with T1 pelvic angle greater than 20 degrees are considered to have severe deformity.[28]

Odontoid Hip Axis (OD-HA)[35]

The angle formed by the highest point of the odontoid process (dens) and acetabulum (bicoxofemoral axis) is known as the odontoid hip axis (OD-HA) **(Fig. 2.11)**. This is a good measure of the overall sagittal balance because it rarely varies and it incorporates the cervical spine, the thoracolumbar spine, and the pelvis and can aid in the evaluation and analysis of the risk of proximal junctional kyphosis following an extended thoracolumbar fusion.[36]

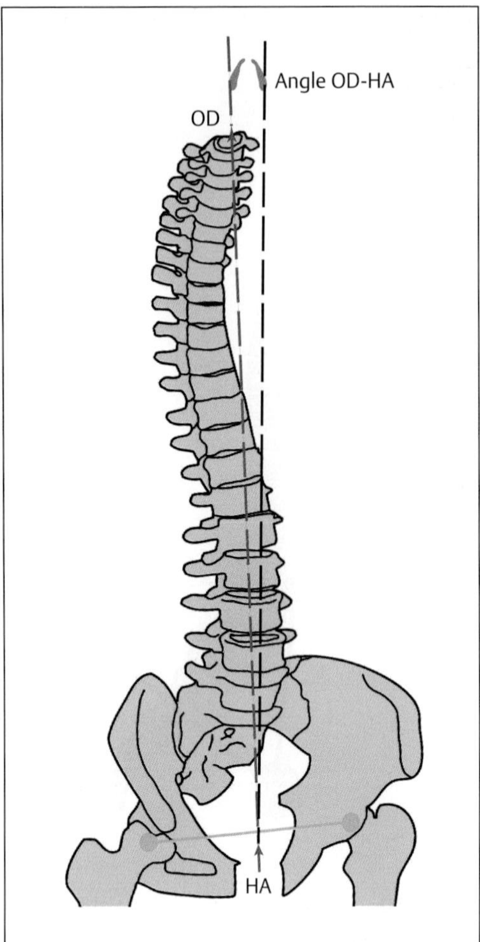

Fig. 2.11 The odontoid-hip axis (OD-HA) angle is the angle between the vertical line crossing the center of the hip axis (HA) and a line between OD and HA. This angle was computed both in sagittal and coronal views.

Sagittal Cervical Parameters

For cervical spine assessment, several radiographic parameters are commonly used. These include cervical lordosis (CL), C2–C7 sagittal vertical axis (C2–C7 SVA), occipito-C2 angle (O-C2), and C7 slope. The cervical spine is separated by two angles (**Fig. 2.12**):

- High cervical angles:
  - The O-C2 is formed by the parallel line to C2 inferior end plate and the McGregor line. The McGregor line is always lordotic and is drawn from the dorsal rostral aspect of the hard palate to the most caudal point on the midline of the occipital curve, with an average value of 15.81 degrees (±7.15 degrees).[37]
- Lower cervical angles:
  - These angles are defined from C2 to C7. The Cobb method was used to evaluate CL from C2 to C7, which involves drawing four lines. There will be two parallel lines: the first line parallels the C2 vertebral terminal plate, and the second line parallels the C7 vertebra. Then two lines are drawn perpendicular to the first two. The angle between the two perpendicular lines is proportional to the amount of cervical curvature.[38]

> **Pearl**
>
> Schwab et al[39] concluded that patients with loss of lumbar lordosis and positive sagittal balance had better postoperative outcomes. Glassman et al,[40] in their study, stated that sagittal balance correction resulted in significant improvement in pain, function, and self-image.

C7 Slope and C2–C7 Sagittal Vertical Axis

An angle formed by a horizontal line and the cranial end plate of the C7 is referred to as the C7 slope (**Fig. 2.12**). The C7 slope can indicate lordosis or kyphosis or neutrality of the cervical spine.[37] Its high value is due to its consideration of the head position. It is therefore closely correlated with SVA and can be used when long films cannot be obtained.[41]

> **Pearl**
>
> The occiput-C2 and C2–C7 angles work inversely.

The C2–C7 SVA is determined by measuring the distance between the C2PL and the

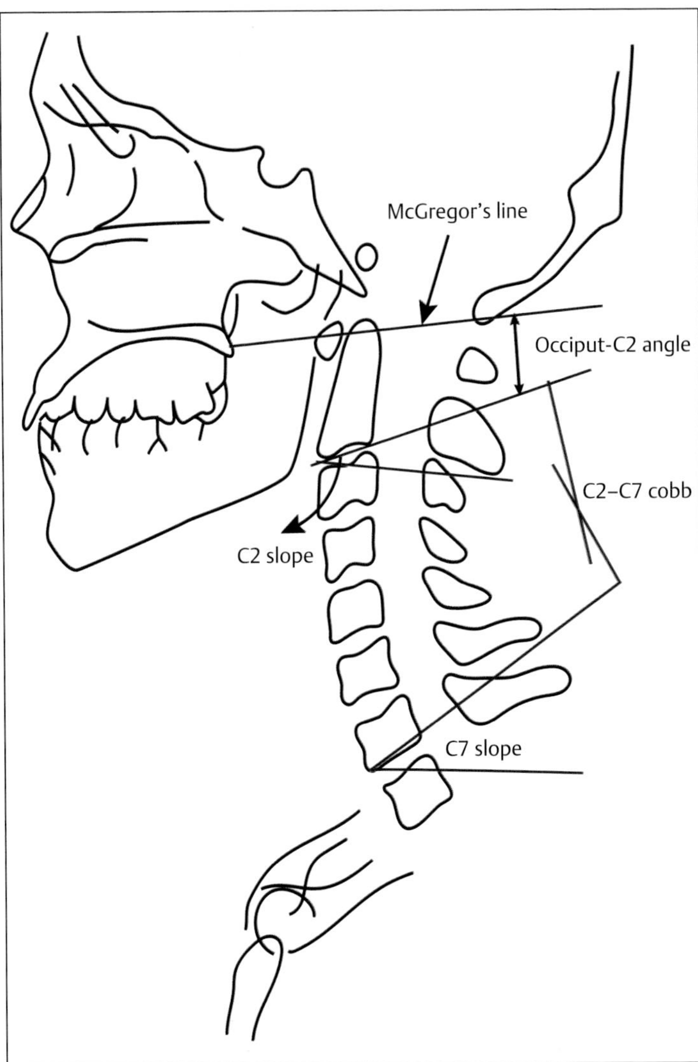

Fig. 2.12 Sagittal cervical parameters: The occiput-C2 angle is the angle between the McGregor line and lower end plate of the C2 vertebra. A positive value indicates lordosis between the occiput and C2, and a negative value indicates kyphosis between the occiput and C2. The C2–C7 Cobb angle was the angle of C2 vertebra lower end plate and C7 vertebra lower end plate, which corresponds to the degree of cervical curvature. The C7 slope is the angle between a horizontal line and the cranial end plate of C7.

vertical line drawn from the posterior superior end plate of C7 (**Fig. 2.13a, b**).

Sagittal Thoracic and Lumbar Spine Parameters

Sagittal balance uses spinal vertical alignment, thoracic kyphosis, and lumbar lordosis (LL) as radiologic parameters. The deformity of kyphosis is characterized by an increase in the posterior convex angle of the spine. The measurement of kyphosis is positive, and that of lordosis is negative.

Thoracic Sagittal Alignment

Thoracic spine posterior convexity is normally 20 to 40 degrees (Cobb method). The T1 to the inferior end plate of T12 is used to measure thoracic kyphosis (**Fig. 2.14**). The proximal thoracic kyphosis is the angle between T2 and T5 (**Fig. 2.15**). Kyphosis in the mid to lower thoracic region is measured from T5 to T12 (**Fig. 2.14**). Thoracolumbar sagittal alignment is measured from T10 to the caudal end plate of L2 using the Cobb method (**Fig. 2.15**).

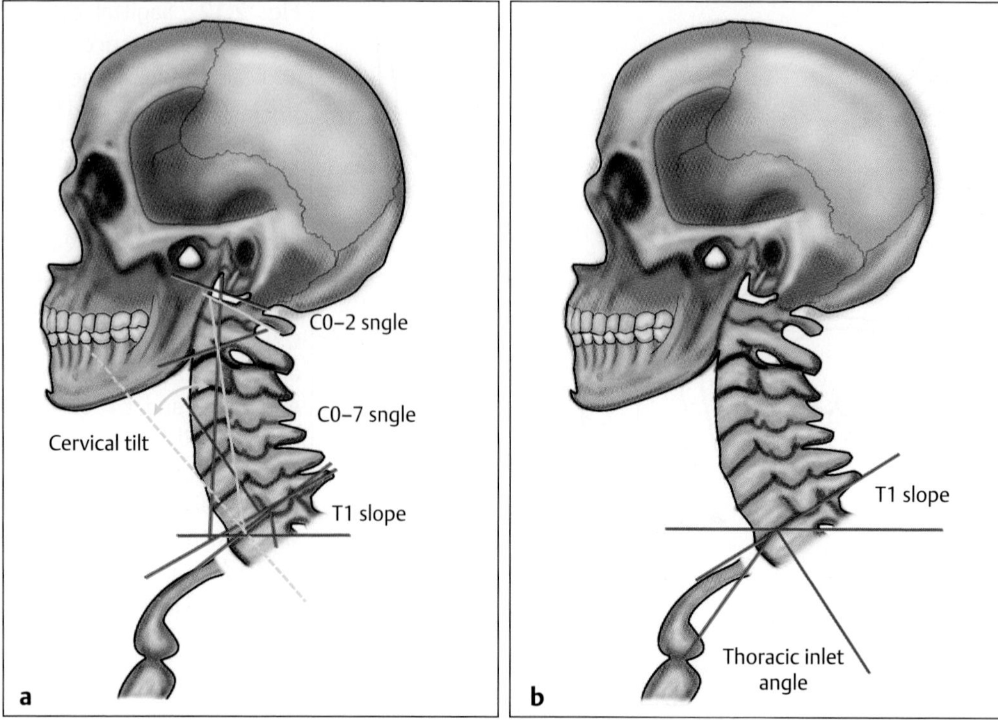

Fig. 2.13 (a, b) C2–C7 sagittal vertical axis (SVA) is the horizontal distance between vertical line from the center of C2 and the posterior superior aspect of C7.

Lumbar Lordosis

Lumbar sagittal alignment is measured from T12 to the end plate of S1. The normal range is 40 to 60 degrees of lordosis (**Fig. 2.16**).

According to Roussouly et al, the LL is measured between LL and thoracic kyphosis, and the upper S1 end plate, at their geometric point of inflexion where LL turns to thoracic kyphosis.[24] This analysis shows that two-thirds of the LL is at the last two levels of the spine.[42,43]

Pearl

The median value of C7 slope is 20 degrees. A lordotic cervical spine is characterized by a C7 slope greater than 20 degrees (lordosis between C2 and C7). A C7 slope of less than 20 degrees indicates a neutral or kyphotic cervical spine.

To understand the spine pathologies, Roussouly et al[44] classified a system that defined four types of spines. This classification can be used to analyze spinopelvic parameters in healthy patients **(Fig. 2.17)**.

- In types 1 and 2, the SS is small (less than 35 degrees):
  - A smaller inferior lordosis arch with the lordosis apex located further below (about L5) characterizes type 1. As a result, the lordosis is "short," while the kyphosis is thoracolumbar.
  - In type 2, also the "flat back," the lower arch is flattened with little curvature.
- In type 3, which is the most balanced type, the lordotic apex is at L4, and the SS is between 35 and 45 degrees. The lordosis is almost evenly distributed between each arch.
- Type 4 is characterized by a steep SS greater than 45 degrees with a lordotic

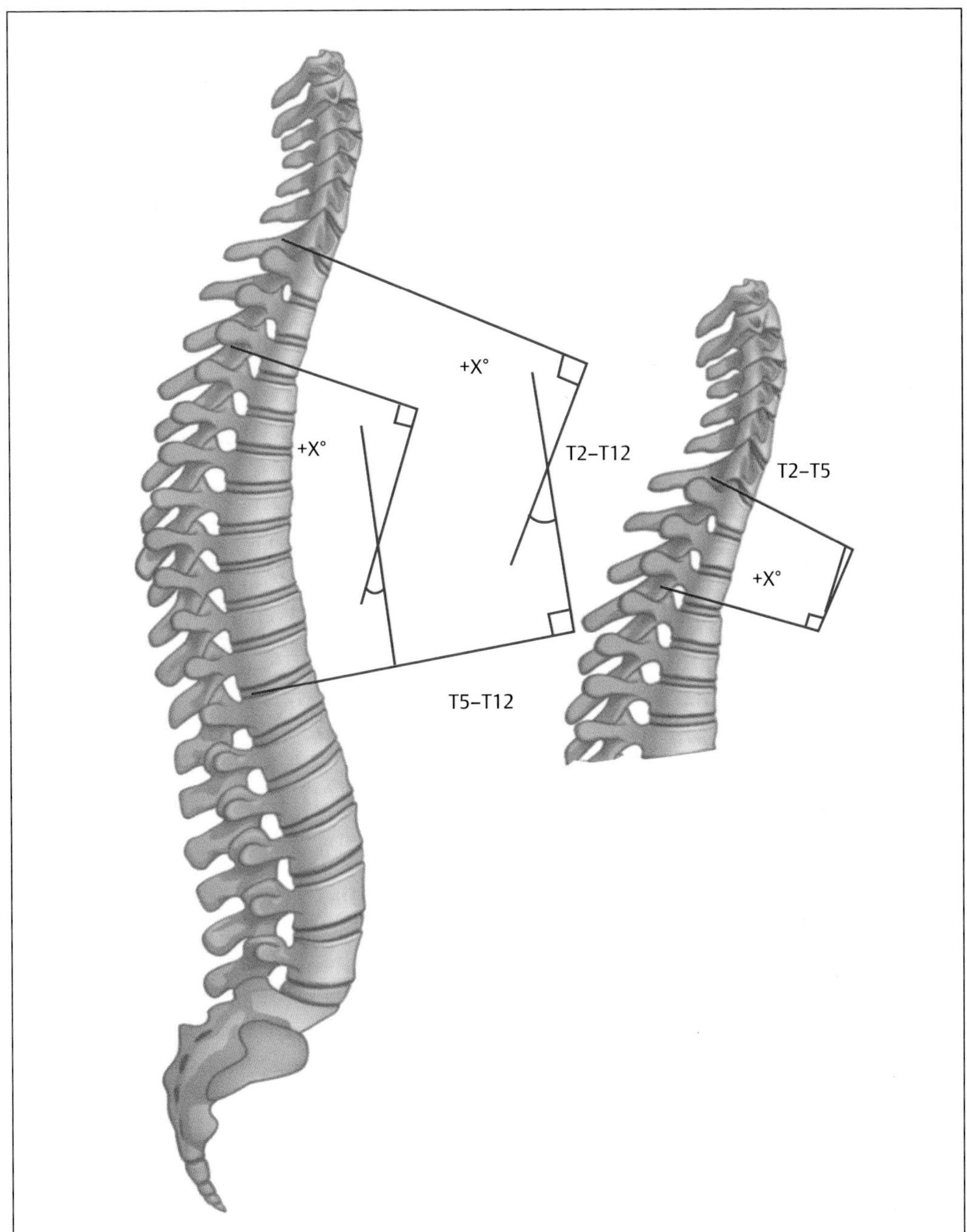

Fig. 2.14 Total thoracic kyphosis is measured from the superior end plate of T1 to the inferior end plate of T12. Mid/lower thoracic kyphosis is measured from the cephalad end plate of T5 to the caudal end plate of T12 using the Cobb method.

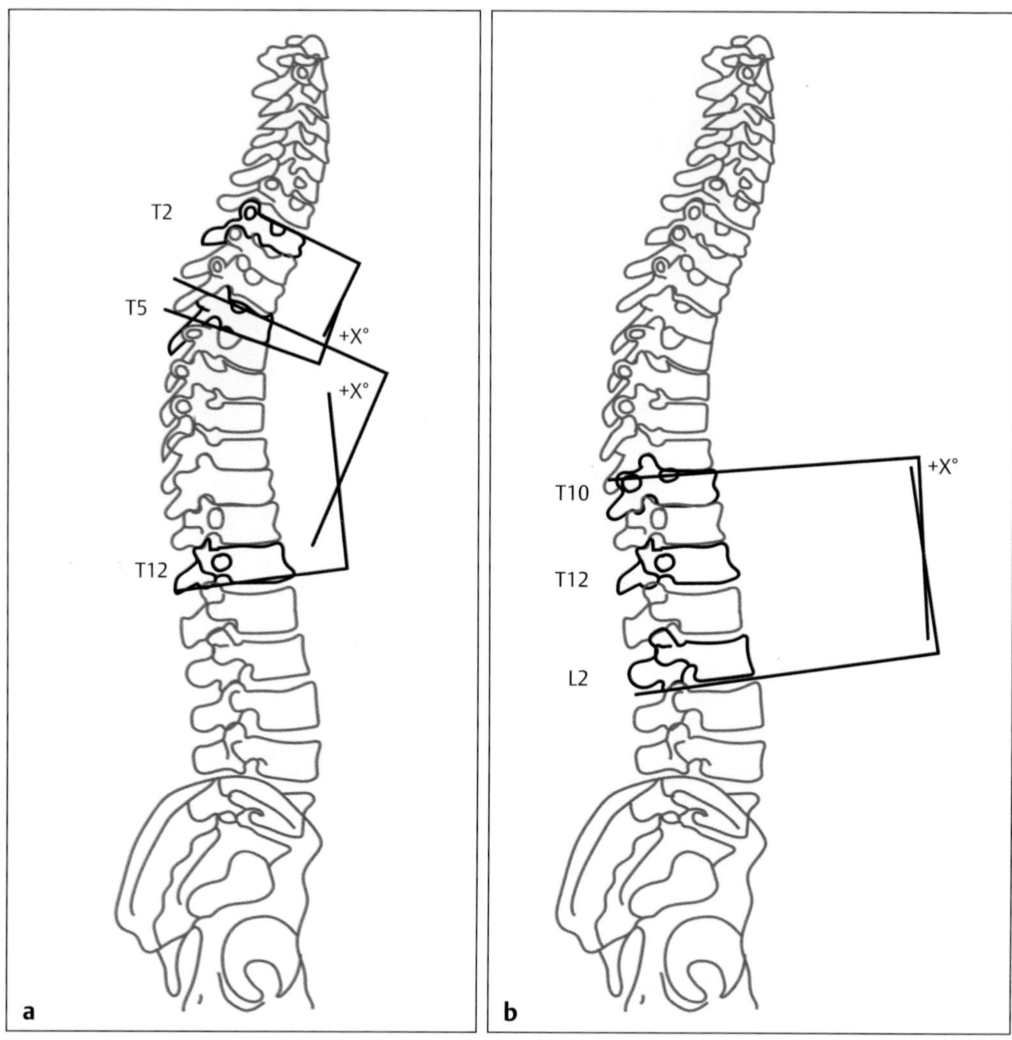

Fig. 2.15 (a, b) Proximal thoracic kyphosis is measured from the cephalad end plate of T2 to the caudal end plate of T5 using Cobb method. Thoracolumbar sagittal alignment is measured from the cephalad end plate of T10 to the caudal end plate of L2 using the Cobb method.

apex at the anterior–inferior corner of L3. The thoracic kyphosis is shorter, and the global lordosis angle consists of more vertebrae than the other types.

Pelvic Parameters

Spinopelvic alignment is critically dependent on the pelvis. Nevertheless, new studies have demonstrated that the pelvis position has been disregarded during the work-up of scoliosis.[45] Postoperative misalignment and treatment failure can result from failing to assess the pelvic parameters for deformity surgery. Specifically, parameters that need consideration are pelvic obliquity, pelvic incidence (PI), PT, SS, and TPA.

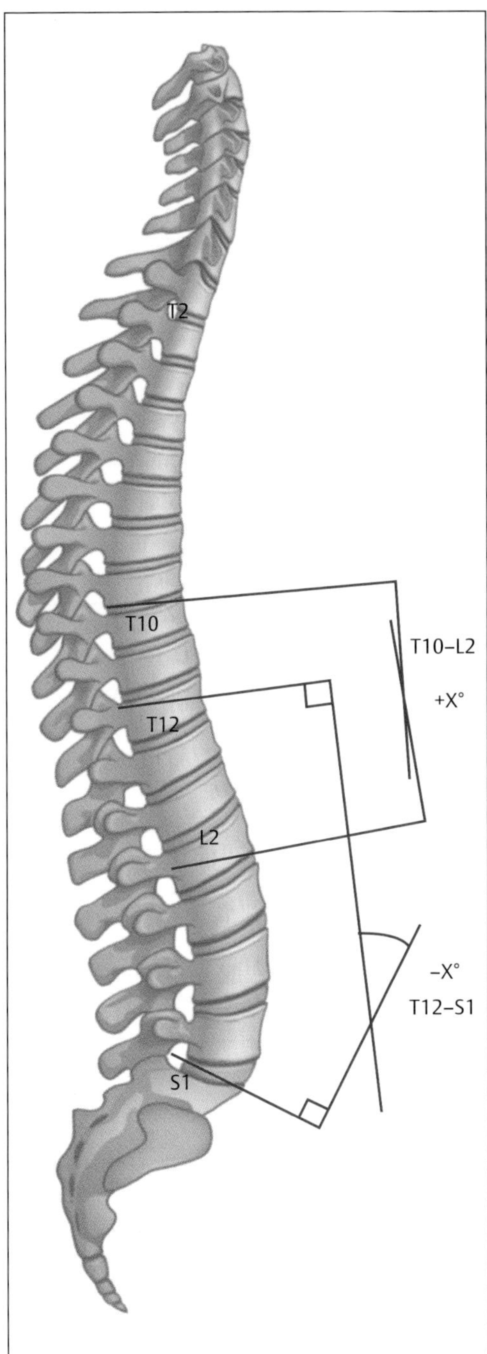

Fig. 2.16 Lumbar sagittal alignment is measured from the cephalad end plate of T12 to the end plate of S1. The normal range is 40 to 60 degrees of lordosis.

Pelvic Obliquity/Leg-Length Discrepancy

Patients with neuromuscular scoliosis or spastic scoliosis have been known to have pelvic obliquity (PO) in scoliosis. Its anatomical origin can be assessed, whether it is caused by a suprapelvic, intrapelvic, infrapelvic problem or a combination of these. Pelvic obliquity is measured using the angle between a horizontal reference line (a parallel line drawn to the floor) and the pelvic coronal line (**Fig. 2.18**).

In cases of suprapelvic spinal deformities, the pelvis may become asymmetrical because of scoliosis. The intrapelvic cause results from morphological changes in the pelvis, which result in hypoplasia of the ilium, the ischium, or the whole hemipelvis. Hip contractures or lower limb length inequality are infrapelvic causes.

Pearl

Both the identification and quantification of pelvic obliquity are important prior to corrective surgery for a patient with idiopathic scoliosis. Stylianides et al reported that the difference in iliac spine geometry was noted in AIS patients with severe scoliosis compared to those without scoliosis or with moderate curves and, therefore, in surgical correction of adolescent idiopathic scoliosis (AIS), the presence of pelvic obliquity could increase the incidence of coronal decompensation particularly when fusion was extended to the lumbar spine.[46]

When assessing leg-length discrepancy, the patient is positioned standing with their legs extended and without blocks under their feet. By creating a horizontal line that is tangent to the highest femoral head, we can create the femoral horizontal reference line (FHRL). The leg-length discrepancy is calculated by measuring the distance between this line and the lower femoral head (**Fig. 2.18**).

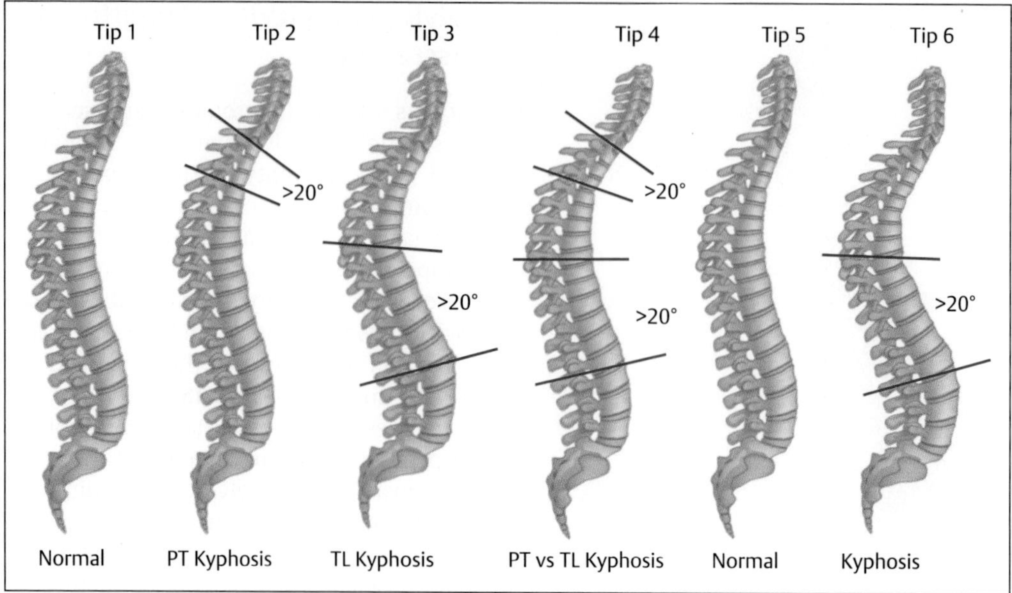

Fig. 2.17 This shows the different types of spine according to Roussouly et al. Types 1 and 2 have a small sacral slope, in which type 1 has a short lordosis, and kyphosis is thoracolumbar. Type 2 has a flattened lower arch also known as flat back. Type 3 shows the most balanced type, with an average sacral slope (between 35 and 45 degrees) and the lordotic apex at L4. Type 4 has a steep sacral slope greater than 45 degrees, the lumbar lordosis is larger, and the thoracic kyphosis is shorter.

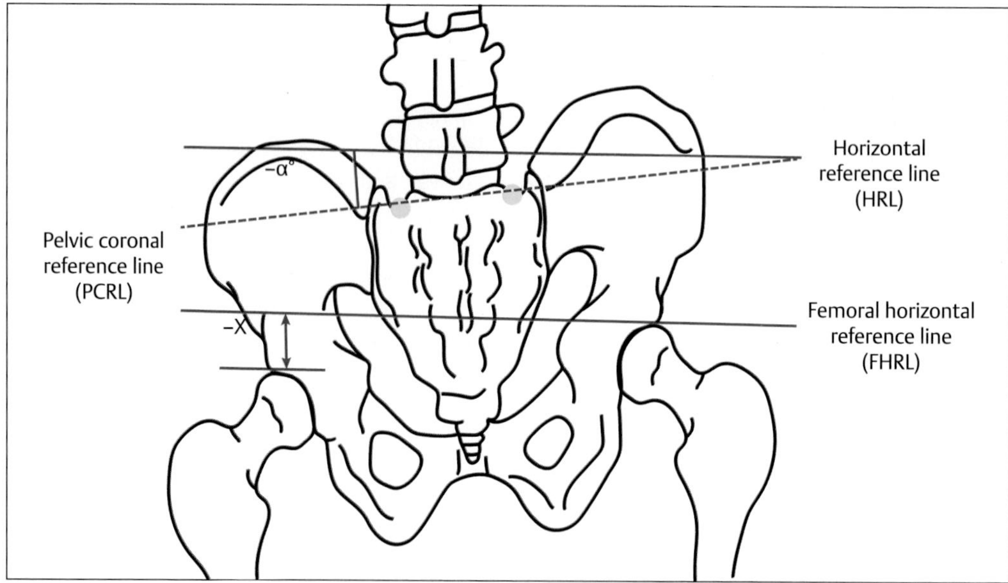

Fig. 2.18 Pelvic obliquity is the angle between the pelvic coronal reference line and a horizontal reference line (a line drawn parallel to the floor). A femoral horizontal reference line (FHRL) will be created by making a horizontal line that is tangent to the top of the highest femoral head. The difference between the height of this line and the height of the lower femoral head will be defined as the leg-length discrepancy.

In a right hip-up position, the value will be negative; in a left hip-up position, the value will be positive (+).

Pearl

The concept of "spinopelvic harmony" suggests lumbar and thoracic shapes are proportional to pelvic shape and shows a better interpretation of how a normal sagittal alignment is achieved (**Fig. 2.19**). Using the formula, LL = PI + 9°, lumbar lordosis could be projected. Research on 125 operated patients demonstrated that those with lumbar lordosis not matching their own pelvic incidence (LL < PI + 9°) had a higher chance of worse clinical outcomes.[46]

Pelvic Incidence

Legaye and Duval-Beaupère described the pearl incidence (PI) as the angle between the perpendicular line passing through the center of upper S1 and the line connecting this point to the axis of the femoral heads (**Fig. 2.20**).[29,48] For each individual, this is a constant anatomical parameter that is independent of how the pelvis is oriented spatially. This angle encompasses the top three sacral vertebrae, the two sacroiliac joints, and the posterior margin of the iliac wings up to the acetabulum. A morphological parameter called PI is determined by adding the SS to the PT: PI = SS + PT.[32]

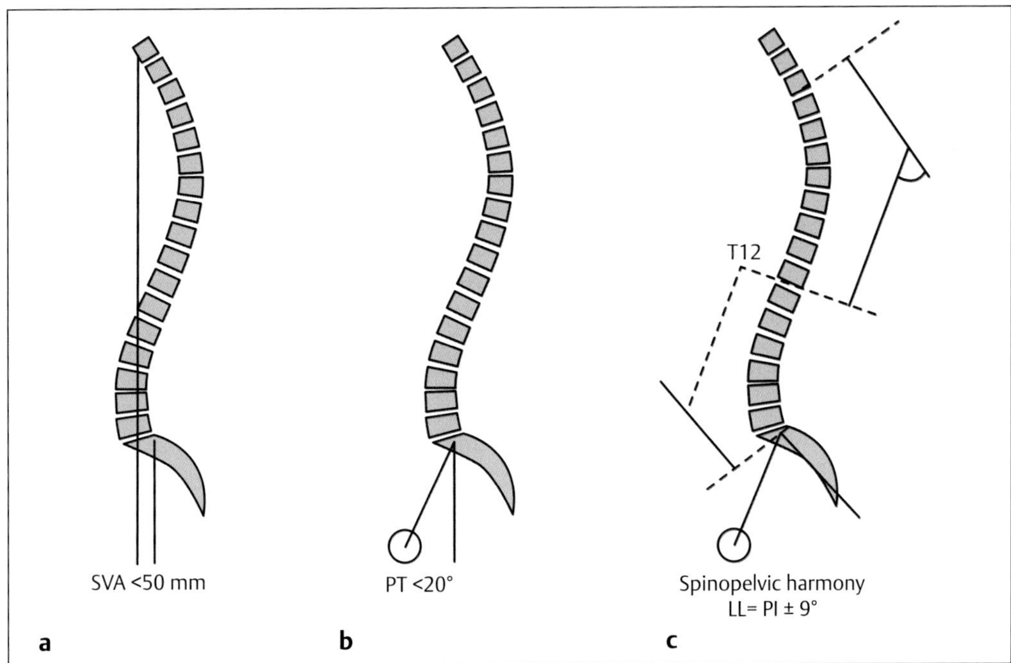

Fig. 2.19 (a-c) Spinopelvic harmony lumbar lordosis could be predicted by the formula LL (lumbar lordosis) = PI (pelvic incidence) + 9 degrees. The concept of "spinopelvic harmony" suggests lumbar and thoracic shapes are proportional to pelvic shape and shows a better interpretation of how a normal sagittal alignment is achieved.

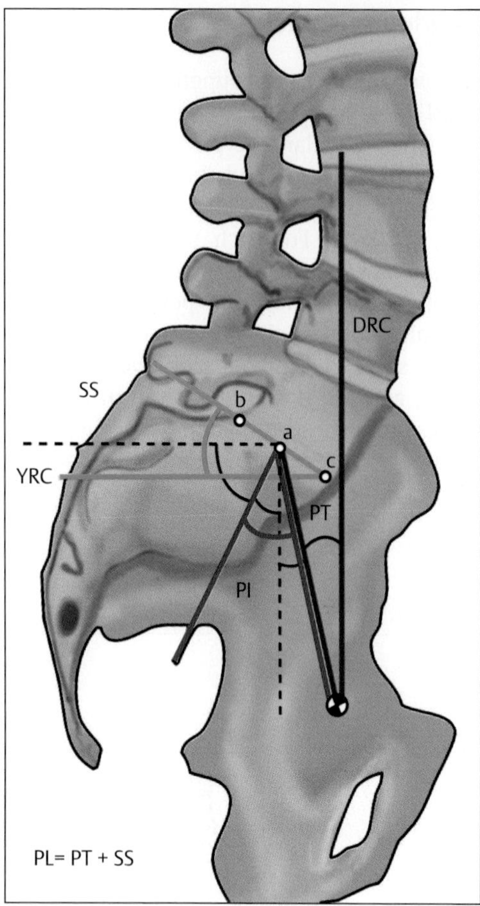

Fig. 2.20 The pelvic incidence corresponds to the angle between the perpendicular to the upper S1 level passing through its center and the line connecting this point to the axis of the femoral heads. The pelvic tilt is the angle created between a line drawn from the midpoint of the femoral heads to the center of the superior end plate of the sacrum and a vertical plumb line through the midpoint of the femoral head. The sacral slope is defined as the angle between a line drawn parallel to the superior end plate of S1 and a horizontal reference line or line drawn parallel to the floor.

Pelvic Tilt

The pelvic tilt (PT) is the angle between a line drawn from the midpoint of the femoral heads to the center of the sacrum superior end plate and a vertical PL through the midpoint of the femoral heads (**Fig. 2.20**).[45,47,49] Degenerative disc disease increases the LL, which in turn increases the spinal vertical alignment. As a natural instinct to restore neutral sagittal balance and patients achieve this by knee flexion and pushing the pelvis posteriorly ("retroversion").[45,47,49] An increase in PT is seen with compensatory pelvic retroversion. This compensation causes poor clinical outcomes if it occurs in postoperative patients due to the additional energy expenditure required.[19,45,47]

Ideally, PT should be greater than 10 degrees and less than 20 degrees. PT greater than 20 degrees indicates compensatory pelvic retroversion. A study by Schwab et al[49] showed that for a negative, neutral (0–5 cm), and positive (>5 cm) spinal vertical alignment, the average PT is 10, 16, and 21 degrees, respectively. In SRS-Schwab Classification, a PT of less than 20, 20 to 30 degrees, and greater than 30 degrees is graded as "0/nonpathological," "+/moderate deformity," "++/marked deformity," respectively.[47,49,50]

Sacral Slope

The sacral slope (SS) also demonstrates the pelvic position and is utilized to identify pelvic retroversion. It is an angle measured between a line drawn parallel to the S1 superior end plate and a horizontal reference line (**Fig. 2.20**). Changes to SS are inversely proportional to changes in the PT[44] **(SS + PT = PI)**. While SS and PT are complementary measurements, the PT is more often used in treatment planning.[51]

Risser Sign

Joseph C. Risser first described Risser sign in 1958.[51] Spinal skeletal maturity is directly related to the degree of iliac apophysis ossification, which is critical to the management of adolescent scoliosis. The iliac apophysis ossification and fusion are divided into six stages (Risser stages 0–5). Stage 0 illustrates the absence of ossification centers in the apophysis on X-ray; in contrast, stage 5 is complete iliac apophysis ossification and fusion. The Risser system has two slightly different versions, where stages 2 to 4 are divided differently. The United States Risser Staging System splits the ossification into quarters, beginning anterolaterally and progressing posteromedially. In contrast, the French Risser system divides the course of the apophysis into thirds (stages 1–3), with stage 4 being complete ossification (**Fig. 2.21** and **Box 2.2**).

Box 2.2 Risser grade of iliac apophysis ossification and fusion

Risser 0: No iliac apophysis visible

Risser 1: Initial appearance of ossification of the iliac apophysis

Risser 2: Migration halfway across the top of the iliac wing

Risser 3: Three-fourths of the distance

Risser 4: Ossification crossing the iliac wing, but not fused to the ilium

Risser 5: Complete ossification of the iliac apophysis with fusion to the ilium

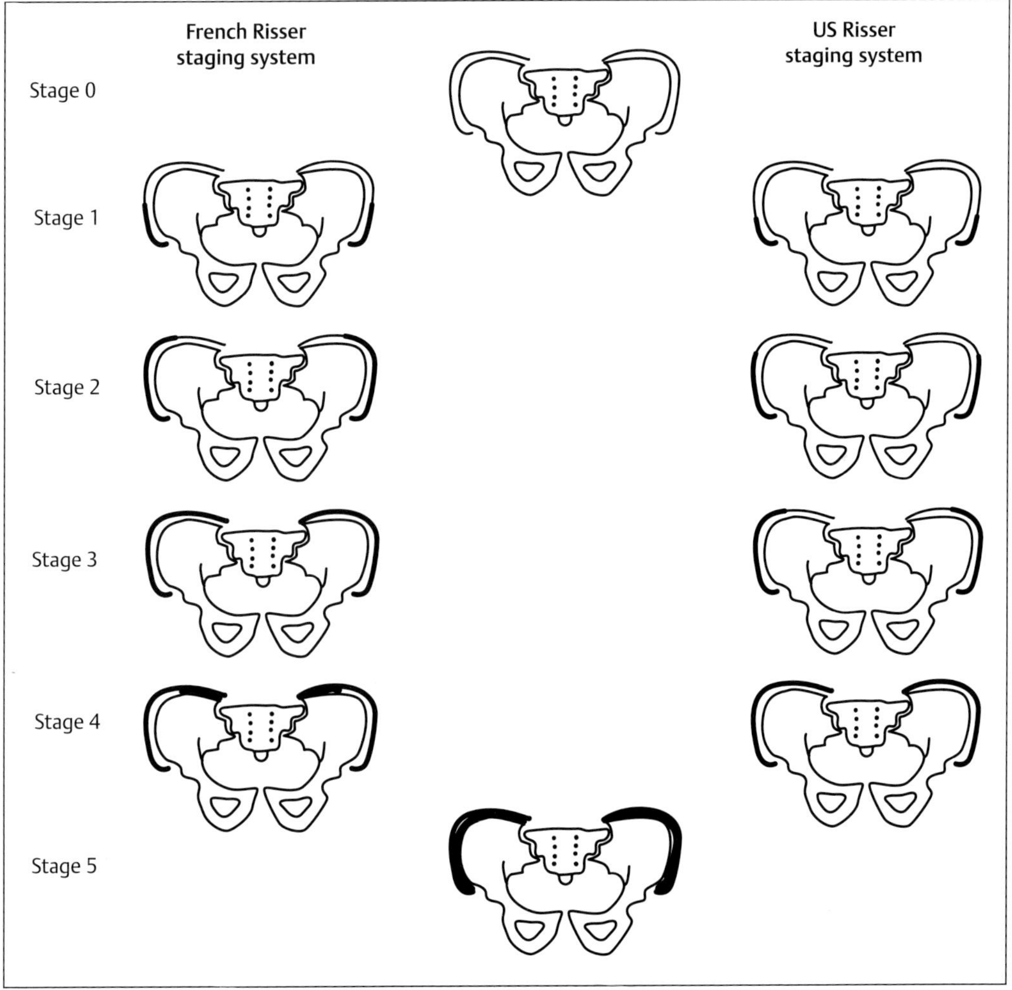

Fig. 2.21 Risser grading, French versus American.

Radiological Imaging

In order to evaluate spinal deformities from the cervicothoracic junction to the pelvis, several factors must be considered for a quality diagnostic film. First, an appropriate distance from the source to the image is important to yield an adequate amount of magnification and distortion, and therefore a distance of 72 inches is recommended. All radiographs, including those for spondylolisthesis, are taken in an upright position to show the true position of the spine.

Posture for Scoliosis X-Rays

Anterior–posterior and lateral radiographs are obtained while standing two meters in the distance. Patients should stand upright with their feet shoulder-width apart, their knees locked and looking straight ahead. If there is a length difference in the lower extremities (the leg-length discrepancy of >2 cm), the lower extremity should be supported from below. If the patient cannot stand in the upright position, radiography can be taken in the unsupported sitting position and only supported sitting position, if necessary. The upper edge of the cassette should be at the level of the ear. While taking lateral radiography, the elbows should be flexed fully, and hands made into a fist over the supraclavicular fossa. In this way, the patient's arms are positioned at an angle of approximately 45 degrees to its vertical axis to prevent overlapping with the spine (**Fig. 2.22a–d**).[1]

Types of X-Rays

- Mandatory radiographs for surgical planning:
  - Standing AP or PA (**Fig. 2.23a, b**–acceptable; **Fig. 2.24a, b**–unacceptable images).
  - Supine side benders: (**Fig. 2.25a–c**–acceptable; **Fig. 2.26**–unsuitable).
    - Two long cassettes or Three 14″ × 17″ (one each for the proximal thoracic, main thoracic, thoracolumbar/lumbar).
    - All three curves must be evaluated for flexibility.
  - Standing lateral (**Fig. 2.27**–acceptable; **Fig. 2.28a, b**–unsuitable).

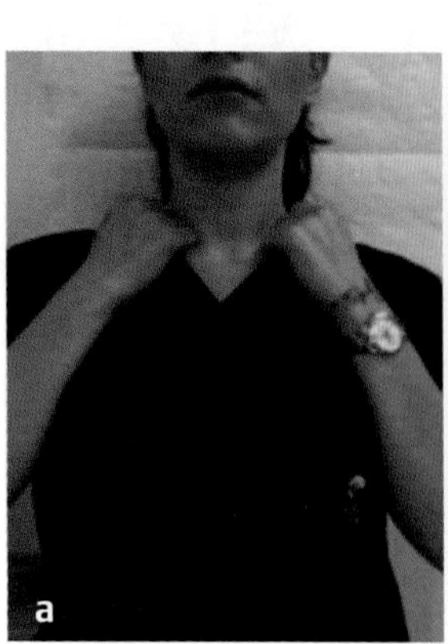
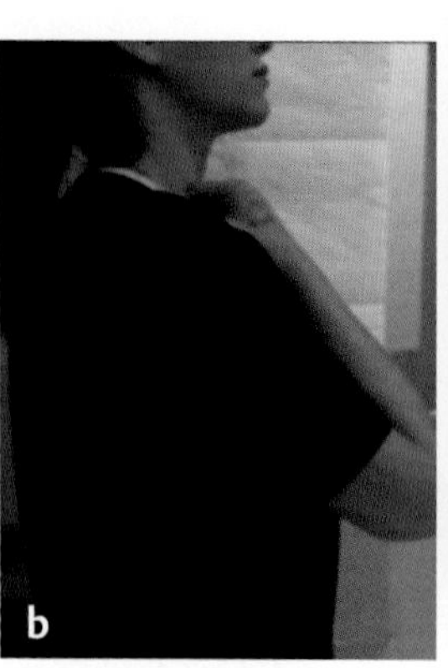
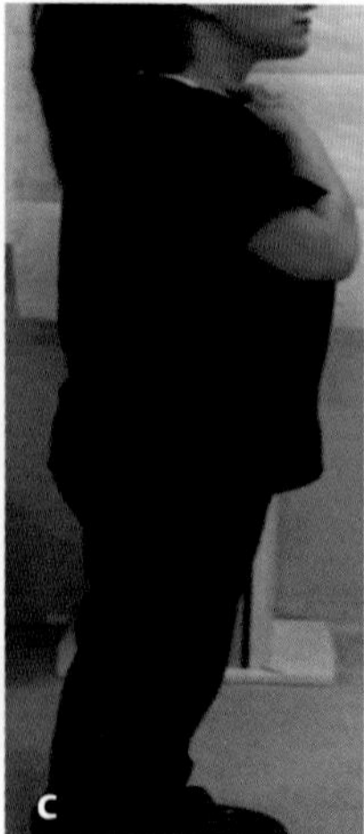
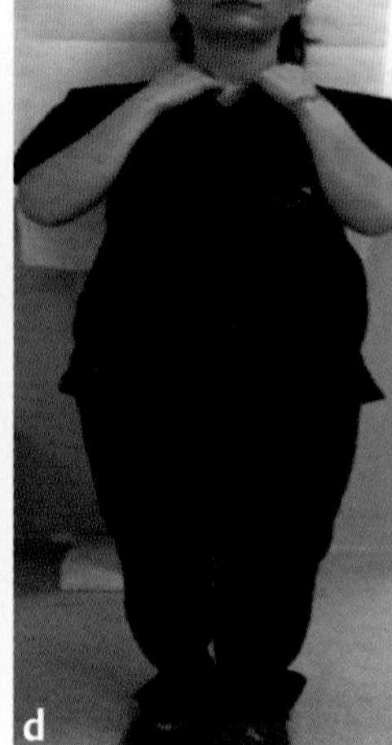

Fig. 2.22 (a-d) Posture for Scoliosis X-rays.

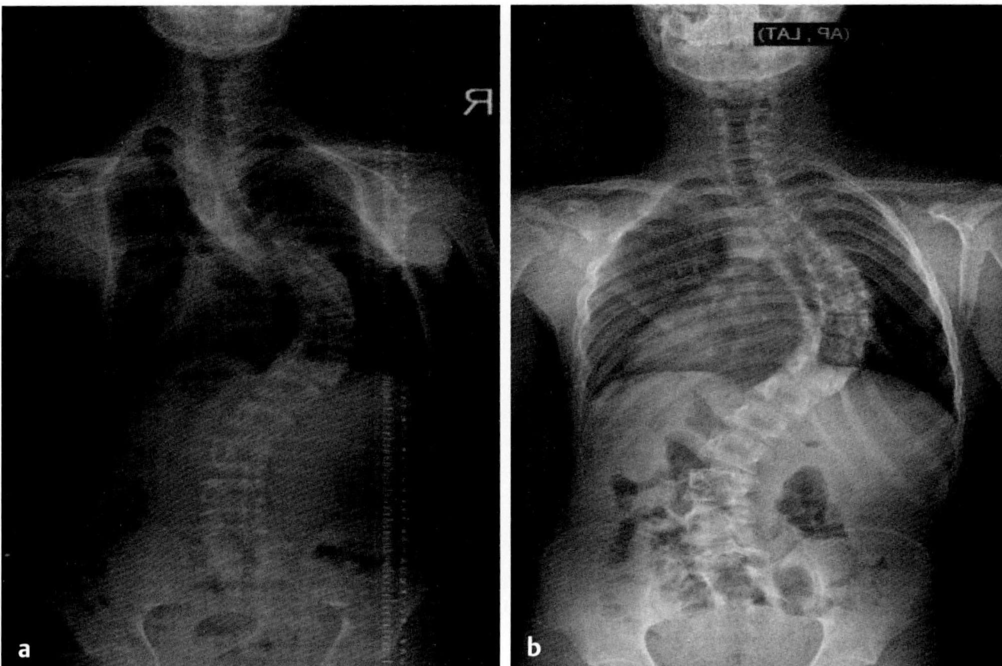

Fig. 2.23 (a, b) Standing anteroposterior (AP) or posteroanterior (PA): quality spinal radiographs should include the area from the C7 to the femoral heads and cover the entire ribcage. It should point from right to left.

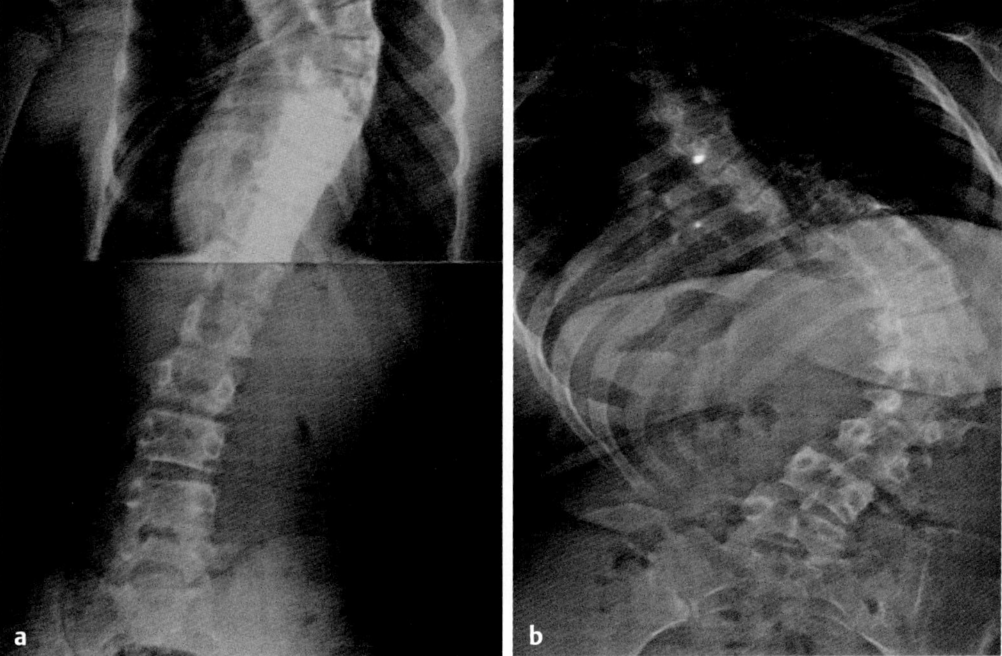

Fig. 2.24 (a, b) Standing anteroposterior (AP) or posteroanterior (PA): pelvis (right and left iliac wings), C7, and S1.

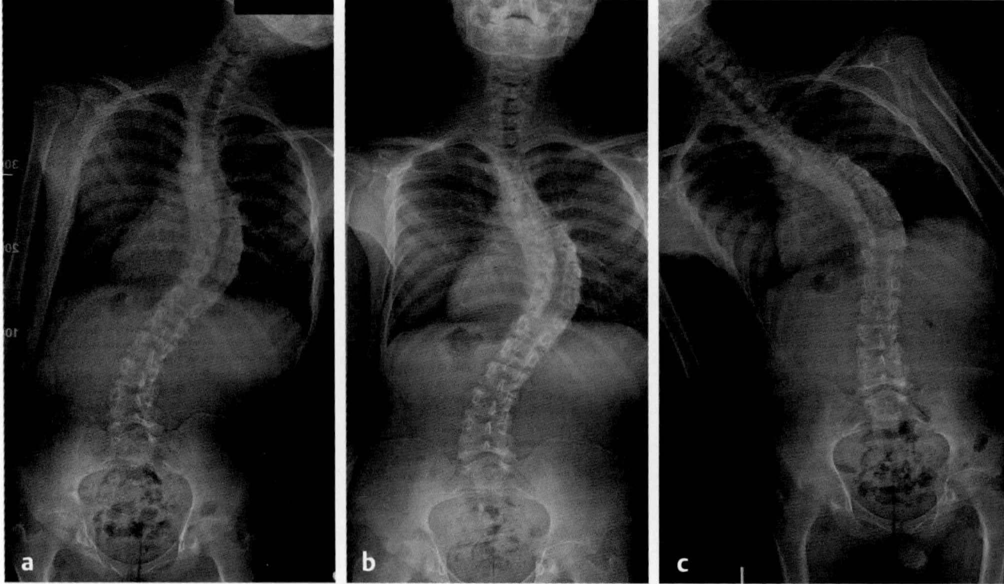

Fig. 2.25 (a–c) Supine side benders: the patient's right, neutral, and left bending radiograph. All vertebras are clearly visible.

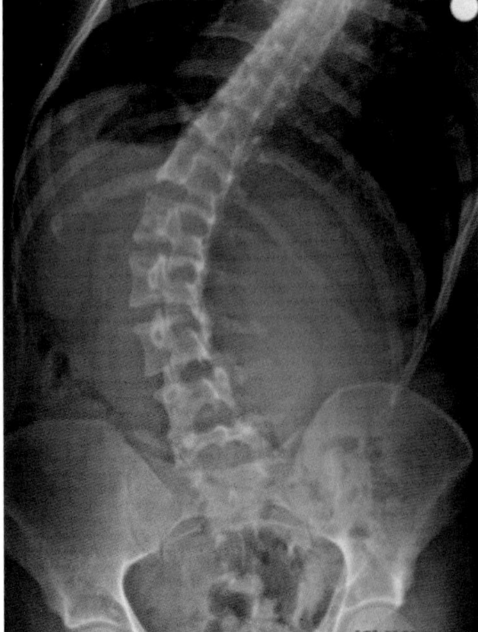

Fig. 2.26 Supine side benders: proximal bend not seen.

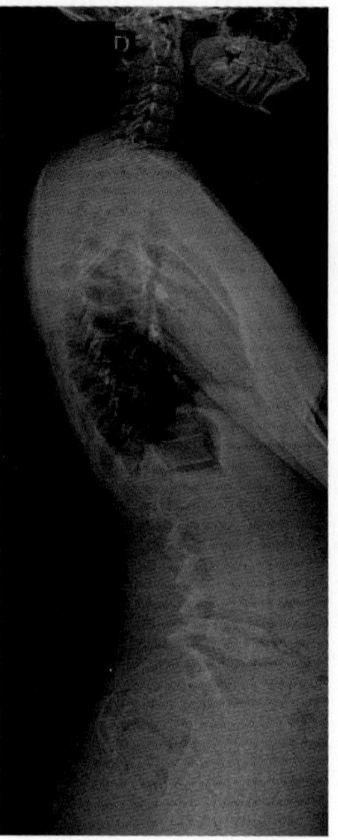

Fig. 2.27 Lateral standing: the radiograph should include C7 to S1. The upper thoracic region can be difficult to image; hence, it is common to have a good quality radiograph where T2 is not clear, but all other landmarks (C7, T5, T10, T12, L2, and the sacrum) are visible.

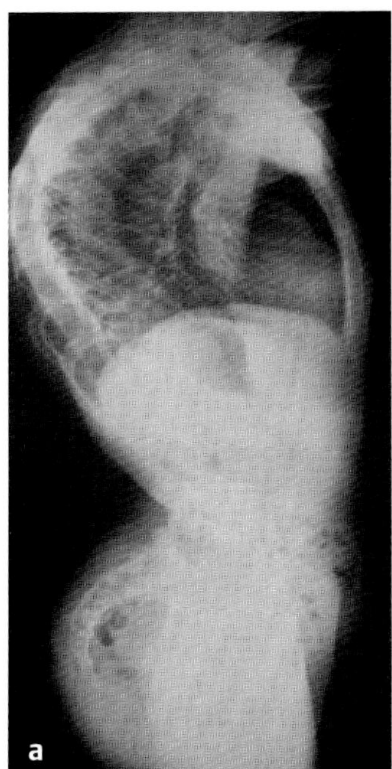

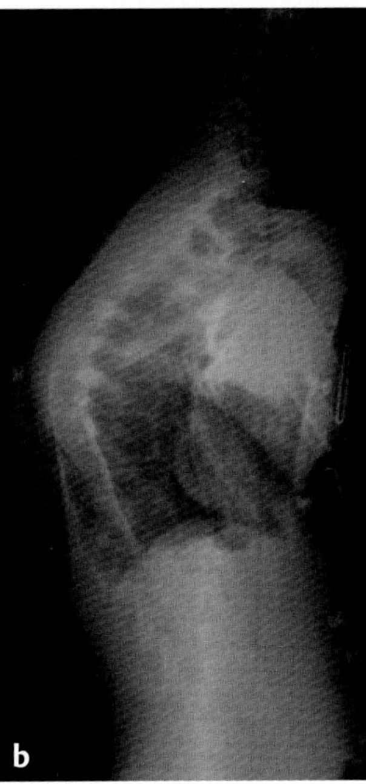

Fig. 2.28 (a, b) Lateral standing: unsuitable lateral images: blurred image and S1 not visible.

References

1. O'Brien M, Kuklo T, Blanke K, Lenke L. Radiographic measurement manual. Spinal Deformity Study Group (SDSG) Medtronic Sofamor Danek USA. Inc; 2008
2. Potter BK, Rosner MK, Lehman RA Jr, Polly DW Jr, Schroeder TM, Kuklo TR. Reliability of end, neutral, and stable vertebrae identification in adolescent idiopathic scoliosis. Spine 2005;30(14):1658–1663
3. King HA, Moe JH, Bradford DS, Winter RB. The selection of fusion levels in thoracic idiopathic scoliosis. J Bone Joint Surg Am 1983;65(9):1302–1313
4. Beauchamp M, Labelle H, Grimard G, Stanciu C, Poitras B, Dansereau J. Diurnal variation of Cobb angle measurement in adolescent idiopathic scoliosis. Spine 1993;18(12): 1581–1583
5. Göçen S, Havitçioglu H. Effect of rotation on frontal plane deformity in idiopathic scoliosis. Orthopedics 2001;24(3):265–268
6. Van Goethem JW, Van Campenhout A. Scoliosis. Spinal imaging. 2007:95–108
7. Malfair D, Flemming AK, Dvorak MF, et al. Radiographic evaluation of scoliosis: review. AJR Am J Roentgenol 2010; 194(3, Suppl) S8–S22
8. Morrissy RT, Goldsmith GS, Hall EC, Kehl D, Cowie GH. Measurement of the Cobb angle on radiographs of patients who have scoliosis. Evaluation of intrinsic error. J Bone Joint Surg Am 1990;72(3):320–327
9. Carman DL, Browne RH, Birch JG. Measurement of scoliosis and kyphosis radiographs. Intraobserver and interobserver variation. J Bone Joint Surg Am 1990;72(3):328–333
10. Pruijs JE, Hageman MA, Keessen W, van der Meer R, van Wieringen JC. Variation in Cobb angle measurements in scoliosis. Skeletal Radiol 1994;23(7):517–520
11. Nash CL Jr, Moe JH. A study of vertebral rotation. J Bone Joint Surg Am 1969;51(2):223–229
12. Vrtovec T, Pernuš F, Likar B. A review of methods for quantitative evaluation of spinal curvature. Eur Spine J 2009;18(5):593–607
13. Jeffries BF, Tarlton M, De Smet AA, Dwyer SJ III, Brower AC. Computerized measurement and analysis of scoliosis: a more accurate representation of the shape of the curve. Radiology 1980;134(2):381–385
14. Obeid I, Berjano P, Lamartina C, Chopin D, Boissière L, Bourghli A. Classification of coronal imbalance in adult scoliosis and spine deformity: a treatment-oriented guideline. Eur Spine J 2019;28(1):94–113
15. Kim H, Kim HS, Moon ES, et al. Scoliosis imaging: what radiologists should know. Radiographics 2010;30(7):1823–1842
16. Holmes C, Brock K, Morgan P. Postural asymmetry in non-ambulant adults with

cerebral palsy: a scoping review. Disabil Rehabil 2019;41(9):1079–1088
17. Shrader MW, Andrisevic EM, Belthur MV, White GR, Boan C, Wood W. Inter- and intraobserver reliability of pelvic obliquity measurement methods in patients with cerebral palsy. Spine Deform 2018;6(3): 257–262
18. Asher M, Lai SM, Burton D, Manna B. The influence of spine and trunk deformity on preoperative idiopathic scoliosis patients' health-related quality of life questionnaire responses. Spine 2004;29(8):861–868
19. Hwang CJ, Lee CS, Lee D-H, Cho JH. Progression of trunk imbalance in adolescent idiopathic scoliosis with a thoracolumbar/ lumbar curve: is it predictable at the initial visit? J Neurosurg Pediatr 2017;20(5): 450–455
20. Floman Y, Penny JN, Micheli LJ, Riseborough EJ, Hall JE. Osteotomy of the fusion mass in scoliosis. J Bone Joint Surg Am 1982; 64(9):1307–1316
21. Trobisch PD, Samdani AF, Pahys JM, Cahill PJ. Postoperative trunk shift in Lenke 1 and 2 curves: how common is it? And analysis of risk factors. Eur Spine J 2011;20(7): 1137–1140
22. Glassman SD, Bridwell K, Dimar JR, Horton W, Berven S, Schwab F. The impact of positive sagittal balance in adult spinal deformity. Spine 2005;30:2024-2029.
23. Diebo BG, Varghese JJ, Lafage R, Schwab FJ, Lafage V. Sagittal alignment of the spine: what do you need to know? Clin Neurol Neurosurg 2015;139:295–301
24. Roussouly P, Berthonnaud E, Dimnet J. [Geometrical and mechanical analysis of lumbar lordosis in an asymptomatic population: proposed classification]. Rev Chir Orthop Repar Appar Mot 2003;89(7): 632–639
25. Kuntz C IV, Levin LS, Ondra SL, Shaffrey CI, Morgan CJ. Neutral upright sagittal spinal alignment from the occiput to the pelvis in asymptomatic adults: a review and resynthesis of the literature. J Neurosurg Spine 2007;6(2):104–112
26. Roussouly P, Nnadi C. Sagittal plane deformity: an overview of interpretation and management. Eur Spine J 2010;19(11): 1824–1836
27. Barrey C, Roussouly P, Le Huec J-C, D'Acunzi G, Perrin G. Compensatory mechanisms contributing to keep the sagittal balance of the spine. Eur Spine J 2013; 22(6, Suppl 6) S834–S841
28. Barrey C, Jund J, Noseda O. Equilibre sagittal pelvi-rachidien et pathologies lombaires dégénératives. Etude comparative à propos de 100 cas. Lyon: Thèse Doctorat-Université Claude-Bernard; 2004
29. Duval-Beaupère G, Schmidt C, Cosson P. A Barycentremetric study of the sagittal shape of spine and pelvis: the conditions required for an economic standing position. Ann Biomed Eng 1992;20(4):451–462
30. Duval-Beaupère G, Legaye J. Composante sagittale de la statique rachidienne. Rev Rhum 2004;71(2):105–119
31. Murtagh RD, Quencer RM, Uribe J. Pelvic evaluation in thoracolumbar corrective spine surgery: how I do it. Radiology 2016; 278(3):646–656
32. Boulay C, Tardieu C, Hecquet J, et al. Sagittal alignment of spine and pelvis regulated by pelvic incidence: standard values and prediction of lordosis. Eur Spine J 2006; 15(4):415–422
33. Ryan DJ, Protopsaltis TS, Ames CP, et al; International Spine Study Group. T1 pelvic angle (TPA) effectively evaluates sagittal deformity and assesses radiographical surgical outcomes longitudinally. Spine 2014; 39(15):1203–1210
34. Protopsaltis T, Schwab F, Bronsard N, et al; International Spine Study Group. TheT1 pelvic angle, a novel radiographic measure of global sagittal deformity, accounts for both spinal inclination and pelvic tilt and correlates with health-related quality of life. J Bone Joint Surg Am 2014;96(19):1631–1640
35. Amabile C, Pillet H, Lafage V, Barrey C, Vital J-M, Skalli W. A new quasi-invariant parameter characterizing the postural alignment of young asymptomatic adults. Eur Spine J 2016;25(11):3666–3674
36. Faundez AA, Richards J, Maxy P, Price R, Léglise A, Le Huec J-C. The mechanism in junctional failure of thoraco-lumbar fusions. Part II: Analysis of a series of PJK after thoraco-lumbar fusion to determine parameters allowing to predict the risk of junctional breakdown. Eur Spine J 2018; **27**(1, Suppl 1)139–148
37. Le Huec JC, Demezon H, Aunoble S. Sagittal parameters of global cervical balance using EOS imaging: normative values from a prospective cohort of asymptomatic volunteers. Eur Spine J 2015;24(1):63–71

38. Hilibrand AS, Tannenbaum DA, Graziano GP, Loder RT, Hensinger RN. The sagittal alignment of the cervical spine in adolescent idiopathic scoliosis. J Pediatr Orthop 1995; 15(5):627–632
39. Schwab FJ, Lafage V, Farcy J-P, Bridwell KH, Glassman S, Shainline MR. Predicting outcome and complications in the surgical treatment of adult scoliosis. Spine 2008; 33(20):2243–2247
40. Glassman SD, Berven S, Bridwell K, Horton W, Dimar JR. Correlation of radiographic parameters and clinical symptoms in adult scoliosis. Spine 2005;30(6):682–688
41. Knott PT, Mardjetko SM, Techy F. The use of the T1 sagittal angle in predicting overall sagittal balance of the spine. Spine J 2010; 10(11):994–998
42. Jackson RP, McManus AC. Radiographic analysis of sagittal plane alignment and balance in standing volunteers and patients with low back pain matched for age, sex, and size. A prospective controlled clinical study. Spine 1994;19(14):1611–1618
43. Roussouly P, Pinheiro-Franco JL. Sagittal parameters of the spine: biomechanical approach. Eur Spine J 2011; 20(5, Suppl 5)578–585
44. Roussouly P, Gollogly S, Berthonnaud E, Dimnet J. Classification of the normal variation in the sagittal alignment of the human lumbar spine and pelvis in the standing position. Spine 2005;30(3):346–353
45. Ames CP, Smith JS, Scheer JK, et al. Impact of spinopelvic alignment on decision-making in deformity surgery in adults: a review. J Neurosurg Spine 2012;16(6):547–564
46. Chan CYW, Naing KS, Chiu CK, Mohamad SM, Kwan MK. Pelvic obliquity in adolescent idiopathic scoliosis planned for posterior spinal fusion: a preoperative analysis of 311 lower limb axis films. J Orthop Surg (Hong Kong) 2019;27(2):2309499019857250
47. Schwab F, Patel A, Ungar B, Farcy J-P, Lafage V. Adult spinal deformity-postoperative standing imbalance: how much can you tolerate? An overview of key parameters in assessing alignment and planning corrective surgery. Spine 2010;35(25):2224–2231
48. Legaye J, Duval-Beaupère G, Hecquet J, Marty C. Pelvic incidence: a fundamental pelvic parameter for three-dimensional regulation of spinal sagittal curves. Eur Spine J 1998;7(2):99–103
49. Schwab F, Lafage V, Boyce R, Skalli W, Farcy J-P. Gravity line analysis in adult volunteers: age-related correlation with spinal parameters, pelvic parameters, and foot position. Spine 2006;31(25):E959–E967
50. Schwab F, Ungar B, Blondel B, et al. Scoliosis Research Society-Schwab adult spinal deformity classification: a validation study. Spine 2012;37(12):1077–1082
51. Risser JC. The Iliac apophysis: an invaluable sign in the management of scoliosis. Clin Orthop 1958;11(11):111–119

3 Scoliosis Case Review

Onur Yaman, Muhammad Yassar Jazaib Ali, and Salman Sharif

Introduction

Scoliosis is a spinal deformity consisting of lateral curvature and rotation of the vertebrae. It can be classified by etiology and by the age of onset (idiopathic, congenital, neuromuscular, and degenerative). The majority of scoliosis cases encountered by the general practitioner is idiopathic.[1] The natural history relates to the etiology and age at presentation and usually dictates the treatment. However, the patient's history, physical examination, and radiographs are critical in the initial evaluation of scoliosis.[2] Most cases of scoliosis are mild and don't need treatment. Treatment is geared toward relieving symptoms and not necessarily fixing the curve. The goal is always to decrease pain and improve function.

This chapter focuses on a few cases dealing with specific types of scoliosis, the preoperative planning of these patients based on scanograms, and proper surgical strategies applied to correct these complex deformities using the Surgimap software.[3–5] These cases are beneficial in developing an understanding of the complex anatomical nature of the scoliotic deformity and the application of various surgical techniques.

Case 1: A Lumbar Degenerative Scoliosis Case

A 72-year-old lady presented to the clinic suffering from back and bilateral leg pain for the last 10 years. She was having neurogenic claudication and used to bend forward on walking. Neurological examination was normal.

Findings of Preoperative Scoliosis Graph Measurements using Surgimap

- Sagittal vertical axis (SVA) = 31.7 cm.
- Lumbar lordosis (LL) = −40 degrees.
- Pelvic tilt (PT) = 41 degrees.
- Pelvic incidence (PI) = 56 degrees.
- Thoracic kyphosis = 14 degree.

Discussion

In this particular case, a PT of 41 degrees indicates that the patient had retroverted her pelvis to decrease the SVA. Also, patient tried to decrease the thoracic kyphosis (14 degrees) to decrease the SVA further. The patient's PI of 56 degrees means that the LL has to be at least 60 degrees following the surgery (**Fig. 3.1**).

Preoperative Planning

Applying a type III (pedicle subtraction osteotomy [PSO]) at L4 is not enough for a proper sagittal alignment (**Fig. 3.2**). A type III at L4 and type II at L3 level also do not suffice for the same patient (**Fig. 3.3**). If a double type II (Ponte) osteotomy combined with a Type III (PSOs) osteotomy is performed, it will balance the sagittal plane but not well enough to correct other parameters (**Fig. 3.4**). Optimal results can be obtained in this case with type IV osteotomy at L4, and

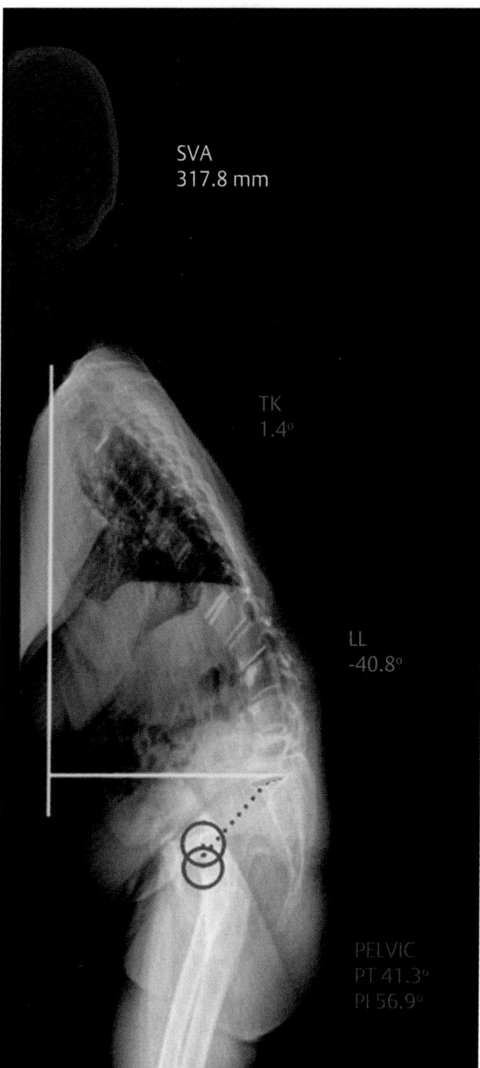

Fig. 3.1 Preoperative radiographs of an adult degenerative scoliosis case with measurements obtained on Surgimap software. Severe sagittal imbalance of 31.7 cm SVA can be noted. Patient has 40-degree kyphosis. PI is 56 degrees. Patient is using compensatory mechanism to balance the spine. Pelvic tilt (PT) is 41 degrees and thoracic kyphosis is only 1 degree. PT, pelvic tilt; PI, pelvic incidence; LL, lumbar lordosis; TK, thoracic kyphosis; SVA, sagittal vertical axis.

type II osteotomy at L2 and L3 is the suitable surgical option to maintain a proper sagittal balance for the patient.

Surgical Intervention

A type IV osteotomy at L4 and type II osteotomies at level L2 and L3 were performed during the surgery. Following the surgical intervention, the patient has a good LL of 38.3 degrees. SVA was 1.7 cm postoperatively. The patient still had a high PT because

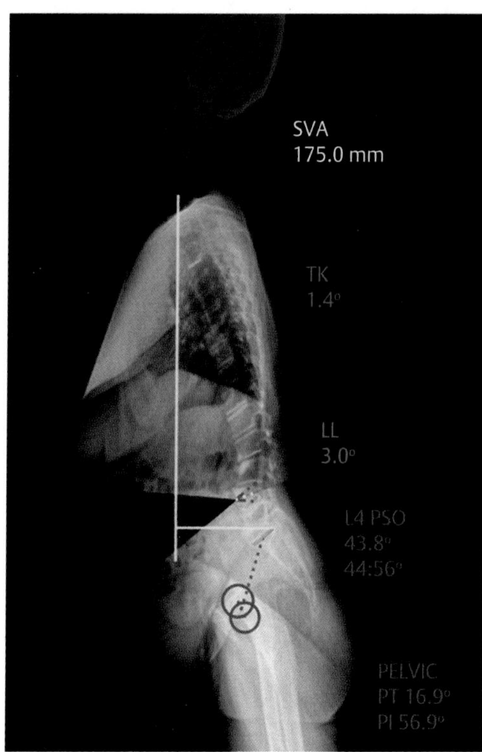

Fig. 3.2 Preoperative radiographs with measurements obtained on Surgimap software, if a Type III PSO at L4 was planned. Applying Type III (PSO) at lumbar 4 vertebra will not be enough to balance the spine. PT, pelvic tilt; PI, pelvic incidence; LL, lumbar lordosis; TK, thoracic kyphosis; SVA, sagittal vertical axis; PSO, pedicle subtraction osteotomy.

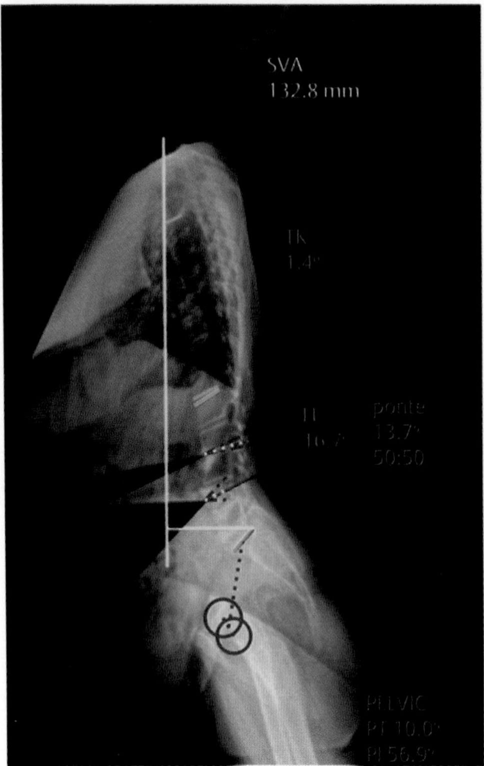

Fig. 3.3 Radiographs with measurements obtained on Surgimap, if a Type III osteotomy at L4, and a Type II osteotomy at L3 level was planned. Applying Type III (PSO) at lumbar 4 vertebra adding a Type II osteotomy (Ponte) at the L3 level will not be enough to balance the spine. PT, pelvic tilt; PI, pelvic incidence; LL, lumbar lordosis; TK, thoracic kyphosis; SVA, sagittal vertical axis.

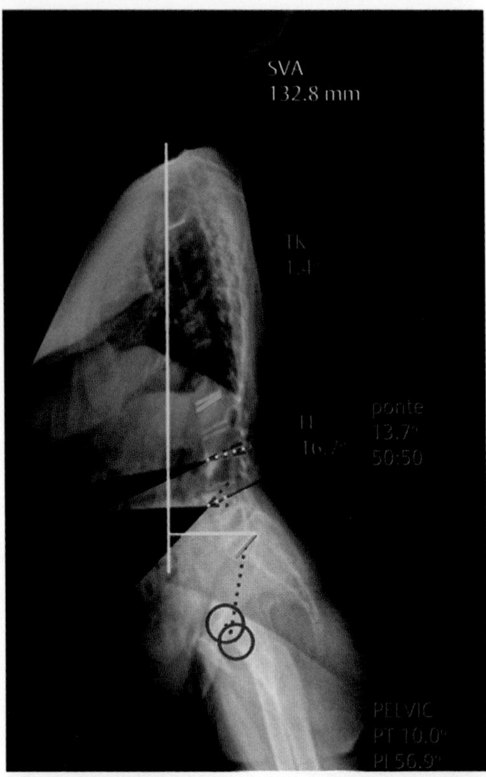

Fig. 3.4 Radiographs with measurements obtained on Surgimap, if a Double Type II (Ponte) osteotomies combined with a Type III (PSO) osteotomy will balance the sagittal plane but it is still not well. PT, pelvic tilt; PI, pelvic incidence; LL, lumbar lordosis; TK, thoracic kyphosis; SVA, sagittal vertical axis. (Surgimap software was used.)

of the lack of anteversion of the pelvis during the surgery (**Fig. 3.5**).

Preoperative and postoperative clinical photo of the same patient is shown in **Fig. 3.6**.

Case 2: A Lumbar Degenerative Scoliosis Case

A 60-year-old female was suffering from back and bilateral leg pain. She was having neurogenic claudication and used to bend forward in a standing posture. Neurological examination was normal.

Findings of Preoperative Scoliosis Graph Measurements using Surgimap

- The patient's SVA was 22.6 cm.
- Lumbar lordosis (LL) was 26 degrees.
- Pelvic tilt (PT) was 36 degrees.
- Thoracic kyphosis was 0 degree.
- Pelvic incidence (PI) was 43 degrees.

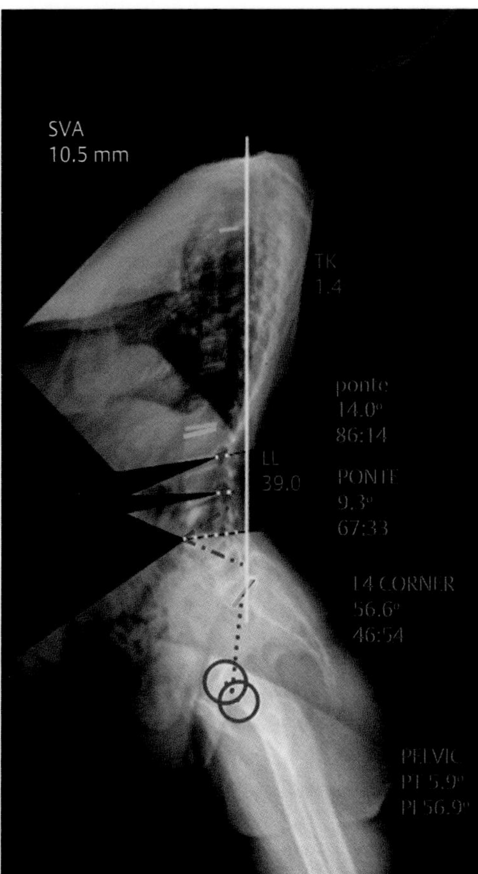

Fig. 3.5 Postoperative radiograph with measurements obtained on Surgimap. Applying Type IV (Corner) at lumbar 4 vertebra adding double Type II osteotomy (Ponte) at the above level is enough for a balanced spine. PT, pelvic tilt; PI, pelvic incidence; LL, lumbar lordosis; TK, thoracic kyphosis; SVA, sagittal vertical axis.

Discussion

Pelvic tilt was 36 degrees which means the patient had retroverted the pelvis to decrease the SVA. Also, patient tried to decrease the thoracic kyphosis to decrease the SVA. Thoracic kyphosis was 0 degree and the patient's PI was 43 degrees. It means that the patient LL has to be at least 50 degrees following the surgery (**Fig. 3.7**).

Preoperative Planning and Surgical Intervention

Applying a Type IV (corner osteotomy) at L4 will maintain a good sagittal balance after the surgery. The patient's SVA is 2.9 cm after the surgery. PT is 1 degree which means that the patient does not need any retroversion now. The patient's sagittal balance is maintained with 57-degree LL and correlated with 43-degree PI (**Fig. 3.8**).

Preoperative and postoperative clinical photos of the same patient are shown in **Fig. 3.9**.

Pearl

Adult degenerative scoliosis

Adult degenerative scoliosis (ADS) is a prevalent disease among old-aged people. ADS is vital to the deformity for surgeon both from a demographic and a clinical perspective. The curve begins to develop during adulthood, secondary to the degeneration of spinal motion segments. Surgical intervention among these patients remains controversial.[6] Proper history, examination, and further work-up can guide regarding the optimal management. Suitable options for the individual patient can be optimized based on clinical and radiographic stability as well as the loss of balance that the patient suffers from. Management options include nonoperative management, decompression alone, instrumentation with posterior spinal fusion, anterior spinal fusion, and osteotomy.[7] In ADS, restoring lumbar lordosis and sagittal balance is the main goal rather than correcting scoliosis itself. The complication rate is high in this age group with other comorbidities; these include infections, cerebrospinal fluid leaks, implant failures, junctional kyphosis, adjacent segment degeneration, and pseudarthrosis. Systemic complications include myocardial infarction, pneumonia, urinary tract infections, and deep vein thrombosis. The high potential complication rates appear to be outweighed by the eventual successful outcomes in patients suitable for surgical intervention.[8]

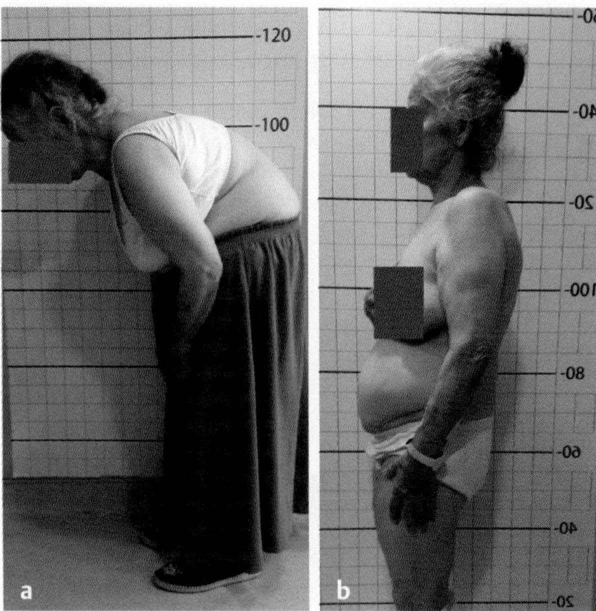

Fig. 3.6 Case of adult degenerative scoliosis. **(a)** Preoperative and **(b)** postoperative clinical photos of the patient. Before the surgery patient had a severe sagittal imbalance. Applying a Type IV (Corner) osteotomy at L4 and Type II (Ponte) at level L2 and L3 balanced the spine in sagittal plane. The marked improvement in bent posture of the patient can be visualized.

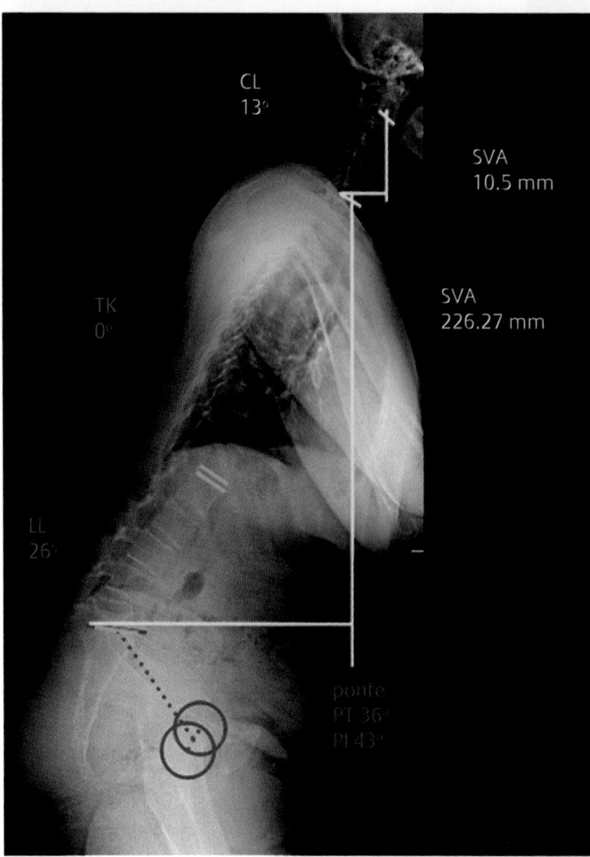

Fig. 3.7 A lumbar degenerative scoliosis case. Preoperative scoliosis graph measurements using Surgimap shows that patient's sagittal vertical axis (SVA) was 22.6 cm. Pelvic tilt (PT) was 36 degrees which means patient had retroverted the pelvis to decrease the SVA. Thoracic kyphosis with 0 degree shows that patient is using compensatory mechanism to balance the spine. Patient's pelvic incidence (PI) was 43 degrees. It means that the patient's lumbar lordosis has to be least 50 degrees following the surgery.

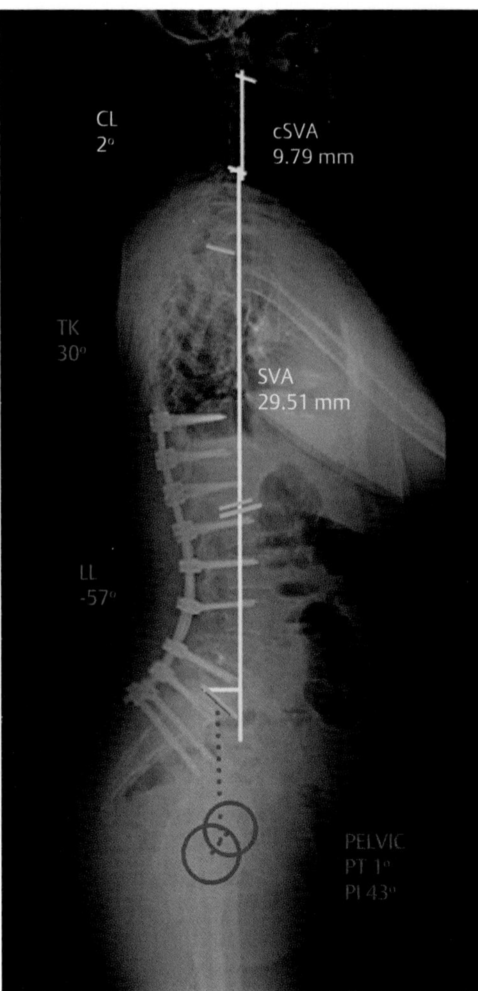

Fig. 3.8 Radiograph showing the post-operative results after applying a Type IV (Corner) osteotomy at L4 and Type II (Ponte) at level L2 and L3 balanced the spine in sagittal plane. Patient pelvic tilt (PT) is in normal range means that the patient is not using any compensatory mechanism.

Case 3: A Case of Neuromuscular Scoliosis

A 10-year-old female presented to the outpatient department with an inability to sit upright and also to suffer from recurrent respiratory infections.

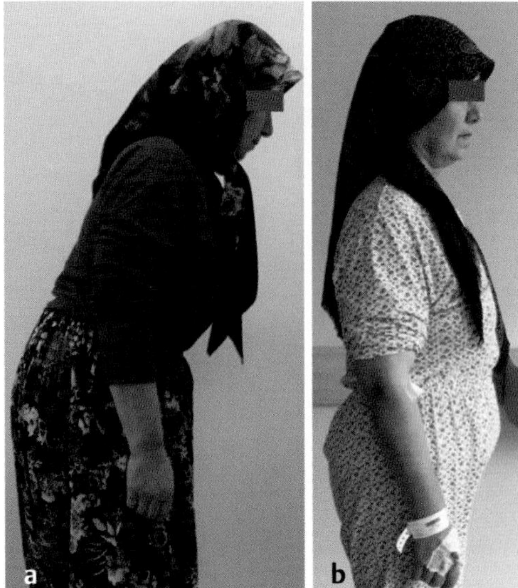

Fig. 3.9 Preoperative and postoperative clinical photos of the patient. **(a)** Before the surgery patient had a severe sagittal imbalance. **(b)** After the surgery patient's sagittal balance is improved.

Findings of Preoperative Scoliosis Graph Measurements using Surgimap

- On the anteroposterior (AP) view, she had large thoracolumbar scoliosis with Cobb's angle of 110 degrees.
- On the lateral view, she had an 11.4-cm sagittal imbalance (**Fig. 3.10**).

Preoperative Planning and Surgical Intervention

The patient was planned to be fixed from the upper thoracic spine to the iliac wings, distracted on the concave side, to enlarge the thoracic chest. Ponte (Type II) osteotomies were applied at the apex and two levels above and below the apex.

After the surgery, Cobb's angle was reduced to 37 degrees, and the height of both iliac wings was brought to the same level. On the other hand, sagittal balance after the

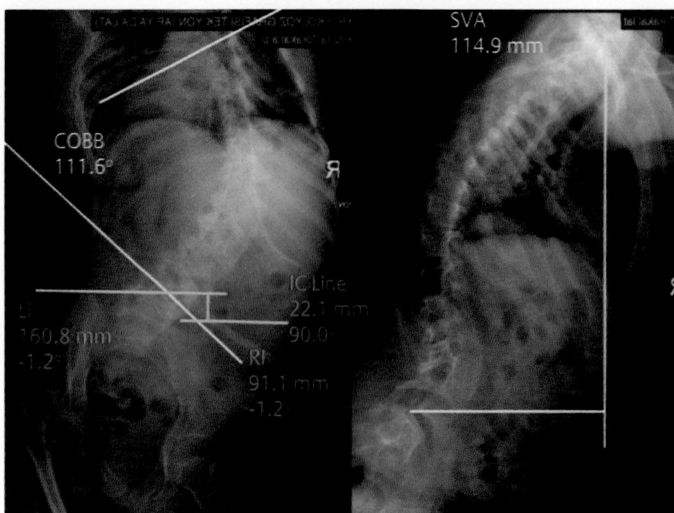

Fig. 3.10 A neuromuscular scoliosis case. A large thoracolumbar scoliosis with 110 degrees and iliac wings were imbalanced. On the lateral view she has 11.4 cm sagittal imbalance.

surgery was better than the preoperative images (**Fig. 3.11**).

Pearl

Neuromuscular scoliosis

Neuromuscular scoliosis, the second most common form of scoliosis, is associated with nerves or muscular system disorders such as cerebral palsy, spina bifida, and spinal cord injury, causing muscles to become weak and spastic or paralyzed.[9,10] Nonsurgical treatments such as bracing, wheelchair modification, physical therapy, and environmental adaptation can help improve mobility. Bracing can prevent further curve worsening during periods of growth but will not correct the curve itself. Stabilizing the spine with *spinal fusion surgery* is the most common treatment, usually necessary when a child reaches adolescence. It is usually necessary to fuse a larger portion of the spine. The goal is to stabilize the curve and stop its progression, balance the spine and pelvis (in patients who are unable to walk), restore the ability to sit upright, and improve/preserve lung function.[11] As these children have a higher rate of complications,[12] preoperative planning all the way through recovery plays a pivotal role.

Case 4: A Case of Adolescent Idiopathic Scoliosis

A 14-year-old male complaining of back pain with no neurological deficit presented to the outpatient department.

Findings of Preoperative Scoliosis Graph Measurements using Surgimap

- A 51-degree thoracic scoliosis.
- The lumbar modifier was type A.
- According to the right and left bending X-ray films, this was a Lenke Type 1A scoliosis (**Fig. 3.12**).
- Thoracic kyphosis was 20 degrees, within normal range (**Fig. 3.13**).

Surgical Intervention

Type II osteotomies were performed at the apex, two levels above and below the apex of the curve, and the spine was fixed from T2 to L3. Preoperative and postoperative X-ray of the patient is shown in **Fig. 3.14(a, b)**. Postoperatively, thoracic scoliosis has been significantly corrected.

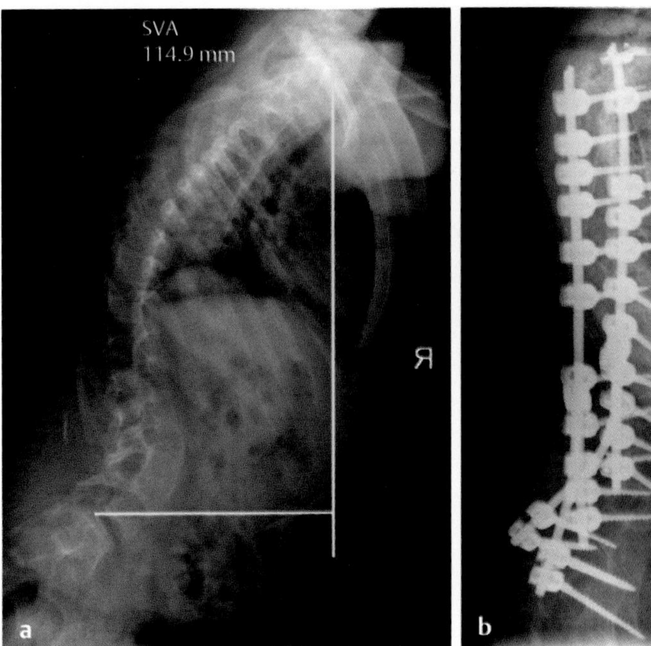

Fig. 3.11 **(a)** Ponte (Type II) osteotomies were applied at the apex and two levels above and below the apex. **(b)** After the surgery, Cobb angle decreases to 37 degrees and the height of both iliac wings is brought to same level. Well-balanced sagittal plane.

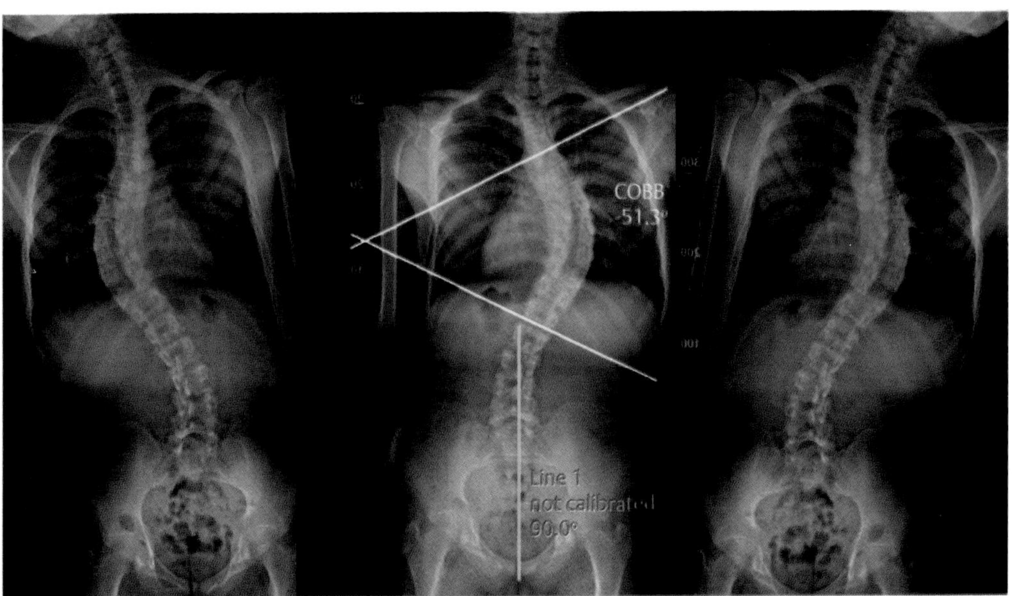

Fig. 3.12 An adolescent idiopathic scoliosis case with 51 degrees thoracic scoliosis on Scanogram. Right and left bending X-ray films. Lumbar modifier was type A.

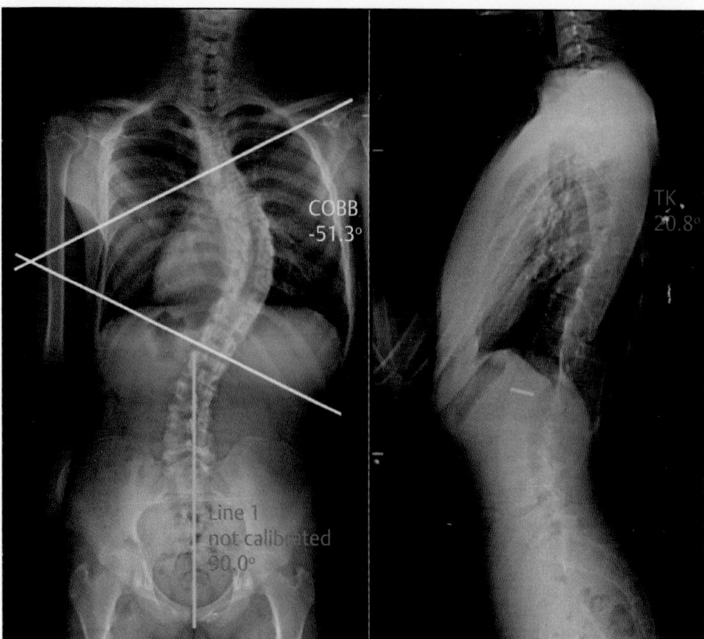

Fig. 3.13 An adolescent idiopathic scoliosis case. Patient's thoracic kyphosis was 20 degrees in normal ranges.

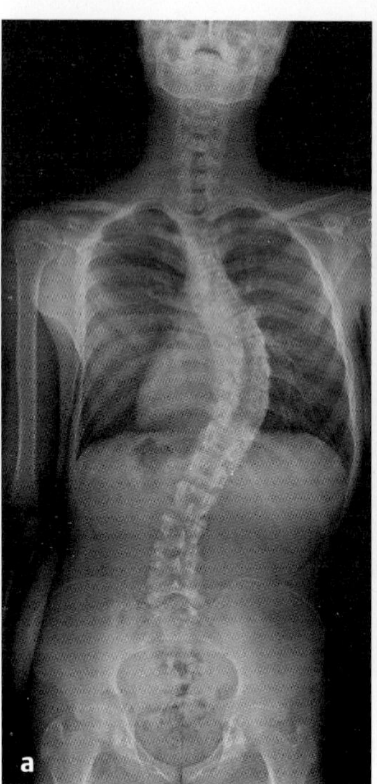

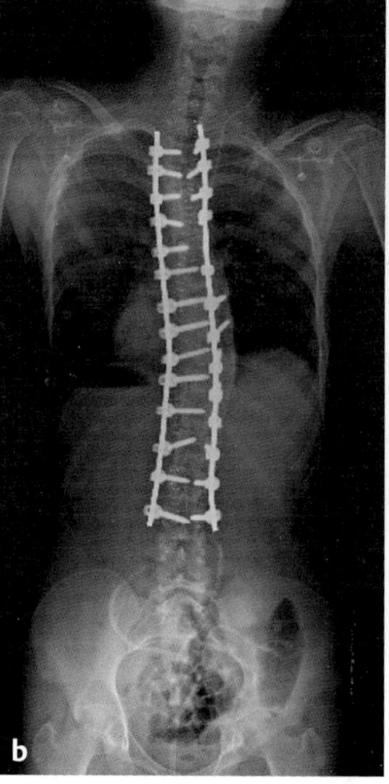

Fig. 3.14 **(a)** Preoperative and **(b)** postoperative X-rays of the patient with adolescent idiopathic scoliosis. Type II osteotomies were performed at the apex, two level above and below of the curve and fixed from T2 to L3.

Pearl

Adolescent idiopathic scoliosis

Adolescent idiopathic scoliosis (AIS) is a coronal plane spinal deformity which most commonly presents in adolescent girls from ages 10 to 18. The three Os can summarize the main treatment options for scoliosis: Observation, Orthosis (bracing), and Operative treatment.[13] The selection of the best treatment is based on the maturity of the patient (age, menarchal status, Risser grading of Iliac apophysis), location, severity, and risk of progression of the curvature. A common protocol used to guide treatment is to observe patients with curves of less than 25 degrees, brace patients between 25 and 45 degrees, and consider surgery on patients with curves of greater than 45 degrees. Advances in biomechanics and technology have led to improvements in the safety and outcomes of surgical and nonsurgical treatments.[14,15]

Conclusion

Scoliosis is a complex anatomical deformity with a deviation of the spine consisting of lateral curvature and rotation of the involved vertebrae. While scoliosis is associated with a variety of diagnoses, the vast majority of patients encountered are idiopathic. A thorough history and physical examination, and radiographs should be completed to identify nonidiopathic causes of scoliosis. The treatment for idiopathic scoliosis is based on age, curve magnitude, and risk of progression and includes observation, orthotic management, and surgical correction. The various surgical treatment strategies should be properly planned for each individual case. These surgical options should further be evaluated on scanograms preoperatively with the aid of Surgimap software[4] to achieve the best results for that individual patient.

References

1. Janicki JA, Alman B. Scoliosis: review of diagnosis and treatment. Paediatr Child Health 2007;12(9):771–776
2. Malfair D, Flemming AK, Dvorak MF, et al. Radiographic evaluation of scoliosis: review. AJR Am J Roentgenol 2010; 194(3, Suppl) S8–S22
3. Helmya NA, El-Sayyad MM, Kattabeib OM. Intra-rater and inter-rater reliability of Surgimap Spine software for measuring spinal postural angles from digital photographs. Bull Fac Phys Ther 2015;20(2):193–199
4. Akbar M, Terran J, Ames CP, Lafage V, Schwab F. Use of Surgimap Spine in sagittal plane analysis, osteotomy planning, and correction calculation. Neurosurg Clin N Am 2013;24(2):163–172
5. Lafage R, Ferrero E, Henry JK, et al. Validation of a new computer-assisted tool to measure spino-pelvic parameters. Spine J 2015;15(12): 2493–2502
6. Kelly A, Younus A, Lekgwara P. Adult degenerative scoliosis: a literature review. Interdisciplinary Neurosurgery 2020;20: 100661
7. Cho K-J, Kim Y-T, Shin SH, Suk SI. Surgical treatment of adult degenerative scoliosis. Asian Spine J 2014;8(3):371–381
8. Kubat O, Ovadia D. Frontal and sagittal imbalance in patients with adolescent idiopathic deformity. Ann Transl Med 2020;8(2):29
9. Murphy RF, Mooney JF III. Current concepts in neuromuscular scoliosis. Curr Rev Musculoskelet Med 2019;12(2):220–227
10. Allam AM, Schwabe ALJP. Neuromuscular scoliosis. PM R 2013;5(11):957–963
11. Vialle R, Thévenin-Lemoine C, Mary P. Neuromuscular scoliosis. Orthop Traumatol Surg Res 2013; 99(1, Suppl)S124–S139
12. Master DL, Son-Hing JP, Poe-Kochert C, Armstrong DG, Thompson GHJS. Risk factors for major complications after surgery for neuromuscular scoliosis. Spine 2011;36(7): 564–571
13. Choudhry MN, Ahmad Z, Verma R. Adolescent idiopathic scoliosis. Open Orthop J 2016; 10:143–154
14. Sud A, Tsirikos AI. Current concepts and controversies on adolescent idiopathic scoliosis: Part I. Indian J Orthop 2013;47(2):117–128
15. Sud A, Tsirikos AI. Current concepts and controversies on adolescent idiopathic scoliosis: Part II. Indian J Orthop 2013;47(3):219–229

4 Biomechanics and Deformity of the Cervical Spine

William J. Kemp, Vikram Chakravarthy, and Edward C. Benzel

Introduction

This chapter summarizes the biomechanics of the intact and diseased cervical spine. The cervical spine has two transition zones at either end: the occipitocervical and cervicothoracic junction. These regions present unique stabilization and instrumentation challenges, particularly considering the close proximity to eloquent neural and vascular tissues. This chapter begins with a brief review of cervical anatomy followed by a discussion of the various biomechanical changes that occur with pathologic and surgically induced states. We discuss both anterior and posterior approaches to the cervical spine. Over time, technology has changed how we evaluate and manage cervical spine pathologies.

Biomechanics is the study of the mechanical laws relating to the movement or structure of living things. As humans, we rely on biomechanically sound spine structures to remain upright and navigate our environment. Specifically, the cervical spine is responsible for balancing the weight of the cranium and maintaining an upright posture. With improved technology, the precision to which we can evaluate the cervical spine continues to evolve. This chapter aims to comprehensively summarize the biomechanical principles associated with the intact and diseased cervical spine.

General Cervical Spine Anatomy and Biomechanics

The cervical spine is composed of seven vertebral bodies and transitional occipitocervical and cervicothoracic zones. These zones facilitate structural support and the containment and protection of the spinal cord and the eight cervical roots. A fibrocartilaginous intervertebral joint lies between the vertebral bodies and is composed of an inner, avascular nucleus pulposus and a circumferential annulus fibrosus. These structures permit a dynamic range of spinal loading and range of motion.[1]

The cervicothoracic junction is a unique transition zone between the dynamic and mobile lordotic cervical spine to the relatively inflexible kyphotic thoracic spine. The C7 vertebra marks the upper boundary of this transition. Anatomically, the size of the pedicles in the cervical spine progressively increase, while the lateral mass decreases, thus transitioning into the robust transverse process of the thoracic spine.[2]

Biomechanics of Occipitocervical Junction (O-C2)

The craniocervical junction is comprised of a unique complex consisting of the occiput, atlas (C1), axis (C2), and the numerous stabilizing ligamentous structures. The atlas is a bony ring consisting of prominent lateral masses without a true vertebral body with which the cranium articulates. Ligamentous structures, including the tectorial membrane (cranial extension of posterior longitudinal ligament), alar ligaments, apical ligament, cruciate ligament, nuchal ligament, anterior and posterior atlanto-occipital membranes, capsular ligaments, and transverse ligament of the atlas (TLA) provide support and maintain the integrity of the complex. The Occiput-C1 (O-C1) joint is primarily responsible for flexion and extension, while the C1–C2 joint permits axial rotation. Translation occurs at both segments during motion. Biomechanically, the alar ligament and TLA are both rate-dependent relative to their resultant instability.

The TLA extends horizontally behind the dens, attaching on the medial aspect of the lateral mass, limiting dorsal translation of the dens into the spinal canal. The "Rule of Spence," which was clinically described by Spence in 1970 and later evaluated biomechanically by Heller et al, confirms that if the combined lateral mass displacement is greater than 7 mm, the TLA is likely ruptured.[3,4] Heller et al used an anterior–posterior (AP) shear injury mechanism and found that 11 specimens failed within the substance of the ligament, and two failed due to bony avulsion. The average load to failure was 692 N (range, 220–1590 N) with the displacement to failure measure as 6.7 mm (2–14 mm). Based on their findings, it was concluded that the AP translation of the C2 dens was dependent on the rate of loading and the integrity of the TLA When the TLA ruptures, the greatest increase in instability occurs in flexion and extension (42% or 22 degrees), followed by lateral bending (5% or 5 degrees). Woods et al recently challenged the "Rule of Spence," citing that biomechanically, the TLA may become incompetent at a shorter length of displacement.[5]

The alar ligaments extend from the superolateral aspects of the C2 dens to the occipital condyles, involved primarily in limiting axial rotation.[6] Child et al found the alar ligaments to be broad and stout.[6] Dvorak et al sectioned 11 specimens and found that the average rotation between occiput and atlas was 4.4 degrees to the right and 5.9 degrees to the left.[7] After sectioning each alar ligament, it was found that the increase in contralateral axial rotation was approximately 29%. The tensile strength (190–290 N) of the alar ligaments was equal bilaterally and failure always occurred at the insertion site. Panjabi et al found that these ligaments failed at 13.6 Nm at 4 degrees per second and at 27.9 Nm at 100 degrees per second.[8]

Radcliff et al evaluated the integrity of the O-C1 and C1–C2 joint capsules by sectioning them sequentially.[9] Sectioning of the O-C1 joint capsule significantly increased translation during flexion-extension. The C1–C2 joint capsule did not act as a significant stabilizer in their study.

Clinical correlations include various radiographic parameters suggesting the presence of craniocervical junction instability. Occipitoatlantal (O-C1) instability should be considered if there is more than 2 mm of translation or 5 degrees rotation of occiput on C1. Atlantoaxial (C1–C2) instability is seen when the atlantodental interval (ADI) is greater than 3 mm in adults and 5 mm in children. If the ADI is greater than 5 mm, the TLA is considered ruptured, and if greater than 9 mm, then both TLA and alar ligaments are likely incompetent. When there is greater than 50% rotation between C1 and C2, this can also be considered a radiographic sign of instability.[10] These measurements on radiographic imaging may be unreliable at times, and should be used as an adjunct to clinical decision-making and can be supplemented with the use of magnetic resonance imaging (MRI).[11] These parameters vary in patients with rheumatoid arthritis, collagen vascular diseases, and other pathologic states of increased ligamentous laxity.

Pearl

The "Rule of Spence," which was clinically described by Spence in 1970, states that if the combined lateral mass displacement is greater than 7 mm, the TLA is likely ruptured.

Biomechanics of Subaxial Cervical Spine

Normally positioned in a lordotic posture, the subaxial cervical spine consists of five vertebral body segments (C3–C7), the cervicothoracic junction. Many groups have studied the various biomechanical limitations of the subaxial cervical spine under tension. Bard and Jones in 1964 evaluated the cervical spine under traction which led Panjabi to evaluate the biomechanics more closely.[10,12,13] In 1978, these authors studied four specimens and axially loaded them in 5 kg increments until failure. They found that ventral injuries with greater than 3.3 mm displacement or greater than 3.8 degree rotation at the disc level were considered unstable. Dorsal injuries causing 27 mm of separation of the interspinous space or an increase in angulation greater than 30 degrees with axial loading were considered unstable.

Dorsal ligamentous structures and their role in cervical spine stability have been comprehensively investigated. Goel et al evaluated the corresponding load-deformation data following multilevel laminectomy at C4–C5 and C5–C6 motion segments (with removal of the supraspinous, interspinous, and flavum ligaments).[14] They found an increase in flexion-extension motion of 10%. Kode et al compared the biomechanics instability caused by multilevel laminectomy versus open and double door laminoplasty at C3–C6 and found almost a 50% decrease in flexion-extension with the performance of a laminoplasty (5.4% open door vs. 57% laminectomy).[15]

The nuchal ligament is a triangular, fibrous superficial membrane that extends from the external occipital protuberance to the spinous process of C7. Takeshita et al utilized a cadaver model with sequential resection of the nuchal ligament and found that complete resection increased the flexion range of the motion (28%) and decreased the stiffness in flexion of the cervical spine.[16] Clinically, the nuchal ligament provides significant structural resistance to flexion.

Kumaresan et al produced an element model of the cervical spine to evaluate the biomechanics of the intervertebral discs within the cervical spine.[17] They found that the ventral region of the disc resisted higher variations in axial force, and the dorsal region transmitted higher shear forces under all loading states. The uncinate processes and the uncovertebral joints (UJs) also contribute to the stability of the cervical spine.[18] The UJ consists of the uncinate processes and the adjacent surfaces on the inferior aspect of the superior vertebrae. The uncinate processes are bony protuberances that extend cranially from the lateral margins of C3–C7, and sometimes T1 and T2. These processes comprise the medial wall of the intervertebral foramen. The vertebral artery typically runs within the intervertebral foramen, usually entering at the C6 level. Utilizing a finite-element model, Clausen et al[18] performed progressive resection of the uncinate processes and UJ, finding that both components affect primary and coupled motions associated with axial rotation and lateral bending.[19] The increase in motion allowed by Luschka joints is balanced by the reduction in motion imposed by the uncinate processes, except in lateral bending. Kotani et al confirmed these findings in an earlier study when evaluating the UJ via sequential UJ resection under all loading modes.[20] Unilateral and bilateral foraminotomies affected the stability primarily during extension, causing a 30% and 36% decrease in stiffness.

In addition to the UJ, the facet joints also provide a site of articulation and motion in the cervical spine. Zdeblick et al evaluated sequential resection of 25, 50, 75, and 100%

of the C5–C6 facet capsules to evaluate the corresponding biomechanical change.[19] Significant hypermobility was seen during both rotation and flexion-extension testing with greater than 50% resection of the facet capsules. This was preceded by the work by Cusick et al who compared unilateral versus bilateral facetectomy and its effect on the instantaneous axis of rotation (IAR).[21] Based on their studies, they found that performing facetectomies moved the IAR anteriorly, decreasing the ability to withstand increased compression-flexion loads. In a finite-element model, Voo et al confirmed that the presence of instability occurs after at least 50% of the facet has been resected.[22]

Anterior cervical discectomies have been performed for many years. Chen et al studied the progressive resection of the anterior column from discectomy to posterior longitudinal ligament transection, finding that each step caused progressively larger increases in instability.[23] With each resection, flexion and extension were the modes of motion that were increased most significantly, suggesting that fixation should limit these motions.

Dens Screw Fixation and Odointectomy

Type II Dens Fractures have long been treated with surgical fixation due to high rate of nonunion caused by instability of the fracture and lack of ample blood supply. Although dorsal fixation provides stability for the fracture, ventral fixation preserves motion. Early work by Wilke et al demonstrated that direct screw fixation of the odontoid under experimental conditions provided sufficient stability for the dens fragment.[24] Initially the placement of two screws was advocated due to the theoretical advantage of increased stability. Sasso et al confirmed that biomechanically there was no difference between the one- and two-screw technique under loading to failure studies.[25] Magee et al compared the biomechanical qualities of a headless, fully threaded variable pitch screw with a partially threaded lag screw and washer in a Cadaver Model. They found that fully threaded variable pitch demonstrated greater stiffness and load to failure.[26] At times, two lag screws are needed for anterior fixation. In formalin-fixed human C-2 dens specimens, Oberkircher et al found the biomechanically optimum location of the screws is as far dorsal to the anterior lower end plate as possible.[27]

Pearls

- Dorsal fixation of Type II Dens fracture provides stability, while ventral fixation preserves motion.
- Biomechanically, there was no difference between the one- and two-screw techniques under loading to failure studies in the anterior treatment of Type II Dens fracture.

Posterior C1 and C2 Instrumentation with and without Occipital Plating

In addition to the anterior approach via odontoid screw fixation, there exist numerous techniques the spine surgeon can utilize to obtain effective instrumented fusion at the C1–C2 junction. These techniques include sublaminar wiring, C1 lateral mass and C2 pars screw, transarticular screws, and translaminar screws.

In the setting of traumatic Type II and Type III odontoid fractures, spine surgeons can often treat either with immobilization or anterior odontoid screws. However, depending on the fracture pattern or the body habitus of the patient, some of these injuries may necessitate posterior instrumentation. In 1939, Gallie[28] first described the posterior C1–C2 fusion via sublaminar steel wire fixation. He reported utilizing a single autograft harvested from the iliac crest to be placed over the C2 spinous process and leaned against the posterior arch of C1. The graft is then secured by a sublaminar wire that passes under arch of C1 and wraps around process of C2. Unfortunately, this technique has a reported nonunion rate as high as 25% considering instability with rotation.[29-31] Brooks-Jenkins later described a sublaminar wiring technique that involved two separate iliac crest autografts placed in between C1 and C2 lamina bilaterally. This approach preserved more rotational stability in addition to flexion and extension stability.

In 1979, Magerl and Jeanneret[32] described a technique for transarticular placement of screws.[32] C1–C2 transarticular facet screws allow for complete elimination of motion at atlantoaxial joint. Another technique utilized is Harms-Goel's C1 lateral mass and C2 pars screw, first described in 1994. Both techniques have been found to have a fusion rate as high as 96.1% and 98.5%, respectively. Regarding complications, both fusion techniques present a risk for serious complications if not done correctly, including iatrogenic spinal cord injury, hypoglossal nerve injury, and vertebral artery injury. A high-riding vertebral artery, anomalous or destructive anatomy of C1 lateral masses, enlargement of the vertebral artery, and presence of a ponticulus posticus increase risk of vertebral artery iatrogenic injury. This risk is higher in Magerl transarticular approach and overall is believed to range between 2.6 and 4.1%. When instrumentation is unable to be placed at C1, occipital-cervical (C2) fusion with occipital plate can be utilized.

Pearls

- Techniques for C1–C2 fusion: sublaminar wiring, C1 lateral mass and C2 pars screw, transarticular screws, and translaminar screws.
- C1–C2 transarticular facet screws: allow for complete elimination of motion at atlanto-axial joint.
- Harms-Goel's C1 lateral mass and C2 pars screw.

Translaminar Screw Fixation of C2: Novel Technique to Avoid Injury to Vertebral Artery

Another method of instrumenting C2 is via translaminar screws. Wright[33] described a technique of placing bilateral crossing laminar screws. Utilizing laminar screws at this site eliminates risk of injury to the vertebral artery while immobilizing C2. The screw is placed in line with the contralateral lamina without violating the spinal canal. After these screws are placed, they can be connected via rods to the C1 lateral mass screws. Prior studies have shown this construct to be biomechanically equal to that described by Harms-Goel.[34]

One advantage with this technique is that neither navigation nor fluoroscopy is required since the screws can be placed under direct visualization. The major risk of this technique is inadvertent penetration into the spinal canal. In addition, the application of laminar screws is helpful when the patient has anomalous anatomy. As described by Chytas et al, such indications include atlas occipitalization, C2–C3 congenital fusion, small pedicles, os odontoideum, dominant side of asymmetric vertebral arteries, or opposite side of vertebral artery occlusion.[35] Chytas et al performed a review that showed more studies are needed to determine the anatomic feasibility of C2 translaminar screws. Most studies presented in this review were focused on Asian populations that questioned the safety and efficacy of this instrumentation. Unfortunately, these results could not be generalized to the general population for application to all ethnicities.

With regard to atlantoaxial instability treatment, another method described in the literature of avoiding risk of injury to the vertebral artery with instrumentation is by placing C1 and C3 lateral mass screws connected by rods and C2 sublaminar wires. Horn et al reported using this technique in patients who had vertebral artery anatomy that was inappropriate for transarticular screw placement in addition to having C2 anatomy that was not suited for C2 pars or pedicle screw placement.[36] This technique requires exposure of C1 posterior arch, C2 lamina, and C3 lateral masses. After placement of C1 lateral mass screws, the C3 lateral mass screws are placed. Rods are placed connecting C1 and C3 bilaterally. Two sublaminar wires are then placed under the axial lamina and secured to the rods on either side. Hip autograft is placed between C1 and C2 lamina and secured with C1 sublaminar wire attached to the C2 spinous process. Between C2 and C3, a cross-link between the two rods is placed in the interlaminar space. This technique spares the C2 pars/pedicle from instrumentation if there is anomalous anatomy. These authors presented a case series of 10 patients with this technique, none of whom incurred vertebral artery injury. The authors had 7/10 patients with good follow-up. Follow-up imaging showed evidence of a stable construct. Perhaps one downside attributed to this method is the loss of motion at C2–C3 motion, though this was believed to be clinically insignificant in the setting of atlantoaxial fusion.

Pearls

- C2 translaminar screws: eliminates risk of injury to the vertebral artery while immobilizing C2.
- Another method described in the literature for avoiding risk of injury to the vertebral artery with instrumentation is by placing C1 and C3 lateral mass screws connected by rods and C2 sublaminar wires.

Pedicle versus Pars Screw at C2

The Goel-Harms technique has been well established as a method of instrumenting C1 lateral mass and C2 pedicle or pars. Differentiating C2 pars and pedicle is important to determine the pros and cons of each technique. As described by Su et al., the C2 pars is trabecular bone lying between the superior and inferior articular processes.[37] In contrast, the C2 pedicle is dense bone connecting the inferior articular facet to the vertebral body. One advantage to utilizing the pars screw at C2 is less risk of iatrogenic injury to a high-riding vertebral artery versus the longer C2 pedicle screw. Su et al report that C2 pedicle screws have increased stiffness and pullout versus C2 pars screws. This is likely due to higher density of bone and bicortical characteristics of the C2 pedicle screw. Typically, C2 pars screws are placed in unicortical fashion as they were in Su's series, thus contributing to less strength. Su et al tested the construct strength and clinical utility of a hybrid construct with a C2 pars screw on the side of a high-riding vertebral artery with a contralateral C2 pedicle screw.

Anterior Instrumentation of the Cervical Spine

Fusion rates after anterior cervical discectomy and fusion (ACDF) increased significantly after surgeons began utilizing rigid plate fixation complexes to enhance stability. While excessive motion can impede fusion, absolute fixation can prevent bone growth as well. Despite the benefit of a rigid plate fixation construct, it can also reduce load sharing through the bone graft, causing loss of micromotion at the graft–end plate interface, impacting bone healing. Yao et al confirmed that with use of anterior plating, there is decreased range of motion.[38] As it pertains to graft size, when an oversized graft is utilized, there is a larger decrease in range of motion in flexion-extension. An undersized graft causes decreased range of motion in lateral bending and axial motion due to locking of the UJs and facet overlap. Other studies have also demonstrated that with graft subsidence, rigid plates bear even more load. Most standard ACDF procedures utilize a four-screw construct for a one-level fusion.

Studies have demonstrated that patients with prior spinal fusion are at increased risk for adjacent segment disease. Prasarn et al compared the adjacent level biomechanics after single versus multilevel ACDF with cadaveric specimens.[39] They found that with multilevel ACDF procedures, there was an increase in sagittal range of motion of 31.30% above and 33.88% below the fused motion segment and an increase in overall stiffness in extension.

Patients undergoing multilevel cervical corpectomies are under greater biomechanical stress compared to the standard ACDF. Standalone anterior plating for the stabilization of long strut graft constructs has been associated with unfavorable biomechanics. Porter et al compared two- versus three-level corpectomy constructs, finding greater stability with two-level corpectomy construct.[40] However, increased stability can be provided in a three-level corpectomy by placing a screw into the graft. Yilmaz et al devised the technique of “skip” corpectomy to enhance stability, especially during lateral bending.[41] Compared to a standard three-level corpectomy, a plated skip corpectomy reduced peak screw pullout forced during axial rotation by 15% (four-screw construct) and 19% (six-screw construct). Isomi et al demonstrated that after 1000-cycle fatigue loading, three-level corpectomy constructs lose their initial stability, while one-level constructs remain stable.[42]

Cunningham et al compared a single-level ACDF, single-level artificial disc replacement (ADR), and an intact spine.[43] The ACDF had a 33% increase in range of adjacent-level motion. The ADR and intact spine had preserved range of motion. In addition, the axis of rotation was preserved in the ADR group, while in the ACDF group it was more variable. Lee et al compared the cervical kinematics between patients with cervical ADR and ACDF for cervical disc herniation.[44,45] During both 1- and 6-month motion analysis, the ADR group retained significantly more range of motion in flexion and extension. With the increased prevalence of ADR, more hybrid constructs are being explored with the use of both ACDF and ADR. Liao compared the biomechanics of three hybrid fusion constructs for three-level fusions.[46] Three-level ACDF was the most restrictive, preventing 65 to 80% of motion. With the use of ADR, the three-level constructs significantly normalized motion at the adjacent segment and were most like the intact spine.

Posterior Instrumentation of Subaxial Cervical Spine

In addition to anterior cervical discectomy and instrumented fusion, the posterior instrumented approach to the subaxial cervical spine is also in the spine surgeon’s armamentarium. Various techniques intended to promote instrumented fusion include wiring, Halifax clamps, and placement of an array of screws with plates. These methods have their disadvantages. The modern standard is lateral mass screw placement at multiple cervical levels connected with a rod system to maintain the biomechanical stability of the cervical spine.

Similar to techniques utilized to achieve C2 instrumentation, these techniques present the risk of iatrogenic injury to neurovascular structures. Magerl, Anderson, and Roy-Camille each developed their own separate techniques. The standard approach is “up and out” to avoid injury to the respective nerve at that level and the vertebral artery between C3 and C6.[47,48] This basic philosophy helps spine surgeons stay clear of iatrogenic injury.

The ability of spine surgeons to utilize a system of lateral mass screws with rods provides for more flexibility in making the construct and allows for more precise screw placement. According to Wu et al, the use of such screws with a plating system made it difficult to contour the instrumentation, limited screw positioning, and made it difficult for future revisions.[48] Thus, this system was suboptimal for treating patients with cervical degenerative spondylosis and kyphosis.

The spine surgeon can also place cervical pedicle screws in the subaxial spine to achieve rigid fixation and has achieved a low complication rate like lateral mass screws. However, there remains a risk of breaching the pedicle wall and causing neurovascular injury.

Instrumentation at C7

The C7 level marks the transition between the cervical and thoracic spine. Placing instrumentation at C7 has significant consequences for the patient. In cases of trauma, degenerative disease, or neoplasm where there is cervical instability, rigid fixation is required across this area.

As previously described, the subaxial cervical spine is best instrumented with lateral mass screws in superior and laterally oriented fashion. In contrast, pedicle screws allow for adequate rigid fixation in the thoracic spine.[2] At C7, the lateral masses are smaller than those at other levels in the subaxial cervical spine, thus making lateral mass screws often unfavorable. The transition point at C7 illustrates that lateral mass screws at C7 will likely not impart the degree of stability seen in upper cervical levels due to decreasing size of the lateral mass as the lateral masses turn into transverse processes traveling down the spinal column.[49] Pedicle screws are more suited for the C7 level. Pedicle screws give the greatest stability and are considered able to withstand higher axial load compared to lateral mass screws. Unfortunately, the small diameter of the C7 pedicle presents the potential for neurovascular injury if there is pedicle wall perforation during instrumentation.

Pearls

- C7: the lateral masses are smaller than at other levels in the subaxial cervical spine.
- C7 pedicle screws give the greatest stability and are considered to be able to withstand higher axial load compared to lateral mass screws.

Conclusion

Biomechanically, the cervical spine is a unique entity. Numerous cadaveric and in vivo studies have been performed over the years to understand how the cervical spine reacts to structural loads and surgical insults. As technology continues to evolve, our understanding of the cervical spine will too evolve and hopefully carry over improved patient centered care and positive clinical outcomes.

References

1. Offiah CE, Day E. The craniocervical junction: embryology, anatomy, biomechanics and imaging in blunt trauma. Insights Imaging 2017;8(1):29–47
2. Bayoumi AB, Efe IE, Berk S, Kasper EM, Toktas ZO, Konya D. Posterior rigid instrumentation of C7: surgical considerations and biomechanics at the cervicothoracic junction. A review of the literature. World Neurosurg 2018;111:216–226
3. Heller JG, Amrani J, Hutton WC. Transverse ligament failure: a biomechanical study. J Spinal Disord 1993;6(2):162–165
4. Spence KF Jr, Decker S, Sell KW. Bursting atlantal fracture associated with rupture of the transverse ligament. J Bone Joint Surg Am 1970;52(3):543–549
5. Woods RO, Inceoglu S, Akpolat YT, Cheng WK, Jabo B, Danisa O. C1 lateral mass displacement and transverse atlantal ligament failure in Jefferson's fracture: a biomechanical study of the "Rule of Spence". Neurosurgery 2018;82(2):226–231
6. Child Z, Rau D, Lee MJ, et al. The provocative radiographic traction test for diagnosing craniocervical dissociation: a cadaveric biomechanical study and reappraisal of the pathogenesis of instability. Spine J 2016; 16(9):1116–1123
7. Dvorak J, Schneider E, Saldinger P, Rahn B. Biomechanics of the craniocervical region: the alar and transverse ligaments. J Orthop Res 1988;6(3):452–461
8. Panjabi MM, Crisco JJ III, Lydon C, Dvorak J. The mechanical properties of human alar and transverse ligaments at slow and fast extension rates. Clin Biomech (Bristol, Avon) 1998;13(2):112–120
9. Radcliff KE, Hussain MM, Moldavsky M, et al. In vitro biomechanics of the craniocervical

junction: a sequential sectioning of its stabilizing structures. Spine J 2015;15(7): 1618–1628
10. Oda T, Panjabi MM, Crisco JJ III, Oxland TR. Multidirectional instabilities of experimental burst fractures of the atlas. Spine 1992; 17(11):1285–1290
11. Roy AK, Miller BA, Holland CM, Fountain AJ Jr, Pradilla G, Ahmad FU. Magnetic resonance imaging of traumatic injury to the cranio-vertebral junction: a case-based review. Neurosurg Focus 2015;38(4):E3
12. Bard G, Jones MD. Cineradiographic recording of traction of the cervical spine. Arch Phys Med Rehabil 1964;45:403–406
13. Panjabi MM, White AA III, Keller D, Southwick WO, Friedlaender G. Stability of the cervical spine under tension. J Biomech 1978;11(4):189–197
14. Goel VK, Clark CR, Harris KG, Schulte KR. Kinematics of the cervical spine: effects of multiple total laminectomy and facet wiring. J Orthop Res 1988;6(4):611–619
15. Kode S, Kallemeyn NA, Smucker JD, Fredericks DC, Grosland NM. The effect of multi-level laminoplasty and laminectomy on the biomechanics of the cervical spine: a finite element study. Iowa Orthop J 2014;34: 150–157
16. Takeshita K, Peterson ET, Bylski-Austrow D, Crawford AH, Nakamura K. The nuchal ligament restrains cervical spine flexion. Spine 2004;29(18):E388–E393
17. Kumaresan S, Yoganandan N, Pintar FA, Maiman DJ. Finite element modeling of the cervical spine: role of intervertebral disc under axial and eccentric loads. Med Eng Phys 1999;21(10):689–700
18. Clausen JD, Goel VK, Traynelis VC, Scifert J. Uncinate processes and Luschka joints influence the biomechanics of the cervical spine: quantification using a finite element model of the C5-C6 segment. J Orthop Res 1997; 15(3):342–347
19. Zdeblick TA, Abitbol JJ, Kunz DN, McCabe RP, Garfin S. Cervical stability after sequential capsule resection. Spine 1993;18(14):2005–2008
20. Kotani Y, McNulty PS, Abumi K, Cunningham BW, Kaneda K, McAfee PC. The role of anteromedial foraminotomy and the uncovertebral joints in the stability of the cervical spine. A biomechanical study. Spine 1998;23(14):1559–1565
21. Cusick JF, Yoganandan N, Pintar F, Myklebust J, Hussain H. Biomechanics of cervical spine facetectomy and fixation techniques. Spine 1988;13(7):808–812
22. Voo LM, Kumaresan S, Yoganandan N, Pintar FA, Cusick JF. Finite element analysis of cervical facetectomy. Spine 1997;22(9): 964–969
23. Chen TY, Crawford NR, Sonntag VK, Dickman CA. Biomechanical effects of progressive anterior cervical decompression. Spine 2001; 26(1):6–13, discussion 14
24. Wilke HJ, Fischer K, Kugler A, Magerl F, Claes L, Wörsdörfer O. In vitro investigations of internal fixation systems of the upper cervical spine. I. Stability of the direct anterior screw fixation of the odontoid. Eur Spine J 1992;1(3): 185–190
25. Sasso R, Doherty BJ, Crawford MJ, Heggeness MH. Biomechanics of odontoid fracture fixation. Comparison of the one- and two-screw technique. Spine 1993;18(14): 1950–1953
26. Magee W, Hettwer W, Badra M, Bay B, Hart R. Biomechanical comparison of a fully threaded, variable pitch screw and a partially threaded lag screw for internal fixation of Type II dens fractures. Spine 2007;32(17):E475–E479
27. Oberkircher L, Bliemel C, Flossdorf F, Schwarting T, Ruchholtz S, Krüger A. Biomechanical evaluation of 2 insertion points for ventral screw fixation of C-2 dens fractures. J Neurosurg Spine 2013;18(6): 553–557
28. Gallie WE. Fractures and Dislocation of the Cervical Spine. AM J Surg 1939;46:495-499.
29. Gautschi OP, Payer M, Corniola MV, Smoll NR, Schaller K, Tessitore E. Clinically relevant complications related to posterior atlanto-axial fixation in atlanto-axial instability and their management. Clin Neurol Neurosurg 2014;123:131–135
30. Ma W, Feng L, Xu R, et al. Clinical application of C2 laminar screw technique. Eur Spine J 2010;19(8):1312–1317
31. Mummaneni PV, Haid RW. Atlantoaxial fixation: overview of all techniques. Neurol India 2005;53(4):408–415
32. Jeanneret B, Magerl F. Primary posterior fusion C1/2 in odontoid fractures: Indications, technique, and results of transarticular screw fixation. J Spinal Disord. 1992;5:464–75.
33. Wright NM, Lauryssen C. Techniques of Posterior C1-C2 Stabilization. Tech in Neurosurg 1998; 4:286-297,1998
34. Park, J., Scheer, J. K., Lim, T. J., Deviren, V., & Ames, C. P. (2011). Biomechanical analysis of Goel technique for C1-2 fusion. Journal of

neurosurgery. Spine, 14(5), 639–646. https://doi.org/10.3171/2011.1.SPINE10446

35. Chytas D, Korres DS, Babis GC, et al. Anatomical considerations of C2 lamina for the placement of translaminar screw: a review of the literature. Eur J Orthop Surg Traumatol 2018;28(3):343–349
36. Horn EM, Hott JS, Porter RW, Theodore N, Papadopoulos SM, Sonntag VK. Atlantoaxial stabilization with the use of C1-3 lateral mass screw fixation. Technical note. J Neurosurg Spine 2006;5(2):172–177
37. Su BW, Shimer AL, Chinthakunta S, et al. Comparison of fatigue strength of C2 pedicle screws, C2 pars screws, and a hybrid construct in C1-C2 fixation. Spine 2014;39(1):E12–E19
38. Yao R, McLachlin SD, Rasoulinejad P, et al. Influence of graft size on spinal instability with anterior cervical plate fixation following in vitro flexion-distraction injuries. Spine J 2016;16(4):523–529
39. Prasarn ML, Baria D, Milne E, Latta L, Sukovich W. Adjacent-level biomechanics after single versus multilevel cervical spine fusion. J Neurosurg Spine 2012;16(2):172–177
40. Porter RW, Crawford NR, Chamberlain RH, et al. Biomechanical analysis of multilevel cervical corpectomy and plate constructs. J Neurosurg 2003; 99(1, Suppl)98–103
41. Yilmaz M, Yüksel KZ, Baek S, et al. Biomechanics of cervical “skip” corpectomy versus standard multilevel corpectomy. Clin Spine Surg 2017;30(3):E152–E161
42. Isomi T, Panjabi MM, Wang JL, Vaccaro AR, Garfin SR, Patel T. Stabilizing potential of anterior cervical plates in multilevel corpectomies. Spine 1999;24(21):2219–2223
43. Cunningham BW, Hu N, Zorn CM, McAfee PC. Biomechanical comparison of single- and two-level cervical arthroplasty versus arthrodesis: effect on adjacent-level spinal kinematics. Spine J 2010;10(4):341–349
44. Lee JH, Kim JS, Lee JH, Chung ER, Shim CS, Lee SH. Comparison of cervical kinematics between patients with cervical artificial disc replacement and anterior cervical discectomy and fusion for cervical disc herniation. Spine J 2014;14(7):1199–1204
45. Pisano A, Helgeson M. Cervical disc replacement surgery: biomechanical properties, postoperative motion, and postoperative activity levels. Curr Rev Musculoskelet Med 2017;10(2):177–181
46. Liao Z, Fogel GR, Pu T, Gu H, Liu W. Biomechanics of hybrid anterior cervical fusion and artificial disc replacement in 3-level constructs: an in vitro investigation. Med Sci Monit 2015;21:3348–3355
47. Mummaneni PV, Haid RW, Traynelis VC, et al. Posterior cervical fixation using a new polyaxial screw and rod system: technique and surgical results. Neurosurg Focus 2002; 12(1):E8
48. Wu JC, Huang WC, Chen YC, Shih YH, Cheng H. Stabilization of subaxial cervical spines by lateral mass screw fixation with modified Magerl’s technique. Surg Neurol 2008; 70(1, Suppl 1):S1, 25–33, discussion S1, 33
49. Horn EM, Reyes PM, Baek S, et al. Biomechanics of C-7 transfacet screw fixation. J Neurosurg Spine 2009;11(3):338–343

5 Harmony of Curves in Sagittal Balance: Concepts to Avoid Proximal Junctional Kyphosis

Emanuele Quarto, Abhishek Mannem, Wendy Thompson, Thibault Cloché, Laurent Balabaud, and Jean Charles Le Huec

Introduction

Adult spinal deformity (ASD) surgery has made great progresses in the past decades but despite the improvement in surgical techniques and the respect of sagittal alignment rules, proximal junctional kyphosis (PJK) is still the most important postoperative mechanical complication not fully understood by the clinicians. PJK is one of the main causes for revision surgery. Understanding the reason for PJK could help to decrease its occurrence by a better surgical planning.[1]

PJK is defined as a change of at least 10 degrees in the first motion segment over the upper instrumented vertebra caused by the failure of either the vertebra, the soft tissue, or the bone–implant interface in thoracolumbar fusion surgeries.[1] This event can occur in the early postoperative period (within 6 weeks) or even after months from the fusion surgery. It is reported that the incidence of PJK varies from 20 to 60% of the cases.[2–5] When the junctional kyphosis becomes symptomatic, it is then called proximal junctional failure (PJF) and it might require revision; the most common reported causes of failure are vertebral fracture, soft tissue failure, and screw pull-out.[6]

Several studies have analyzed the risk factors associated with these complications and correlations were found both with patient's related factors and with the postoperative sagittal alignment achieved.

The most important patient-related factors are the magnitude of the deformity, age, body mass index (BMI), bone mineral density, and paravertebral muscle quality.[7] Concerning age, it is reported that patients older than 55 years have higher risk of developing a PJK[8,9]; patients with higher BMI might have greater mechanical stress on their implants[10] and a bad bone quality might increase the risk of screw pull-out and hardware failure.[9]

Finally, a fatty infiltration of the thoracolumbar spine extensor muscles has been advocated as possible cause of PJK.[11]

Two radiological parameters are very often reported to have an influence on the postoperative mechanical complication, namely, sagittal vertical axis (SVA) and the mismatch between the pelvic incidence (PI) and the lumbar lordosis (LL). An SVA >50 mm and a PI-LL mismatch >10 degrees are both correlated to bad clinical outcomes and higher rates of postoperative mechanical failures; on the other hand, it is also known that LL and SVA overcorrections are also related to higher incidences of PJK.[7]

Despite the knowledge of these risk factors and careful preoperative surgical planning following the principal sagittal spinal alignment rules,[12,13] the incidence of PJK in ASD surgery is still consistent.[14–16]

Knowing that it is difficult or sometimes impossible to modify patient's risk factors like age, BMI, bone mineral density, and paravertebral muscle quality, we propose to analyze the PJK risk paying attention to the biomechanical analysis as this factor can be studied and controlled on the basis of physics knowledge. In this biomechanical analysis, the authors suggest that a PJK could be the consequence of an excessive lever arm on the upper instrumented vertebra that might overcome the mechanical resistance of the vertebral osteoligamentous complex at the two cephalad junctional noninstrumented vertebrae. The hypothesis is that PJK is due to an exceeding load on the anterior column overcoming its compression forces resistance and/or the posterior column tension band strength.[1] To evaluate this stress force on each thoracic vertebral body, the cervical inclination angle (CIA) has been described: this angle is measured tracing a line going from the tip of the odontoid (C2) to the center of the superior end plate of the last instrumented vertebra and a horizontal line traced from this point. This angle was calculated in an asymptomatic adult population with a constant result from T1 to T12 (range: 74.83–83.82 degrees) (**Fig. 5.1**).[1] This parameter is very important because it includes the craniocervical complex in the spine sagittal balance evaluation and can predict the risk of PJK in postoperative patients; nevertheless, always keep in mind that patient-related factors might also play a role.

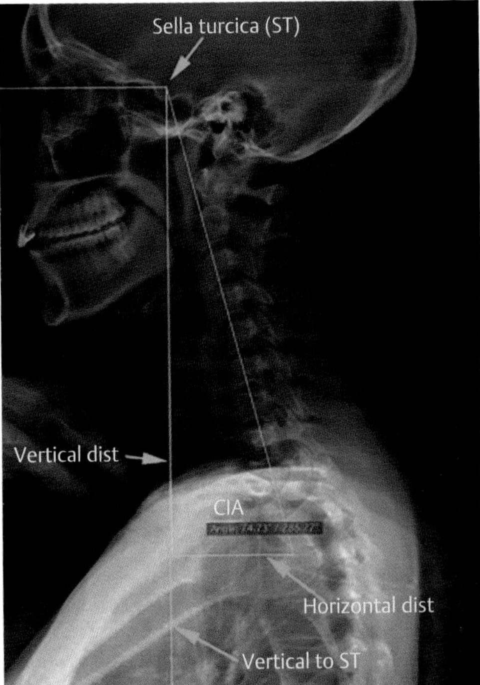

Fig. 5.1 Measurement of cervical inclination angle. dist, distance; CIA, cervical inclination angle.

In order to try to define a strategy for preoperative surgical planning, the authors propose to define the key parameters to be analyzed to keep an economical balance or a compensated balance. They will describe how to analyze the global balance and how to evaluate the segmental alignments that contribute to keeping the balance. The conus of economy defined by Dubousset is the base.[17] Furthermore, the three-conus theory recently published allows to analyze segment by segment the behavior of the craniocervical complex, thoracolumbopelvic complex, and the lower limb complex.[12]

Pearls

- The patient-related risk factors associated with PJK are age >55, BMI >25, poor bone quality, and fatty infiltration of thoracolumbar extensor muscles.
- Radiological parameters having an impact on the postoperative sagittal complication are sagittal vertical axis (SVA) >50 mm, pelvic incidence (PI) and the lumbar lordosis (LL) >10 degrees. CIA angle of 80 degrees reduces the risk of proximal mechanical failure.
- Conus of economy is defined as an upright static position with minimal muscular effort, which is only possible when each subject's center of mass projects at the center of a polygon situated between the two feet.

Global Sagittal Balance Analysis

When the spinal surgeon faces ASD, he must globally analyze the spinal balance of the patient; considering the large number of PJK after long thoracolumbar fusion, it seems that the commonly used SVA or PI-LL mismatch target values can't be considered enough anymore.[18,19]

The first important concept to keep in mind is the "conus of economy" that was first described in 1994 by Jean Dubousset: maintaining an upright static position with minimal muscular effort is only possible when each subject's center of mass projects at the center of a polygon situated between two feet. When walking, his conus of economy enlarges but the upright position is still possibly maintained with small muscular rebalancing efforts. On the contrary, if a patient has an anterior sagittal imbalance his conus will be much wider, and the muscular effort needed to maintain the upright position will be greater (**Fig. 5.2**).[12,17] To obtain an economic posture, it is then important that

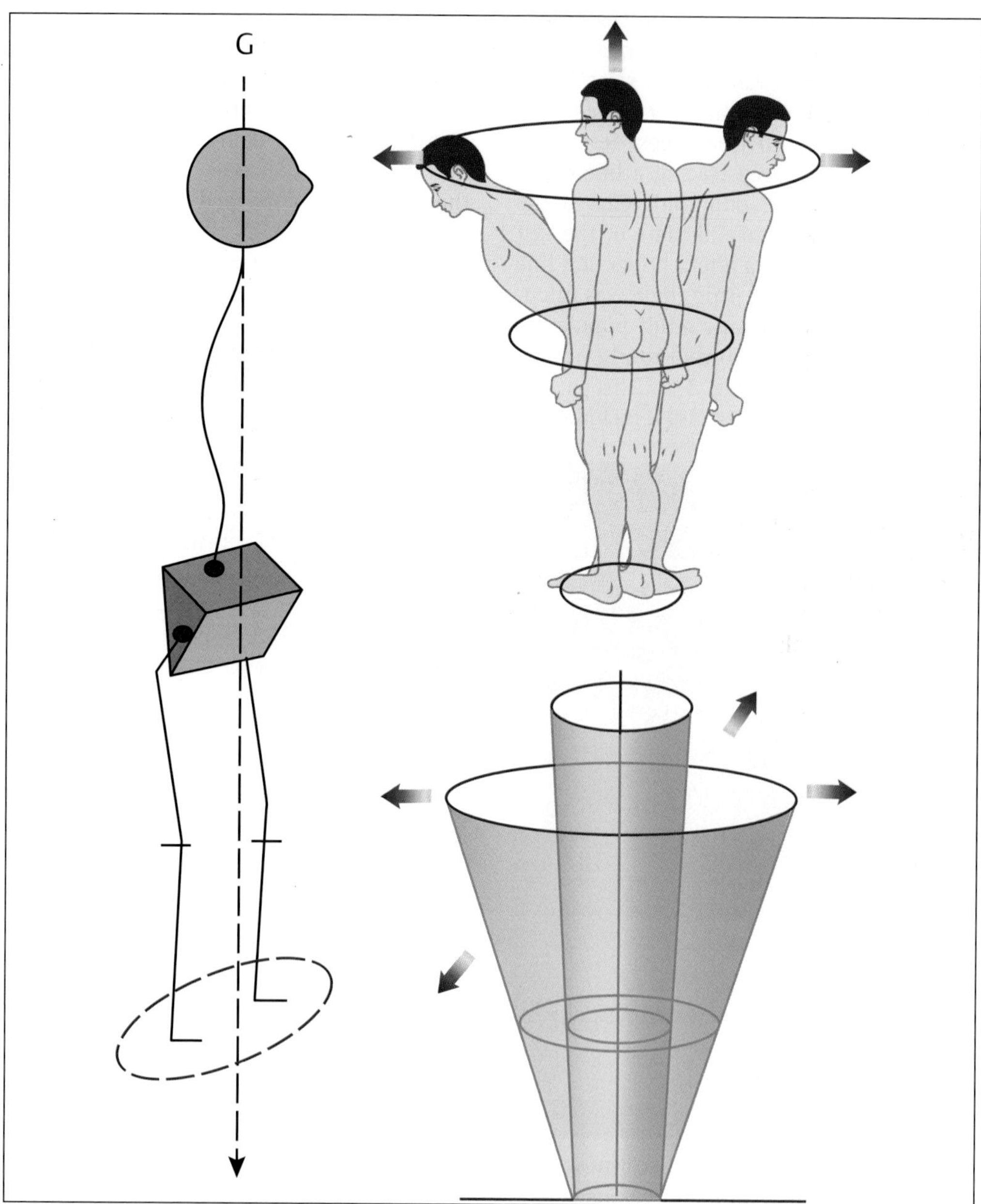

Fig. 5.2 Efficiency conus of Dubousset.

the head be aligned over the pelvis and the feet. It sounds normal then to include the head and cervical spine in the analysis of the global sagittal balance.

It is well known that with the aging process, even in asymptomatic subjects, the authors can see a progressive loss of lumbar lordosis due to multiple level degenerative disc disease: this activates a series of compensatory mechanisms such as hyperextension of the adjacent lumbar discs, thoracic hypokyphosis, increase in cervical lordosis, pelvic retroversion. Hip extension reserve and knee flexion are the ultimate mechanisms to be recruited (**Fig. 5.3**). All those mechanisms have the only goal of maintaining the subject in an ergonomic balance within his conus of economy.[20]

To simplify we will suppose that the lower limbs are straight in the following analysis, with the knee flexion and ankle hyperextension being the last compensation phenomenon. In the analysis of the head-cervical-thoracic-lumbar-pelvic complex, a new angle known as the odontoid hip axis angle (OD-HA) is described: this angle has been demonstrated to be constant despite the age, with a mean value ranging from −5 to 2 degrees.[21] This OD-HA angle is the C2 tilt taking the femoral head as a reference.

The analysis of global sagittal balance then starts with the evaluation of the OD-HA angle and then continues with the analysis of regional possible compensatory mechanisms that may be used to maintain the head over the hips.

In the lumbopelvic region, it is mandatory to analyze each patient's pelvic incidence (PI) and, on this basis, his real and theoretical pelvic tilt (PT; theoretical PT = PI × 0.44 – 11.4), sacral slope (SS) and LL (theoretical LL = PI × 0.54 + 27.6) angles.[13] One of the most powerful compensatory mechanisms is the pelvic retroversion and hip extension. Pelvic retroversion possibility is higher for those who have a high pelvic incidence angle.

At the thoracic level the angle of global kyphosis (T1–T12) should be calculated. As described previously, with aging the kyphosis should increase but in cases of loss of LL, the paravertebral thoracic extensor muscles may activate and reduce the thoracic kyphosis (TK) to re-establish a global sagittal alignment. Knowing the rigidity of the thoracic segment is mandatory when planning the levels of fusion because an excessively rigid thoracic spine might not adapt at the new postoperative alignment, raising the risk of PJK. It is then important to complete the preoperative evaluation with dynamic flexion-extensions X-rays of the spine and an analysis of muscular capacities.

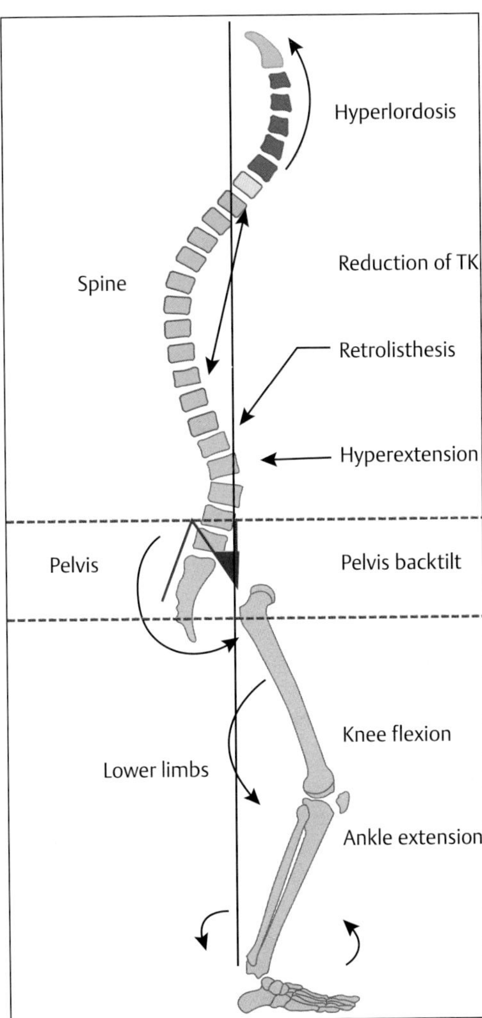

Fig. 5.3 Compensatory mechanisms occurring over aging process. TK, Thoracic kyphosis.

Analyzing the craniocervical complex is also very important. In a compensated imbalance, the authors might see an increase in the cervical lordosis that has the objective of bringing back the center of mass of the head reducing consequently the lever arm on the thoracic vertebrae: this can be analyzed measuring the CIA angle that should be approximately 80 degrees to reduce the risk of proximal mechanical failure.[1]

Finally, in very important imbalance, the surgeon should also analyze the lower limbs and especially verify the residual capacity of extension of the hips, flexion of the knees, and ankle extension.

Pearls

- New angle known as the odontoid hip axis angle (OD-HA) is described;[22] this angle has been demonstrated to be constant despite the age, with a mean value ranging from −5 to 2 degrees.
- The most powerful compensatory mechanisms for the sagittal balance are the pelvic retroversion and hip extension.
- Analyze the lower limbs and especially verify the residual capacity of extension of the hips, flexion of the knees, and ankle extension.

Surgical Planning

First, the surgeon should analyze the severity of the deformity he is facing and the presence of a more or less severe degree of sagittal imbalance.

Pearls

- The principal parameters to be analyzed for the surgical planning are:
  - Pelvic incidence (PI).
  - Pelvic tilt (PT).
  - Lumbar lordosis (LL).
  - Thoracic kyphosis (TK).
  - Cervical lordosis (CL).
  - Odontoid hip axis angle (OD-HA).
  - Cervical inclination angle (CIA).
  - Flexion of knees.
- Once the deformity is well studied, the surgeon should calculate the theoretical balance parameters of his patient given his PI:
  - PT = PI × 0.44 −11.4.
  - LL = PI × 0.54 + 27.6.
  - TK = 0.75 LL.
- The objective is to keep harmony of curves avoiding hypo- or hypercorrection. We should keep in mind that the final goal is to keep the head over the pelvis.

Once the degree of lordosis correction needed is known, it is important to understand the distribution of the lordosis based on each patient type according to Roussouly.[24] In all cases, it is important to restore approximately 60% of the lordosis in the lower lumbar spine, defined as the lumbar spine below the apex of the lordosis (to simplify the L4–S1 segments). Actually, an overcorrection of the upper lumbar lordosis (ULL; T12–L4), even if achieving the goal of global lordosis calculated on the basis of the PI, has been reported as an important risk factor for PJK.[23] In daily practice, the authors can remember that ULL between inflexion point and lordosis apex at L4 is approximately 20 degrees.[24]

Once the amount of correction needed is established and the levels where to correct are chosen, then it is important to analyze if the patient still has some compensatory mechanism reservoir or not, and whether this can be used to find the ideal postoperative balance. If the patient still has some degree of pelvic retroversion possibility this can be eventually utilized in the corrective strategy planning. The objective is to keep harmony of curves avoiding hypo- or hypercorrection. We should keep in mind that the final goal is to keep the head over the pelvis. Fixed segments have no possibility of adaptation and will create abnormal shift and therefore create inadequate lever arm from the part of the body localized on top of them. For this reason, analyzing the thoracic kyphosis between T1 and T12 is of major importance. This kyphosis can be fixed, due to arthrosis or fusion, or mobile, and in case of a mobile thoracic spine the quality of the muscles must be evaluated to know whether the patient is able to compensate and how much he can reduce or increase his kyphosis.

Furthermore, it is important to evaluate the global status of the patient considering his sex, age, BMI, bone mineral density, and spine extensors muscle power. In the case of a middle-aged male with a normal BMI and good muscular quality, a more aggressive correction can be attempted to obtain the theoretical ideal balance parameters; on the other hand, facing a deformity in an osteoporotic elderly, with fatty infiltration of her spine extensors muscles, the surgical strategy should be adapted and the final goal would be the good global balance (OD-HA between −5 and 2 degrees) that can be obtained with a lesser correction of her LL and TK using her pelvic retroversion as a compensatory mechanism. In all cases, the postoperative CIA angle at the upper instrumented vertebra should be in a range of normality (close to 80 degrees) to reduce the risk of PJK. This planning simulation is possible today, but it also requires that during surgery, the surgeon must control the correction performed to fit the preoperative planning. This point is very important as only few spine surgeons do this per-operative check.

Case Examples

Case 1: Planning for Compensated Harmonious Correction

A 65-year-old woman presenting back pain for a degenerative lumbar scoliosis; her preoperative parameters were PI 65 degrees, PT 32 degrees, SS 33 degrees, and LL 27 degrees (**Fig. 5.4**). She needed a spinal canal decompression and stabilization due to L3–L4 degenerative listhesis and scoliosis.

She underwent a first-stage L5–S1 Anterior lumbar interbody fusion (ALIF) fusion followed by a second-stage posterior T12–Ilium fusion with L4–L5 transforaminal lumbar interbody fusion (TLIF). Her postoperative parameters were PI 70 degrees, PT 34 degrees, SS 36 degrees, LL 40 degrees, CIA 79.8 degrees, and OD-HA 0 degree (**Fig. 5.5**). The planning was to avoid a pedicle subtraction osteotomies (PSO) which was considered too aggressive due to her general health status. The accepted compromise was to plan a final LL of 40 degrees instead of 62 degrees (according to Le Huec formula) and to accept a PT at 32 degrees as postoperative.

The postoperative result was satisfactory as we could obtain a good global balance (OD-HA 0 degree) with a mild correction of her LL and using her pelvic retroversion to obtain the final balance.

Case 2: PJK Following Lumbar Lordosis Hypercorrection at the Wrong Level: Disharmonious Curves Distribution

A 69-year-old woman presenting with back pain and claudication due to multiple level degenerative disc disease with loss of lumbar lordosis; her preoperative parameters were PI 65 degrees, PT 39 degrees, SS 25 degrees, LL 36 degrees, and lower lumbar lordosis (LLL) 5 degrees (**Fig. 5.6**).

She underwent in another center a T11–Ilium fusion with correction of the hypolordosis. The postoperative parameters were PI 65 degrees, PT 36 degrees, SS 27 degrees, LL 83 degrees, LLL 45 degrees. Three months after her first surgery the patient consulted for severe back pain due to a PJK (**Fig. 5.7**).

She was then treated with a posterior wedge osteotomy correction at T11 and the fusion was extended to T3 (**Fig. 5.8**); unfortunately the patient presented a few months later with back pain and a new PJK and hardware failure at the thoracolumbar junction (**Fig. 5.9**).

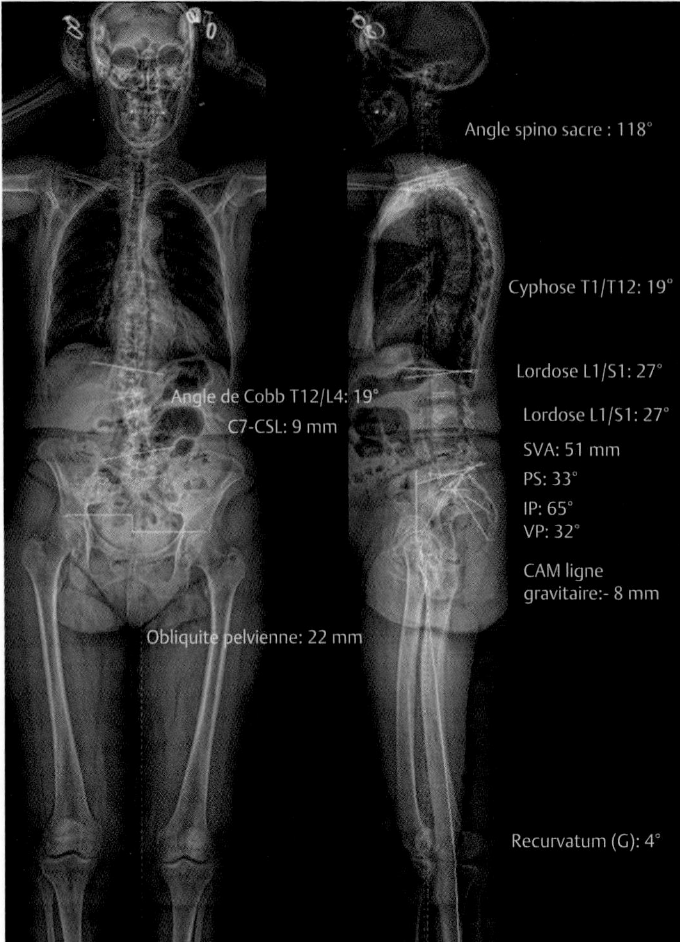

Fig. 5.4 Planning for compensated harmonious correction in Case 1.

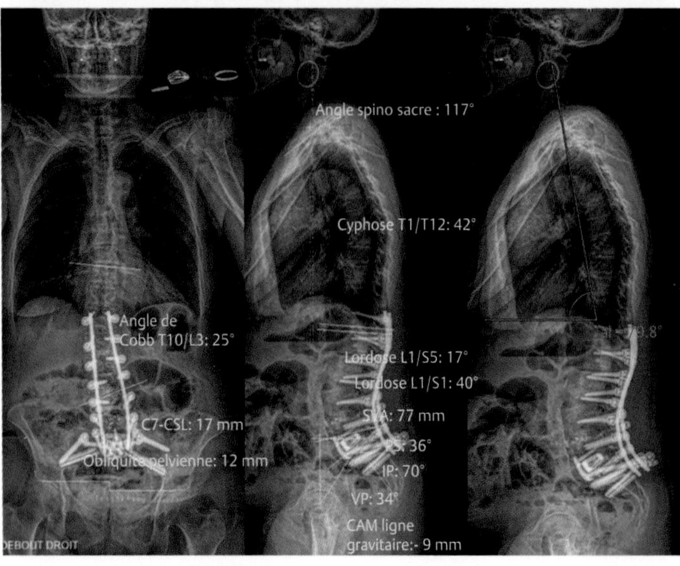

Fig. 5.5 Case 1 postoperative results after two-stage procedure.

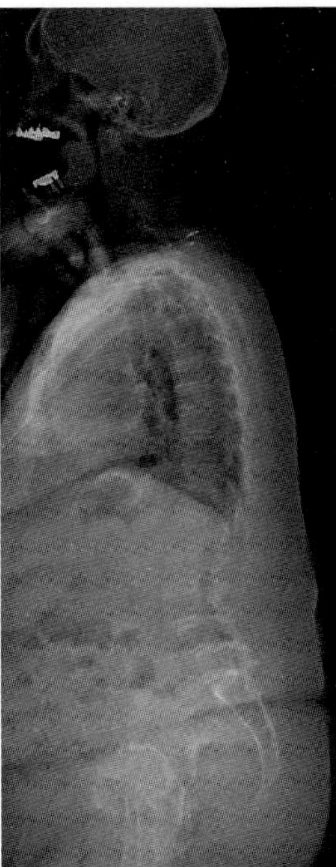

Fig. 5.6 Lateral radiograph of a Case 2 patient planned for lumbar lordosis correction.

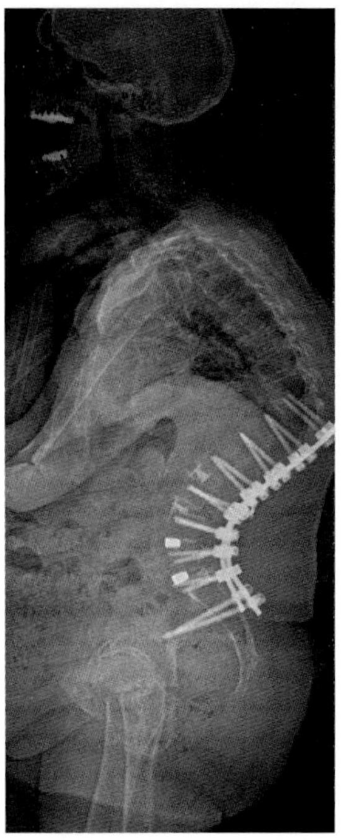

Fig. 5.7 Hypercorrection of lumbar lordosis leading to proximal junctional kyphosis.

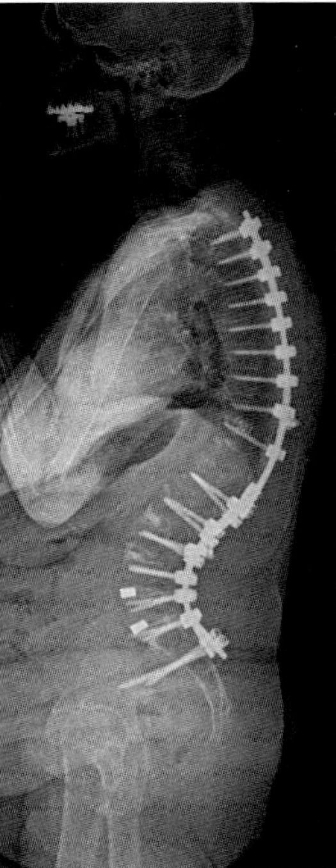

Fig. 5.8 T11 postosteotomy and extension of instrumentation to correct proximal junctional kyphosis.

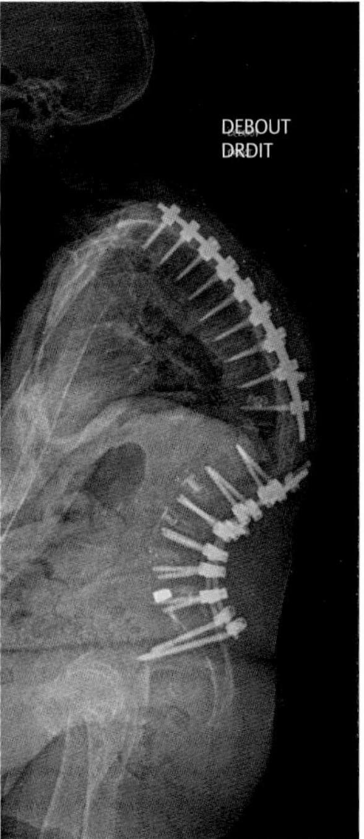

Fig. 5.9 Hardware failure with rod breakage at thoracolumbar junction.

In this case, the problem was the excessive LL correction given during the first surgery with disharmonious distribution of lordosis. The LL obtained (83 degrees) was too high in relation to her PI due to an excessive ULL. According to the theoretical LL by Le Huec and Hasegawa, her optimal lordosis would have been LL = 65 × 0.54 + 27.6 = 62.7 degrees and two-third of this lordosis should have situated between L4 and S1 (41.8 degrees) with only 20.9 degrees in the ULL, but instead the patient had a ULL of 38 degrees.

Considering this excess in the ULL she was finally treated with a posterior opening wedge osteotomy (POWO) at L3 that reduced her ULL by 16 degrees with a good clinical and radiological postoperative follow-up at 3 years (**Fig. 5.10**).

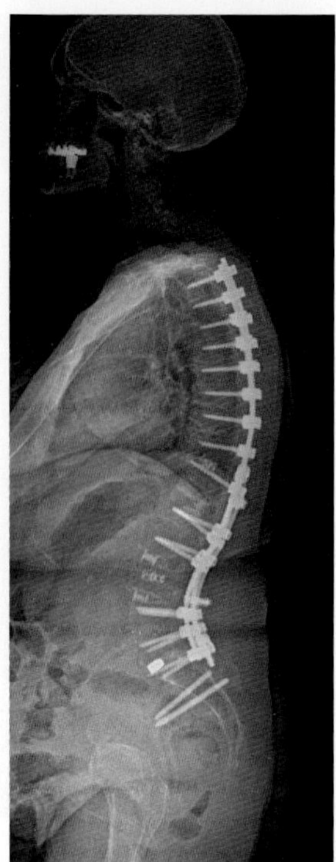

Fig. 5.10 Reducing the lumbar lordosis and revising hardware leading to favorable outcome.

Case 3: Harmonious Correction of a Severe Adult Scoliosis Using a PSO Osteotomy

A 73-year-old woman presenting with severe coronal and sagittal imbalance causing her back pain and bad life quality. Preoperatively, she had an OD-HA angle of 6 degrees and 81-mm coronal imbalance; her segmental parameters were: PI 42 degrees, PT 24 degrees, SS 18 degrees, LL 1 degree (kyphosis), and TK –11 degrees (lordosis) (**Fig. 5.11**). The deformity was stiff on flexion (**Fig. 5.12**) and lateral bending X-rays (**Fig. 5.13**).

The preoperative planning consisted of a first-stage L5–S1 ALIF followed by a second-stage posterior surgery with an L4 PSO, multiple PSO, and a T4–Ilium fusion (**Fig. 5.14**). In this case, a PSO was necessary, considering the severe preoperative sagittal and coronal rigid imbalance. The L4 PSO enabled to re-establish the correct LLL angle. Postoperatively, the patient parameters were: PI 49 degrees, PT 13 degrees, SS 36 degrees, LL 50 degrees, TK 42 degrees, OD-HA 0 degree, CIA 75.1 degrees.

The postoperative result was very satisfactory with a harmonious distribution of the curves and a good clinical result at 1-year FU.

Conclusion

Global balance analysis is well performed by measuring the OD-HA angle. Patient's general condition and self-parameters (age, BMI, muscular conditioning, osteoporosis, etc.) must be well evaluated as they can be limiting factors. Compensatory mechanisms must be evaluated in order to plan a final postoperative perfect balance or a compensated balance. Perioperative control of the correction is mandatory. The planning must pay attention to preserve harmony of the curves and avoid hypercorrection.

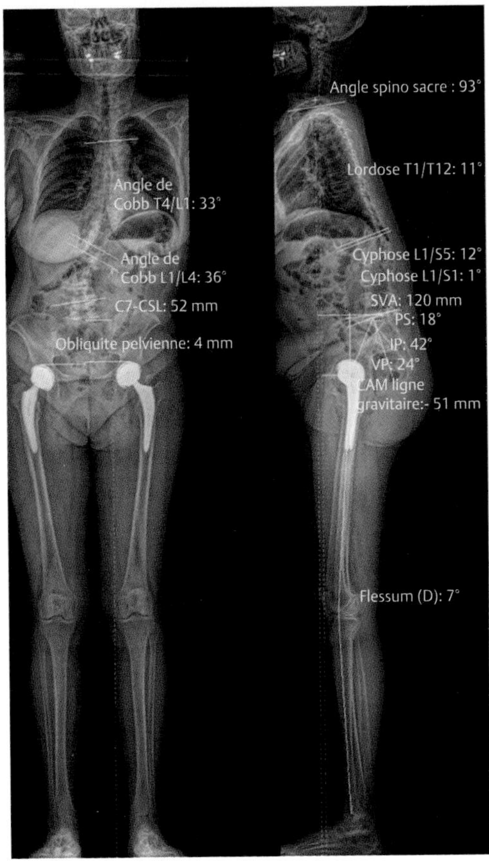

Fig. 5.11 Case 3: A 73-year-old female presenting with dorsolumbar back pain and coronal imbalance.

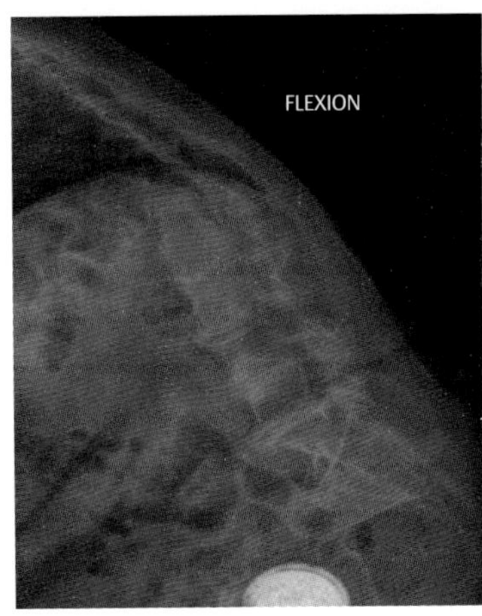

Fig. 5.12 No movement observed on flexion X-rays.

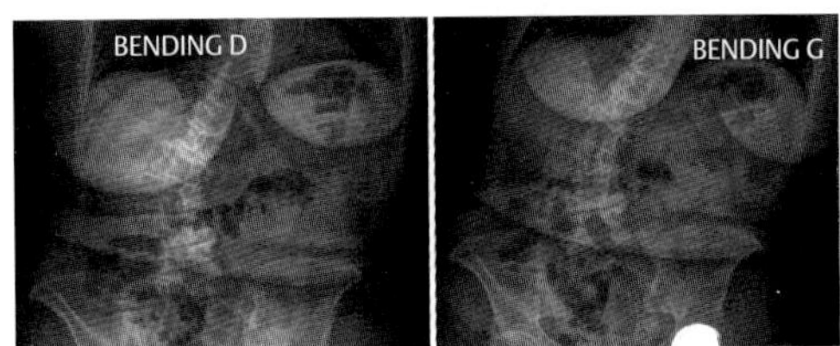

Fig. 5.13 No movement seen on lateral bending X-ray dynamic films.

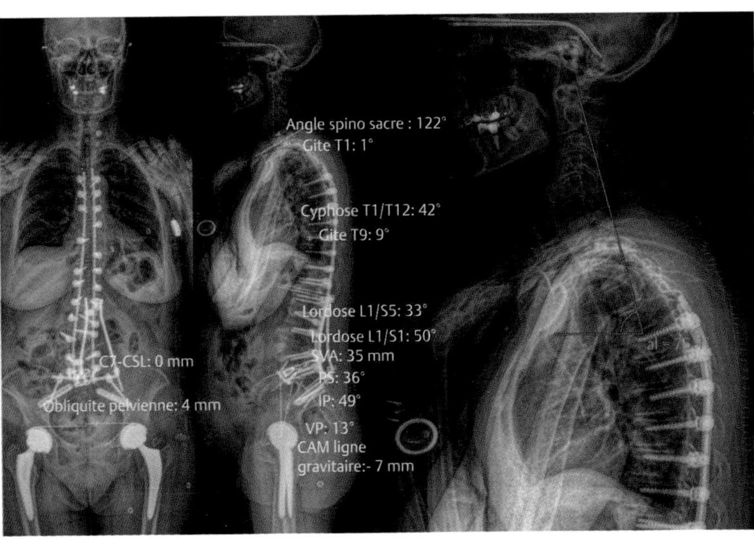

Fig. 5.14 Correction of deformity following two-stage procedure.

References

1. Le Huec JC, Richards J, Tsoupras A, Price R, Léglise A, Faundez AA. The mechanism in junctional failure of thoraco-lumbar fusions. Part I: Biomechanical analysis of mechanisms responsible of vertebral overstress and description of the cervical inclination angle (CIA). Eur Spine J 2018;27(Suppl 1):129–138
2. Diebo BG, Henry J, Lafage V, Berjano P. Sagittal deformities of the spine: factors influencing the outcomes and complications. Eur Spine J 2015;24(Suppl 1):S3–S15
3. Han S, Hyun S-J, Kim KJ, Jahng TA, Lee S, Rhim SC. Rod stiffness as a risk factor of proximal junctional kyphosis after adult spinal deformity surgery: comparative study between cobalt chrome multiple-rod constructs and titanium alloy two-rod constructs. Spine J 2017;17(7):962–968
4. Jain A, Naef F, Lenke LG, et al. Incidence of proximal junctional kyphosis in patients with adult spinal deformity fused to the pelvis: analysis of 198 patients. Spine J 2016;16: 311–312
5. Scheer JK, Osorio JA, Smith JS, et al; International Spine Study Group. Development of validated computer based preoperative predictive model for Proximal Junction Failure (PJF) or clinically significant PJK with 86% accuracy based on 510 ASD patients with 2-year follow-up. Spine 2016;41(22): E1328–E1335
6. Hostin R, McCarthy I, O'Brien M, et al; International Spine Study Group. Incidence, mode, and location of acute proximal junctional failures after surgical treatment of adult spinal deformity. Spine 2013;38(12): 1008–1015
7. Diebo BG, Shah NV, Stroud SG, Paulino CB, Schwab FJ, Lafage V. Realignment surgery in adult spinal deformity: prevalence and risk factors for proximal junctional kyphosis. Orthopade 2018;47(4):301–309
8. Lau D, Clark AJ, Scheer JK, et al; SRS Adult Spinal Deformity Committee. Proximal junctional kyphosis and failure after spinal deformity surgery: a systematic review of the literature as a background to classification development. Spine (PhilaPa1976) 2014; 39(25):2093–2102
9. Liu F-Y, Wang T, Yang S-D, Wang H, Yang DL, Ding WY. Incidence and risk factors for proximal junctional kyphosis: a meta-analysis. Eur Spine J 2016;25(8):2376–2383
10. Kim DK, Kim JY, Kim DYK, Rhim SC, Yoon SH. Risk factors of proximal junctional kyphosis after multilevel fusion surgery: more than 2 years follow-up data. J Korean Neurosurg Soc 2017;60(2):174–180
11. Hyun S-J, Kim YJ, Rhim S-C. Patients with proximal junctional kyphosis after stopping at thoracolumbar junction have lower muscularity, fatty degeneration at the thoracolumbar area. Spine J 2016;16(9):1095–1101
12. Le Huec JC, Thompson W, Mohsinaly Y, Barrey C, Faundez A. Sagittal balance of the spine. Eur Spine J 2019;28(9):1889–1905
13. Le Huec JC, Hasegawa K. Normative values for the spine shape parameters using 3D standing analysis from a database of 268 asymptomatic Caucasian and Japanese subjects. Eur Spine J 2016;25(11):3630–3637
14. Quarto E, Zanirato A, Ursino C, Traverso G, Russo A, Formica M. Adult spinal deformity surgery: posterior three-column osteotomies vs anterior lordotic cages with posterior fusion. Complications, clinical and radiological results. A systematic review of the literature. Eur Spine J 2021;30(11):3150–3161
15. Wu HH, Chou D, Hindoyan K, et al. Upper instrumented vertebra-femoral angle and correlation with proximal junctional kyphosis in adult spinal deformity. Spine Deform 2021; Online ahead of print.
16. Lord EL, Ayres E, Woo D, et al. The impact of global alignment and proportion score and bracing on proximal junctional kyphosis in adult spinal deformity. Global Spine J 2021; Online ahead of print.
17. Dubousset J. Three-dimensional analysis of the scoliotic deformity. In: Weinstein S, ed. The pediatric spine: principles and practice. New York: Raven Press; 1994:479–496
18. Diebo BG, Ferrero E, Lafage R, et al. Recruitment of compensatory mechanisms in sagittal spinal malalignment is age and regional deformity dependent: a full-standing axis analysis of key radiographical parameters. Spine 2015;40(9):642–649
19. Ferrero E, Guigui P, Khalifé M, et al. Global alignment taking into account the cervical spine with odontoid hip axis angle (OD-HA). Eur Spine J 2021;30(12):3647–3655 10.1007/s00586-021-06991-1 Online ahead of print

20. Barrey C, Roussouly P, Le Huec J-C, D'Acunzi G, Perrin G. Compensatory mechanisms contributing to keep the sagittal balance of the spine. Eur Spine J 2013; 22(Suppl 6):S834–S841
21. Amabile C, Pillet H, Lafage V, Barrey C, Vital JM, Skalli W. A new quasi-invariant parameter characterizing the postural alignment of young asymptomatic adults. Eur Spine J 2016; 25(11):3666–3674
22. Amabile C, Le Huec JC, Skalli W. Invariance of head-pelvis alignment and compensatory mechanisms for asymptomatic adults older than 49 years. Eur Spine J 2018;27(2): 458–466
23. Faundez AA, Richards J, Maxy P, Price R, Léglise A, Le Huec JC. The mechanism in junctional failure of thoraco-lumbar fusions. Part II: Analysis of a series of PJK after thoraco-lumbar fusion to determine parameters allowing to predict the risk of junctional breakdown. Eur Spine J 2018;27(Suppl 1): 139–148
24. Roussouly P, Pinheiro-Franco JL. Sagittal parameters of the spine: biomechanical approach. Eur Spine J 2011;20(Suppl 5):578–585

6 Spinal Sagittal Balance

Onur Yaman, Çağrı Canbolat, and Salman Sharif

Evolution and Equilibrium

Equilibrium is a state when the resultant force vector acting on the object and the corresponding moment vector are both zero. In this situation, a stationary object retains its equilibrium state as long as no force is applied to it. The most fundamental problem of motion in the evolutionary process has been gravity, which is a constant and continuous force. The anatomy of every living subgroup is based on gravity. While reptiles and fish from vertebrates have developed the ability to move in the coronal plane, mammals have gained the ability to move in the sagittal plane.[1] When we examine the movements of higher animals, we can see how important locomotion and organs are in evolution. Without designed or adaptive motive forces, it is safe to suppose that life would never have developed beyond the plant kingdom.[2] Bipedalism is one of the most distinctive features of humanity. It is characterized by an ergonomically optimal position, thanks to a narrow support base and the pelvis between the lumbar and cervical inclinations. Upright posture and bipedal movement necessitate coordination of the spine, pelvis, head, and lower extremities. This alignment differs significantly from that offered by quadrupedal nonhuman hominoids.[3,4] The growth of the spinopelvic functional unit was aided by changes in the sagittal architecture of the pelvis and spine.[5]

Pearls

- Equilibrium is a state when the resultant force vector acting on the object and the corresponding moment vector are both zero.
- The most fundamental problem of motion in the evolutionary process has been gravity, which is a constant and continuous force.
- Bipedalism is one of the most distinctive features of humanity.

Bipedalism and Balance

Maintaining the body's center of gravity within the acceptable region of the foot's sole provides the foundation for standing straight. To stand erect against gravity, the opposing forces exerted to the joints, which are the moment points, must be coordinated. It provides this coordination because of perceiving the sensory system and coordinating the locomotor system in this direction. Sensory signals are integrated in the central nervous system and modified by impulses from the reticular formation, extrapyramidal system, cerebellum, and cortex.[6]

Ideal spinal alignment can be characterized as the harmonious balancing of the trunk on the pelvis, requiring least energy expenditure to place the weight-bearing axis in a balanced physiological posture.[7]

The assessment of spinal balance in adults is mainly based on the evaluation of pelvic parameters, spinal parameters, and global sagittal balance.

The spine integrity has different curvature in bipedal stance. Lordosis occurs in the cervical and lumbar regions, while kyphosis occurs in the thoracic and sacral regions. These curvatures work in collaboration with the pelvis to hold the trunk above the pelvis. Lordosis diminishes as the pelvis tilts backward; conversely, when lordosis increases, the pelvis tilts forward and seeks to maintain balance. Curvatures in the spine work together to adjust the orientation of the pelvis in certain situations. While sitting, the pelvis rotates backward and the lumbar lordosis decreases, but when the pelvis rotates forward, the lumbar lordosis increases and regulates the body position.

With the deterioration of a systemic or functional unit, compensation mechanisms develop to restore sagittal balance against changes in the spine. When the spine begins to deform on the pelvis, some compensatory changes occur in the pelvis, which tries to maintain sagittal balance. These changes in the spine are evaluated through spinopelvic parameters.[8,9]

Pearls

- Maintaining the body's center of gravity within the acceptable region of the foot's sole provides the foundation for standing straight.
- Ideal spinal alignment can be characterized as the harmonious balancing of the trunk on the pelvis, requiring least energy expenditure to place the weight-bearing axis in a balanced physiological posture.

Radiographic Evaluation and Measurements

Scoliosis radiography is the most fundamental evaluation tool in the measurements that comprise a substantial portion of today's practice. Images in a normal scoliosis radiograph should be taken at an adequate distance, at the proper dose, and with precautions to preserve the patient's health, in order to clearly show the complete spine from the Cranio-cervical junction to the femoral heads. Nowadays, with various technologies, systems have been developed that create images from the vertex to the soles of the feet, boosting the quality and protecting the patient by exposing them to less X-ray photons.

While measurements are done on photos that are acceptable for the direct graphy shooting technique, measurements can be made with quick measurement periods and high accuracy by using various paid and free applications. Images for scoliosis X-rays are taken in the Anterior Posterior (P-A) and lateral positions. Both side bending and traction radiographs are included in coronal curves, as are supplementary radiographs of push-prone, inpatient A-P, fulcrum radiograph, traction A-P, hyperextension, and hyperflexion to aid in surgery planning.

Pearl

Images in a normal scoliosis radiograph should be taken at an adequate distance, at the proper dose, and with precautions to preserve the patient's health, in order to clearly show the complete spine from the cranial cervical junction to the femoral heads.

Basic Measurements

Static measurements are made on photographing the patient in a fixed position and on X-ray images. Measurements are made on static images, and although the measurements made in this way reflect the static balance, we believe that the future will be built on understanding and interpreting the dynamic balance. Appropriate images must be obtained at the correct positions for accurate measurement. If the images are not suitable, it means that the measurements are also not suitable.

Cervical Lordosis/Thoracic Kyphosis/ Lumbar Lordosis

Cervical lordosis is the Cobb angle value between C2 lower end plate and C7 lower end plate. Thoracic kyphosis is the Cobb angle value between T2 upper end plate and T12 lower end plate. Lumbar lordosis is the Cobb angle value between the L1 upper end plate and the S1 upper end plate (**Fig. 6.1a** and **b**).

Sagittal Vertical Axis (SVA)

It can be defined as the shortest distance from the midpoint of the C7 vertebra corpus in the sagittal plane to the posterior point of the S1 vertebra corpus upper end plate of the vertical line drawn perpendicular to the ground. The vertical line is expressed as plus (+) if it is anterior to this point, and minus (–) if it remains posterior to this point (**Fig. 6.2**).

Spinosacral Angle

Global determination of the thoracic and lumbar spine is made with the spinosacral angle. It is the angle between the line drawn from the midpoint of the C7 corpus to the midpoint of the upper end plate of the sacrum (**Fig. 6.3**). It affects the entire spine and is linked to sacral slope. When the spine bends forward with age, the pelvis rotates backward as a compensatory mechanism, and the spinosacral angle decreases, while the sacral tilt angle (SS) falls but the pelvic tilt increases. Attempts are made to maintain normal pelvic parameters. Knee joints flex in an attempt to compensate and maintain the spine erect.

Spinopelvic Parameters

Sacral slope (SS), pelvic tilt (PT), and pelvic incidence (PI) are the most used spinopelvic parameters. Since the sacrum carries the entire mobile vertebral arm, these values also significantly affect the alignment of the vertebral arm. The angle formed by the upper end plate of the S1 vertebra, and an imaginary line drawn parallel to the ground is known as the sacral slope. It is the angle formed by the imaginary line drawn perpendicular to the ground and the line

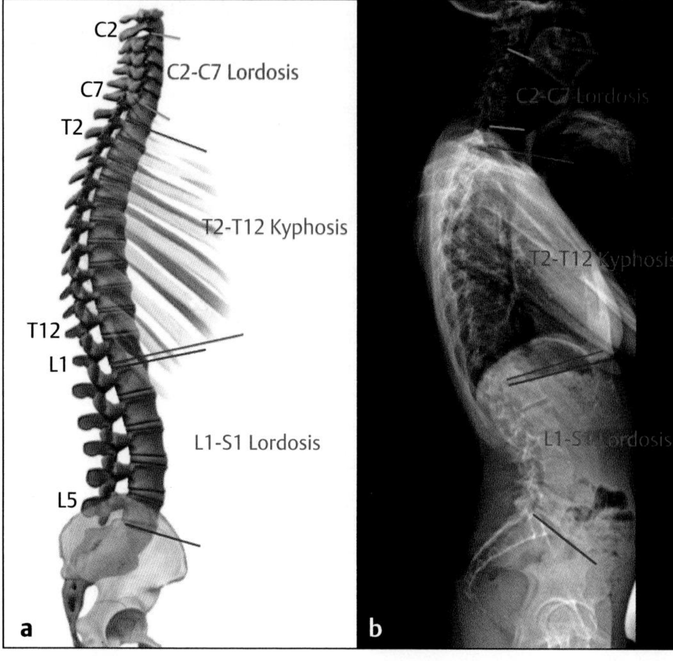

Fig. 6.1 Cervical lordosis, **(a)** thoracic kyphosis, and **(b)** lumbar lordosis measurements.

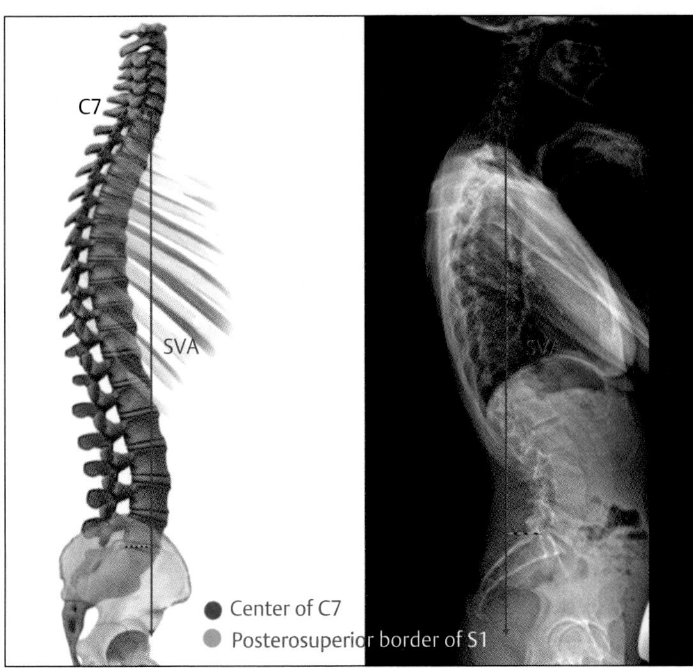

Fig. 6.2 Sagittal vertical axis (SVA) measurement.

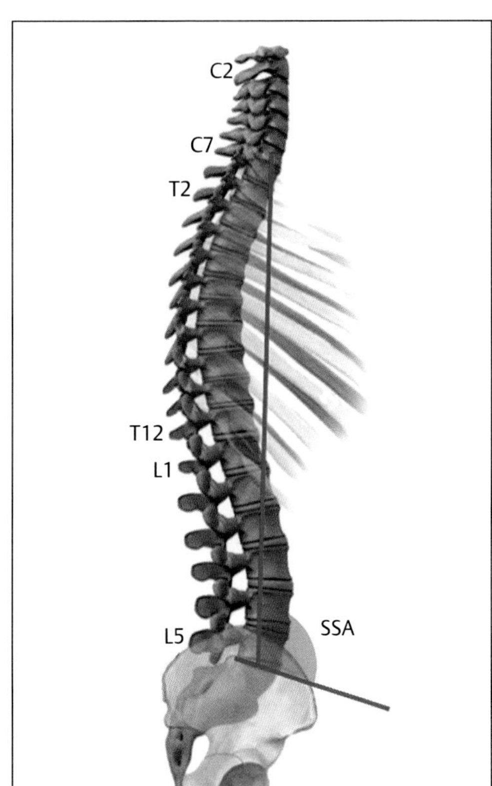

Fig. 6.3 Spinosacral angle (SSA) measurement.

drawn from the middle of the imaginary line connecting the midpoints of the PT femoral heads to the midpoint of the superior end plate of the S1 spine. PI is the angle between the line drawn from the middle of the imaginary line connecting the midpoints of the femoral heads to the midpoint of the upper end plate of the S1 vertebra and the imaginary line drawn perpendicular to the S1 superior end plate (**Fig. 6.4**). The equation PI = PT + SS is invariant. Although PT and SS change positionally, their sum shows the PI value (**Fig. 6.5**).

Pearl

The equation PI = PT + SS is invariant. Although PT and SS change positionally, their sum shows the PI value.

Clinic and Balance

The sacrum is the basis of the erect spine. With Jean Dubousset's idea of "pelvic vertebra," spinopelvic balance has become a focus.[10] While Legaye et al defined the PI

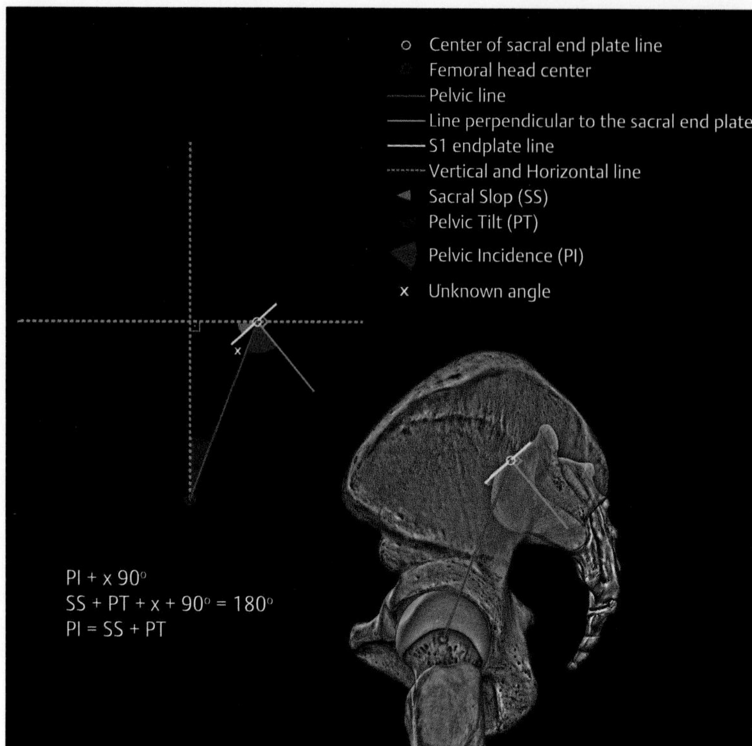

Fig. 6.4 Spinopelvic parameters. SS, sacral slope; PT, pelvic tilt; PI, pelvic incidence.

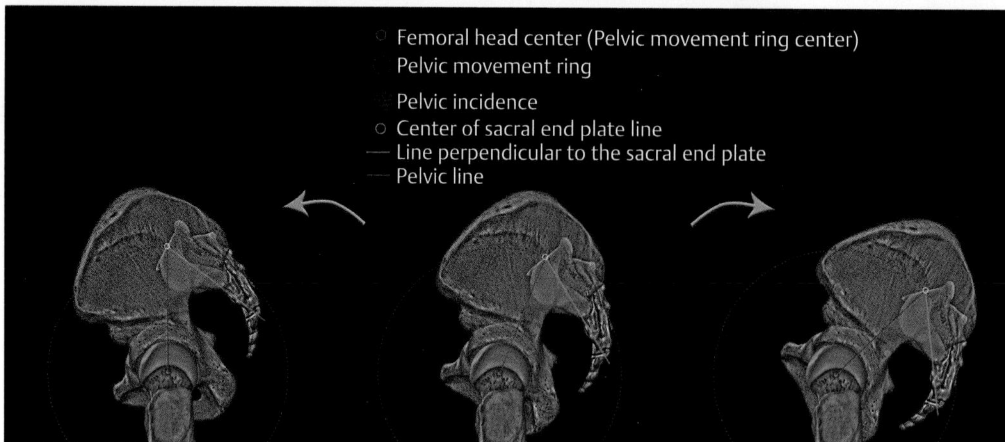

Fig. 6.5 As the sacral slope (SS) angle decreases in pelvic restoration, the pelvic tilt (PT) increases at the same rate (pelvic incidence [PI] = PT + SS).

angle using the Duval-Beaupere method,[11] Jackson et al introduced the pelvic radius technique in 1998 to measure the lumbar lordosis angle for the study of pelvic morphology.[12] The sacrum is part of the pelvic ring through the sacroiliac joints; it is a minimally mobile diarthrodial joint, thus comprising a single functional unit with the pelvis articulating with the femoral heads via the acetabulum. Roussouly et al stated that there are different variations in the shape of the spine in a significant part of the population and they studied the importance of having a posture in which an optimal harmony between the pelvis and the spine was seen.

Mehta et al reported mean values of asymptomatic adults (**Table 6.1**).[13] This study found an appropriate range of LL values for PI, which is a morphological measure used to preserve sagittal equilibrium. Patients with an abnormal PI value may cause problems such as isthmic spondylolysis, spondylolisthesis, degenerative spondylolisthesis, spinal deformity, adolescent idiopathic scoliosis, hip arthrosis, and fixed sagittal imbalance.[14] On the contrary, degenerative spinal pathologies due to disc degeneration that occur with aging cause flattening in the lumbar lordosis and cannot provide adequate compensation as a result of deterioration of balance with muscle atrophy and the deterioration process accelerates. It is critical to maintain or give enough lumbar lordosis (LL) for existing pelvic parameters during surgical intervention for any spinal disease, and to recognize that patients with high PI require greater LL.

The relationship between lumbar lordosis and sacral inclination was first noted by et al.[15] The greater the sacral slope, the greater is the LL; conversely, the lumbar curvature flattens as the SS becomes horizontal. According to the orientation of the sacral slope, Roussouly et al described four different types of lumbar lordosis in nonsymptomatic adults (**Fig. 6.6**).[16]

Table 6.1 Spinopelvic parameters and values in asymptomatic adults

Parameter	Definition	Values in asymptomatic adults, degrees
Pelvic incidence	See Fig. 6.4	48–55
Sacral slope	See Fig. 6.4	36–42
Pelvic tilt	See Fig. 6.4	12–18
Lumbar lordosis	Angle from the superior end plate of L1 to the caudal L5 end plate	43–61
Thoracic kyphosis	Angle from the superior end plate of T4 to the inferior end plate of T12	41–48

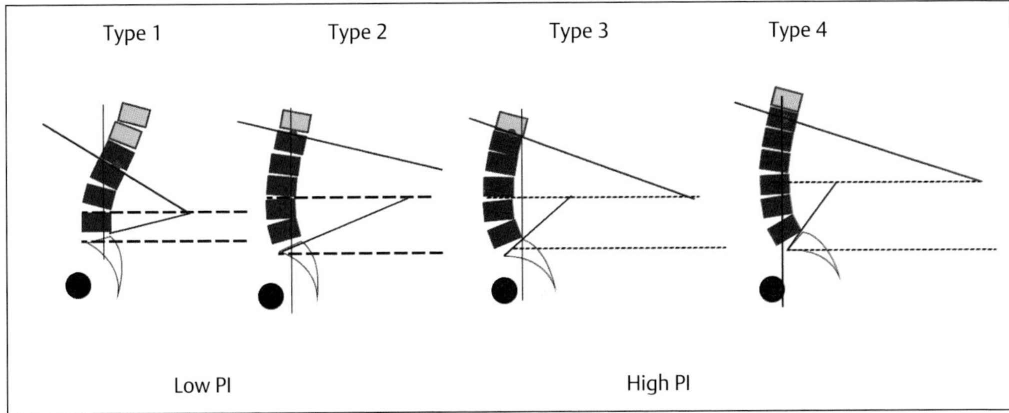

Fig. 6.6 The four types of spine shapes described by Roussouly et al.

Roussouly's classification basically outlined four different forms of sagittal examination of the human spine. Sacral inclination causes these various types of lumbar lordosis. According to a related study, Type 1 spine shape was observed in 5% of the population, Type 2 in 23%, Type 3 in 47%, and Type 4 in 25%.[13,17]

In Type 1 lumbar lordosis, the SS is less than 35 degrees, the apex of the lordosis is localized to the midpoint of the L5 vertebral body, and the lower curvature of the lordosis is small. The anterior edge of the upper end plate of the first lumbar spine is bent posteriorly according to the perpendicular line drawn from the sacral promontory. The lordosis is short, and the kyphosis is in the thoracolumbar.

Type 2 is characterized with an SS of less than 35 degrees, the peak of the LL located near the base of the L4 vertebral body, and a relatively flat lower arch of the lordosis. The anterior border of the superior end plate of the first lumbar vertebra is relatively posterior to the perpendicular line drawn from the sacral promontory, but it is closer to the vertical line and slightly greater than Type 1 lordosis; the lordosis slope is positive.

In Type 3 lumbar lordosis, the SS is between 35 and 45 degrees, the LL angle is localized to the midpoint of the L4 vertebral body, the lower arch of the lordosis is more prominent, and the lordosis slope is around 0 degrees. It is the most balanced type.

In Type 4 lumbar lordosis, the SS is greater than 45 degrees, and there is an abnormal rise in pelvic anteversion. The lumbar crest of lordosis is placed at or above the L3 vertebral base, the lordosis lower arch is prominent, and the lordosis slope is 0 or negative. Thoracic kyphosis is reduced.

Roussouly indicated in his study that it is possible to determine which form of spine will have which kind of ailment. The Type 1 spine was dubbed the nonconsonant spine by Roussouly. High pressure is given to the posterior parts of the lumbar area in this type of spine, and the spinous processes may come into touch with each other. These modifications ultimately increase the likelihood of developing spondylolisthesis as a result of hyperextension, as well as the risk of developing thoracolumbar discopathies in this type of spine. Type 2 spine has a harmonious alignment, but the person has a flat waist. In this type of spine, high pressure is applied to the discs and the risk of early degeneration and disc herniation is high. Type 3 spine has the most harmonious arrangement. However, with aging, the disc tissue collapses, and changes in the shape of the spine occur. Over time, a Type 3 spine might evolve into a Type 1 or 2 spine. Type 4 spines are also in an extreme lordotic alignment and have a harmonic alignment. The load is transferred mostly through the facet joints in this type. As a result, early facet arthropathies can be observed. Again, the risk of developing lumbar stenosis and spondylolisthesis is higher in this type of spine than in others.[16,17]

Depending on the correlation between SS and PI, Type 1 and 2 will usually have low-level PI, and Type- 3 and 4 will generally have high-level PI. The first and second types of lumbar lordosis are accompanied by changes in the anterior vertebral column segment (decreased disc height, wedging, osteophytes at L3, L4, L5 levels). These alterations must be observed in order for an intervertebral disc protrusion in the lumbar vertebrae to occur. The third and fourth forms of lordosis (hyperlordotic posture) cause degenerative-destructive alterations in the posterior complex, resulting in spinal canal narrowing and accompanying neurological findings.[16]

In a multicenter prospective study by Schwab et al, it was shown that the greatest correlation between radiographic parameters and deterioration in quality of life was the difference between LL and PI and sagittal measurements.[18] The Scoliosis Research Society (SRS)-Schwab adult spinal deformity classification is a widely used classification system that includes three classifications, one of which specifies the type of curvature and three of which include the sagittal spinopelvic variation classification (PI-LL, SVA, PT) (**Fig. 6.7**).[19]

Coronal Curve Types	Sagittal Modifiers
T: Thoracic only with lumbar curve <30°	PI-LL 0 [PI-LL < 10°] + [10° < PI-LL < 20° ++ [PI-LL > 20°]
L: T1/Lumbar only with thoracic curve <30°	Pelvic tilt (PT) 0 [PT < 20°] + [20° < PT < 30°] ++ [PT > 30°]
D: Double curve with T and TL/lumbar curves >30°	Global Alignment (SVA) 0 [SVA < cm] + [4 cm < SVA < 9.5 cm] ++ [SVA > 9.5 cm]
N: No major coronal deformity all coronal curves <30°	

Fig. 6.7 Scoliosis Research Society (SRS)-Schwab classification system. SVA, sagittal vertical axis; PI, pelvic incidence; LL, lumbar lordosis.

Pearls

- The greater the sacral slope, the greater is the LL; conversely, the lumbar curvature flattens as the SS becomes horizontal.
- It was shown that the greatest correlation between radiographic parameters and deterioration in quality of life was the difference between LL and PI and sagittal measurements.

Conclusion

Spinopelvic parameter analysis aids in guiding surgical approach in spinal surgery. Corrective operations that alter sagittal alignment and spinopelvic balance are extremely complicated and will continue to be the domain of specialized spine surgeons for the foreseeable future. All spine surgeons will need to understand and use these fundamental concepts in order to prevent iatrogenic abnormalities, even in short-level fusions. Whether or not the sagittal balance is affected, sagittal balance must be considered before any operation, especially if the L4-L5-S1 levels at the lumbar level are included in the fusion.

References

1. Rockwell H, Evans FG, Pheasant HC. The comparative morphology of the vertebrate spinal column. Its form as related to function. J Morphol 1938;63(1):87–117
2. Cope ED. The relation of animal motion to animal evolution. Am Nat 1878;12(1):40–48
3. Jenkins FA Jr. Chimpanzee bipedalism: cineradiographic analysis and implications for the evolution of gait. Science 1972; 178(4063):877–879
4. Lovejoy CO. The natural history of human gait and posture. Part 1. Spine and pelvis. Gait Posture 2005;21(1):95–112
5. Tardieu C, Hasegawa K, Haeusler M. How did the pelvis and vertebral column become a functional unit during the transition from occasional to permanent bipedalism? Anat Rec (Hoboken) 2017;300(5):912–931
6. Means KM, Rodell DE, O'Sullivan PS. Use of an obstacle course to assess balance and mobility in the elderly. A validation study. Am J Phys Med Rehabil 1996;75(2):88–95
7. Barrey C, Jund J, Noseda O. (2004) Equilibre sagittal pelvi-rachidien et pathologies lombaires dégénératives. Etude comparative à propos de 100 cas. Lyon: Thèse Doctorat-Université Claude-Bernard
8. Le Huec JC, Saddiki R, Franke J, Rigal J, Aunoble S. Equilibrium of the human body and the gravity line: the basics. Eur Spine J 2011; 20(5, Suppl 5):558–563

9. Ali Fahir Ozertk, Caglar Bozdogan. Sagittal balance in the spine. Turk Neurosurg 2014; 24(1):13–19
10. Dubousset J (1984) Le bassin «os intercalaire». Monographie du GES:15–22
11. Legaye J, Duval-Beaupère G, Hecquet J, Marty C. Pelvic incidence: a fundamental pelvic parameter for three-dimensional regulation of spinal sagittal curves. Eur Spine J 1998;7(2):99–103
12. Jackson RP, Peterson MD, McManus AC, Hales C. Compensatory spinopelvic balance over the hip axis and better reliability in measuring lordosis to the pelvic radius on standing lateral radiographs of adult volunteers and patients. Spine 1998;23(16): 1750–1767
13. Mehta VA, Amin A, Omeis I, Gokaslan ZL, Gottfried ON. Implications of spinopelvic alignment for the spine surgeon. Neurosurgery 2012;70(3):707–721
14. Yoshimoto H, Sato S, Masuda T, et al. Spinopelvic alignment in patients with osteoarthrosis of the hip: a radiographic comparison to patients with low back pain. Spine 2005;30(14):1650–1657
15. Stagnara P, De Mauroy JC, Dran G, et al. Reciprocal angulation of vertebral bodies in a sagittal plane: approach to references for the evaluation of kyphosis and lordosis. Spine 1982;7(4):335–342
16. Roussouly P, Gollogly S, Berthonnaud E, Dimnet J. Classification of the normal variation in the sagittal alignment of the human lumbar spine and pelvis in the standing position. Spine 2005;30(3):346–353
17. Le Huec JC, Thompson W, Mohsinaly Y, Barrey C, Faundez A. Sagittal balance of the spine. Eur Spine J 2019;28(9):1889–1905
18. Schwab FJ, Blondel B, Bess S, et al; International Spine Study Group (ISSG). Radiographical spinopelvic parameters and disability in the setting of adult spinal deformity: a prospective multicenter analysis. Spine 2013; 38(13):E803–E812
19. Kyrölä K, Repo J, Mecklin J-P, Ylinen J, Kautiainen H, Häkkinen A. Spinopelvic changes based on the simplified SRS-Schwab adult spinal deformity classification: relationships with disability and health-related quality of life in adult patients with prolonged degenerative spinal disorders. Spine 2018;43(7):497–502

7 Congenital Scoliosis

Stacey Darwish

Introduction

Congenital spinal deformity occurs in approximately 1 in 1,000 live births, with scoliosis being the most commonly identified deformity (80%). The deformities usually arise sporadically and the rate of transmission is quoted as 1%. There occurs an association with the Homeobox genes of the Hox class.[1,2]

Congenital scoliosis is defined as a lateral curvature with associated rotation of the spine caused by vertebral anomalies that produce a coronal plane deformity. The anomalies are present at birth but it may take several years for the curvature to develop.

The anomalies result in a spectrum of deformity from a very benign curve with low potential for progression to a much more severe curve that can rapidly progress and cause significant functional and cosmetic complications.

Embryology and Etiology

Vertebral anomalies form around 4 to 6 weeks gestation. Embryologic development of the spine occurs around the same time as many organs and therefore it is not surprising that vertebral anomalies are often associated with abnormalities in other organ system.[3,4] Sixty percent of patients with a vertebral anomaly will have another issue.[5] Most commonly, the genitourinary tract is affected with issues such as renal agenesis, ectopic or duplex kidney, and reflux. Other spinal cord problems can also coexist; the most common being a tethered cord, diastematomyelia (present in 5–20%), and syringomyelia. Around 50% patients with a unilateral unsegmented bar and same level contralateral vertebra have an associated neural axial abnormality.

The acronym VACTERL (V—vertebral anomalies, A—anal atresia, C—cardiac defect, TE—tracheoesophageal fistula, R—renal defects, L—limb defect) is a group of anomalies which are all linked. These systems should all be investigated as part of the routine work-up of a new patient presenting with a congenital scoliosis.

Environmental factors have been linked with the development of congenital scoliosis in animal studies; hypoxia and vitamin A deficiency have predominantly been seen.[6] Further investigation is being undertaken in this field.

Pearls

- Scoliosis genetics are not fully understood.
- Both genetic and environmental factors are considered to be involved.

Classification

Two main types of vertebral anomaly occur: failure of formation (type I) and failure of segmentation (type II) (**Fig. 7.1**). A third group is often included in this classification—a mixed pattern. We will discuss these further.

This, commonly used, classification system[7] focusses on the anterior anatomy only, and therefore when deciding to operate, an understanding of the posterior anatomy is essential, which can be achieved with three-dimensional imaging (discussed later).

Failure of formation can be partial or complete causing either a wedged vertebra

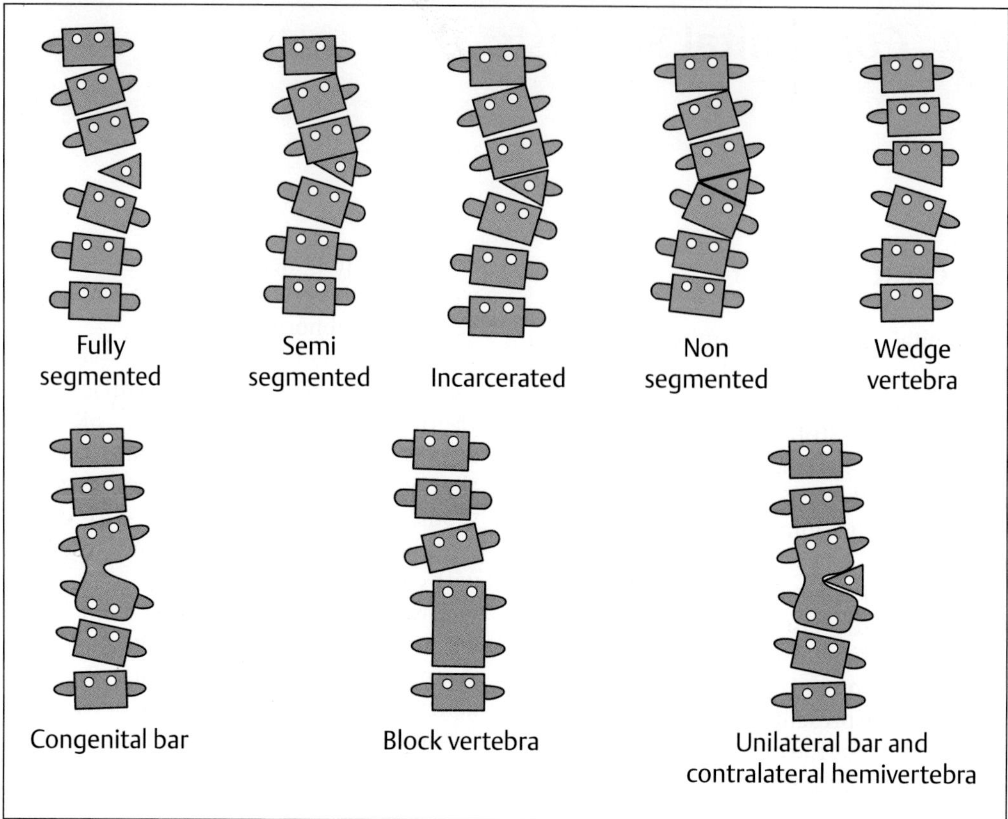

Fig. 7.1 Pictorial representation of the types of formation/segmentation deformities.

with intact pedicles or a hemivertebra with a single pedicle.

Wedge vertebra: This can produce asymmetrical growth.

Fully segmented hemivertebra: The adjacent vertebrae shape is normal and both the superior and inferior end plates of the hemivertebra have growth potential. Rate of progression is approximately 1 to 2 degrees per year.

Semisegmented hemivertebra: The hemivertebra is fused at one end with the adjacent vertebra and so there is only growth potential at the opposite end. This produces a tilting of the spine and a more slowly progressing curve.

Incarcerated hemivertebra: The hemivertebra has growth potential both superiorly and inferiorly but this is compensated for by the adjacent levels. There are abnormal looking vertebrae on either side of the hemivertebra. There is very little deformity associated with this type of anomaly.

Nonsegmented hemivertebra: There is no growth potential in these cases as the hemivertebra is fused with the adjacent levels on either side; therefore, there is no progression in deformity.

Failure of segmentation can again be either partial or complete. Partial cases have a congenital bar (anterior, posterior, lateral, or mixed) whereas completed cases have a block vertebra. The location of the bar will determine the type of deformity that develops; kyphosis, lordosis, scoliosis, or kyphoscoliosis. Block vertebra tend to cause the spine to shorten but have limited progression in the coronal plane.

Many cases have complex vertebral anomalies with both failures of segmentation and formation across several levels giving a mixed deformity (Type III).

A unilateral unsegmented bar with a contralateral hemivertebrae is the most progressive with around 6-degree progression per year.

These anomalies cause an unbalanced spine. The number of unbalanced healthy growth plates determines the degree of deformity and rate at which the deformity will progress (**Table 7.1**). Other risk factors for progression of the deformity include the age of the patient (they progress more through periods of rapid growth, i.e., first 2 years of life and adolescent growth spurt) and the location of the anomalies—lumbosacral hemivertebra causes a far greater imbalance than that of a mid-thoracic.

Assessment

History and Physical Examination

Patients with suspected congenital scoliosis should be referred early to a specialist in pediatric deformity for assessment and management of this condition. These patients are often referred to deformity surgeons by a pediatrician who may be responsible for their care due to an associated issue.

A detailed history including birth history and achievement of developmental milestones should be noted during the standard history taking.

Clinical examination should be performed at each visit beginning with an assessment of the patient's height (sitting or standing dependent on ability) and weight. This should then progress to assessing sagittal and coronal balance clinically. Shoulder and waist asymmetry should be documented as well as any listing of the trunk from the center of pelvis. Gait should be checked if possible and any leg length discrepancy quantified.

Neurological status should be documented but may have to be adjusted depending on patient age and ability to cooperate with examination. Reflexes and any evidence of muscle atrophy should be noted.

Note should also be made at each assessment of the flexibility of the deformity—this can be done by a simple stretch (lifting the child under their arms and viewing how the deformity corrects).

Other anomalies should be examined for such as neck motion, short neck, and low hairline (congenital anomalies are also found with Klippel-Feil syndrome) as well as other deformities in the extremities (in particular, radial malformation and foot deformities such as pes cavus). Cutaneous markings or dimpling of the back should also be noted (signs of diastematomyelia).

Imaging

Imaging should make up part of the initial assessment of a congenital scoliosis and a plain radiograph is the first step. Ideally initial radiographs should be taken before

Table 7.1 Risk of progression by deformity

Risk of progression (highest to lowest)	Curve progression
Unilateral unsegmented bar with contralateral hemivertebra	Rapid and constant
Unilateral unsegmented bar	Rapid
Fully segmented hemivertebra	Steady
Partially segmented vertebra	Slow
Incarcerated vertebra	May progress slowly
Unsegmented vertebra/block vertebra	Little progression

the age of 4 years as after this stage they are too ossified and classification is more challenging. This allows the type of anomaly to be categorized. Whole spine posteroanterior (PA) and lateral films should be taken to check the type and location of the abnormality as well as Cobb angles should be measured to determine the size of the curve.[8] These films also allow the surgeon to assess pedicle size and presence as well as any rib abnormalities such as fusion or absence. Stretch films or suspended should be performed to assess for flexibility of the curve.

Subsequent radiographs should be compared with the original and one should not rely solely on Cobb angle measurements as these are known to have a higher rate of measurement error due to the irregular spinal landmarks.[9] Studies have shown inter- and intraobserver variance of anywhere between 2 and 10 degrees.[10] Awareness of the development of a compensatory curve as well as the assessment of the original curve can confirm the progression. Compensatory curves are made up of normal vertebrae and can be more reproducibly measured. If the compensatory curve does not progress, it is unlikely that the congenital curve will progress significantly.

Previously magnetic resonance imaging (MRI) was only considered in those patients who had neurological symptoms or those likely to proceed to surgery. Now, it is highly unusual to not perform MRI scanning of the whole spine in these children. A 30% associated with intraspinal anomaly is too high to ignore and so this should also be part of the initial investigation of these patients.[11] It is worth noting that in young children this is likely to require a general anesthetic and if possible could be combined with another procedure to avoid multiple anesthetics.

Computerized tomography (CT) with three-dimensional reconstructions allows the surgeon a better understanding of the structural deformity. These deformities can be difficult to interpret on plain radiographs due to overlying structures or the severity of the deformity. These reconstructions can now also allow three-dimensional printing of models of the spine which can be very useful in preoperative planning stage of treatment or, in certain centers, can even allow for patient-specific implants/guides to be created for theater.

Other investigations should include a renal ultrasound and urinalysis to look for renal anomalies—although these are often performed prior to visiting a spinal specialist. A cardiac assessment should also be requested in the form of an echocardiogram. Onward referral to the appropriate specialists should occur based on findings of these investigations.

Pulmonary function tests should be performed in patients who are being considered for surgical intervention as a thoracic height less than 22 cm will have a percent predicted FEV1 (forced expiratory volume in one second) and FVC (forced vital capacity) of <50%.[12]

Pearls

- Investigations should be completed before embarking on a treatment path.
- A multidisciplinary approach is required.
- MRI scan must be performed in all cases of congenital deformity.

Treatment

The treatment of congenital scoliosis is different from idiopathic scoliosis and should be adapted on a patient-by-patient basis. Treatment should be based on a thorough understanding of the deformity and the risk of progression. Surgery is often indicated early to prevent significant progression and the development of permanent large deformities at skeletal maturity.

Nonoperative

This can be in the form of observation alone or bracing.

All scoliosis patients require close clinical observation during periods of rapid growth. These regular assessments allow for the evaluation of curve progression.

Bracing has a limited role in the congenitally abnormal spine as it does not prevent progression of the structural curve but may be useful in controlling the compensatory flexible curve. In specific cases of a long flexible curve, progression can be slowed by bracing.[13] The other problem with bracing is the considerable period of time between onset of deformity and skeletal maturity and therefore bracing is merely a temporary measure. Compliance remains an issue in this group as it does in the idiopathic scoliosis group.

The use of rigid bracing to correct may actually be detrimental in some cases as it can exacerbate chest wall deformities.

That being said, the main stay of nonoperative treatment is clinical monitoring of a static curve.

Operative

The decision to operate or not is usually not debated. The type of surgery and timing is more difficult to determine. In adolescent idiopathic scoliosis it is usual to aim to delay surgery to close to skeletal maturity, allowing improved patient height. This is not the case in congenital scoliosis patients; surgery is often performed early to prevent the decompensation associated with structural curves and to allow fusion of the fewest levels.

The loss of height by early operative intervention is irrelevant in these cases as the growth that occurs is abnormal—increased rotation and development of compensatory curves.

That being said, the aim of achieving as much thoracic height as is safely possible prior to surgery is important because when scoliosis causes chest wall deformity it can cause cardiopulmonary failure. Decrease in thoracic height and width is associated with a reduction in exercise tolerance and poor or deteriorating pulmonary function.

As with all surgeries, complications and risks should be fully discussed with the patient (if applicable) and parents/guardian.[4]

Surgery for congenital scoliosis carries all the usual risks but neurological injury is known to be higher than for other scoliosis types and as such intraoperative neurophysiology (both somatosensory- and motor-evoked potentials) should be used.

Nutritional status should be fully optimized prior to embarking on any surgical intervention as soft tissue healing is paramount and this can be compromised by undernutrition. Superior mesenteric artery syndrome is associated with any spinal deformity surgery.[14] A multidisciplinary approach involving gastroenterology and pediatric surgeons is often required in its management, so it is useful to have these teams involved prior to embarking on any surgery.

The aim of operative treatment in all scoliosis surgery is to achieve a balanced spine.[15] In congenital scoliosis one side of the spine is growing more quickly that the other and balance can be achieved either with or without reduction of the deformity by altering growth.[16]

Multiple ways to achieve this have been described but we will focus on the most common ones:

- Posterior spinal fusion (with or without instrumentation).
- Combined anterior and posterior spinal fusion.
- Hemiepiphysiodesis.
- Hemivertebra excision.
- Guided growth systems.

Posterior Spinal Fusion

The decision of whether to fuse the spine is based on curve size and risk of progression. In the small curve that is anticipated to worsen (i.e., a unilateral unsegmented bar) the decision to proceed with an uninstrumented in situ fusion may be appropriate whereas larger curves which require some correction will need instrumentation. It is worth noting that the rigid congenital deformity will not correct with a posterior-only fusion but the surrounding flexible levels will allow some improvement in the overall curve.

Posterior spinal fusion is the simplest and safest way to halt growth. The approach is a standard posterior midline approach although care must be taken to avoid neurological injury as there may be unrecognized laminar defects. The introduction of CT scanning preoperatively has reduced this risk. Intraoperative imaging should be available from the start of the case to ensure the anomaly level can de targeted. Levels should be confirmed both prior to incision and prior to fusion to ensure all levels of the involved vertebrae in the congenital curve can be included in the fusion. The fusion should extend laterally as far as the transverse processes.

Postoperative bracing is required to achieve fusion and should be in place for 4 to 6 months.

As the anterior spine is untouched, anterior spinal growth remains active and therefore there is an increased risk of rotational deformity with bending of the fusion mass, known as crankshaft phenomenon. The risk is increased in the younger patient and in larger curves at the time of correction. Studies quote 15% crankshaft incidence in patients undergoing posterior spinal fusion before the age of 10 years with curves greater than 50 degrees.[17]

The use of instrumentation is now widely accepted and the development of smaller implants aimed at the pediatric population has reduced the risk of implant prominence and subsequently reduced reoperation rates.[18] As with all instrumentation the risk of neurological injury remains, although current intraoperative spinal cord monitoring and careful preoperative planning (anticipating difficult anatomy with 3D imaging) has again reduced this risk and makes instrumentation more feasible in the young population.

Combined Anterior and Posterior Spinal Fusion

The advantage of performing an anterior surgical procedure is that it allows a full discectomy and removal of the end plates resulting in a better deformity correction.

Bone graft is used to aid the fusion and this can be allograft, autograft, or synthetic.

The combined anterior and posterior spinal fusion versus posterior-only fusion reduces the risk of pseudoarthrosis.[19] Anterior approach obviously carries its own risks and in patients with multiple anomalies it is important to be aware of the potential vascular anomalies to the spinal cord which could result in cord ischemia after vessel ligation during the approach.

In areas such as the thoracolumbar junction the anterior spine may be approached laterally or from the back as retroperitoneal dissection can allow enough visualization of the spine.

More modern techniques such as endoscopy allow the anterior spine to be prepared through a minimally invasive approach.

Hemiepiphysiodesis

This is a concept taken from other forms of pediatric orthopaedic surgery, (i.e., long bones). This involves slowing the growth on the convex side of the curve to allow the deformity to correct as the concave side grows.[20] This results in gradual correction of the deformity.

The same prerequisites as that of long bone surgery apply here—there must be enough remaining growth to allow for correction (i.e., a young patient—usually under 6 yrs of age), specific to the spine is that it should be a short curve (less than 7 levels), no pathologic kyphosis or lordosis, curve <70 degrees and there must be enough growth potential on the concave side (i.e., functioning growth plates).

This technique obviously requires a combined anterior and posterior approach and again requires a significant period of immobilization with bracing postoperatively.

Anteriorly the convex discectomy, end plate preparation, and bone grafting are performed while posteriorly a unilateral facetectomy and fusion with bone graft are performed at each level. This technique can provide up to 20 degrees of correction by skeletal maturity. Convex compression with instrumentation posteriorly can improve immediate correction.

Hemivertebra Excision

This procedure traditionally involved a combined anterior and posterior surgical exposure, followed by excision of the hemivertebra and anterior and posterior fusion. Anterior structural bone graft is utilized on the concave side to maintain correction. If the patient is old enough (>5 yrs) and has a large curve, instrumentation should be used to improve the rate of fusion. It has been shown that patients undergoing posterior hemivertebrae excision before the age of 6 years (with pedicle screw fixation) have better deformity correction without compromising growth when compared with their older peers (6–10 yrs).[21]

The use of instrumentation allows a brace to be used in the postoperative period rather than a nonremovable cast.

More commonly now this is being performed through a single posterior approach.[22]

This procedure is usually reserved for patients with an unacceptable deformity such as a fixed lateral translation of the trunk. This procedure is safest in the lumbar and lumbosacral regions.

Guided Growth Procedures

Concern regarding thoracic insufficiency syndrome was the driving factor in the development of growth-preserving surgical techniques. The use of guided growth rods and vertical expandable prosthetic titanium rib (VEPTR) devices aims to allow continued spinal growth and relive constriction on the concave hemithorax in patients with congenital scoliosis.

Allowing patients to achieve maximum spinal height before definitive fusion optimizes thoracic volume and therefore pulmonary function.[23–25]

VEPTR has a role in patients who not only require guided growth but also have associated rib fusions. The main aim of VEPTR is to improve thoracic volume and maintain correction until skeletal maturity. It can be used to expand the concave hemithorax at 6 monthly intervals. VEPTR can use hooks as either a rib-to-rib or a rib-to-spine construct. When VEPTR is used before the age of 2 years it has been shown that pulmonary function at 5-year follow-up is significantly better than compared with children who undergo surgery later.[26]

These procedures are not the holy grail of scoliosis surgery and are associated with multiple complications; therefore, patients and their families need to be appropriately counselled before embarking on this route of treatment.

Traditional growing rods are inserted through a posterior approach and require lengthening at 6 monthly intervals under general anesthetic.[27] There has been debate on the use of single- and dual-rod constructs; studies have shown that dual-rod constructs achieve greater overall growth and curve correction.

The most recent addition to the guided growth armamentarium is the magnetic growing rods. These are based on the same principle of the traditional growth control rods but allow the rods to be lengthened in the outpatient setting. This obviously has significant impact on the children with less hospital stays, reduced anesthetic time, less time off school, etc.

The MAGEC system has been shown to be more cost effective than conventional growth rods. Estimated cost saving after 6 years is approximately £12,000. The MAGEC system (NuVasive, introduced in 2009) is recognized in the National Institute for Clinical Excellence (NICE) guidelines for scoliosis as an effective surgical option in children who require surgery for scoliosis.[28]

MAGEC rods have been controversial in recent years with reports of metallosis and concerns regarding metal ions, but the British Spine Society, the British Orthopaedic Association, and the UK Spine Societies Board are of the opinion that although there are problems with the MAGEC rods they remain the optimal choice in many children with severe, progressive spinal deformity.

Guided growth procedures require conversion to definitive fusion either when adequate correction has been achieved or the patient is old enough for this—usually when they have reached double-digit age.

Pearls

- These are difficult cases to treat with many options available to the surgeon; this is a condition that is very different to adolescent idiopathic scoliosis.
- Cases need to be taken on an individual basis.
- Aim is to prevent deformity and preserve respiratory function.
- Nonoperative treatment is of limited value in a progressive curve.

Conclusion

Patients with congenital scoliosis are complex who require a multidisciplinary management approach with significant surgical planning.

References

1. Karlin LI. Congenital spinal deformities 42. *Spine Secrets Plus E-Book* 2011:291
2. Tsirikos AI. Congenital deformities of the spine. In: *Non-idiopathic spine deformities in young children.* Springer; 2011: 45–72
3. Johal J, Loukas M, Fisahn C, Chapman JR, Oskouian RJ, Tubbs RS. Hemivertebrae: a comprehensive review of embryology, imaging, classification, and management. Childs Nerv Syst 2016;32(11):2105–2109
4. Poorman GW, Jalai CM, Diebo B, et al. Congenital etiology is an independent risk factor for complications in adolescents undergoing corrective scoliosis surgery: comparison of in-hospital comorbidities using Nationwide KID's Inpatient Database. J Pediatr Orthop 2019;39(8):406–410
5. Jog S, Patole S, Whitehall J. Congenital scoliosis in a neonate: can a neonatologist ignore it? Postgrad Med J 2002;78(922):469–472
6. Li Z, Yu X, Shen J. Environmental aspects of congenital scoliosis. Environ Sci Pollut Res Int 2015;22(8):5751–5755
7. McMaster MJ, Ohtsuka K. The natural history of congenital scoliosis. A study of two hundred and fifty-one patients. J Bone Joint Surg Am 1982;64(8):1128–1147
8. Shands AR Jr, Bundens WD. Congenital deformities of the spine: an analysis of the roentgenograms of 700 children. Bull Hosp Jt Dis 1956;17(2):110–133
9. Loder RT, Urquhart A, Steen H, et al. Variability in Cobb angle measurements in children with congenital scoliosis. J Bone Joint Surg Br 1995;77(5):768–770
10. Facanha-Filho FA, Winter RB, Lonstein JE, et al. Measurement accuracy in congenital scoliosis. J Bone Joint Surg Am 2001;83(1): 42–45
11. Gettys FK, Carpenter A, Stasikelis PJ. The role of MRI in children with congenital limb deficiencies with associated scoliosis. J Pediatr Orthop 2020;40(5):e390–e393
12. Theologis AA, Smith J, Kerstein M, Gregory JR, Luhmann SJ. Normative data of pulmonary function tests and radiographic measures of chest development in children without spinal deformity: is a T1–T12 height of 22 cm adequate? Spine Deform 2019;7(6):857–864
13. Winter RB, Moe JH, MacEwen GD, Peon-Vidales H. The Milwaukee brace in the nonoperative treatment of congenital scoliosis. Spine 1976;1(2):85–96
14. Moyer K, Thompson GH, Poe-Kochert C, Splawski J. Superior mesenteric artery syndrome complicated by gastric mucosal necrosis following congenital scoliosis surgery: a case report. JBJS Case Connect 2019;9(3):e0380
15. Loughenbury PR, Gummerson NW, Tsirikos AI. Congenital spinal deformity: assessment,

natural history and treatment. Orthop Trauma 2017;31(6):364–369
16. Tikoo A, Kothari MK, Shah K, Nene A. Current concepts: congenital scoliosis. Open Orthop J 2017;11:337–345
17. Kesling KL, Lonstein JE, Denis F, et al. The crankshaft phenomenon after posterior spinal arthrodesis for congenital scoliosis: a review of 54 patients. Spine 2003;28(3):267–271
18. Wiggins GC, Shaffrey CI, Abel MF, Menezes AH. Pediatric spinal deformities. Neurosurg Focus 2003;14(1):e3
19. Andrew T, Piggott H. Growth arrest for progressive scoliosis. Combined anterior and posterior fusion of the convexity. J Bone Joint Surg Br 1985;67(2):193–197
20. Winter RB, Lonstein JE, Denis F, Sta-Ana de la Rosa H. Convex growth arrest for progressive congenital scoliosis due to hemivertebrae. J Pediatr Orthop 1988;8(6):633–638
21. Chang D-G, Suk S-I, Kim J-H, Ha K-Y, Na K-H, Lee J-H. Surgical outcomes by age at the time of surgery in the treatment of congenital scoliosis in children under age 10 years. Spine J 2015;15(8):1783–1795
22. Ruf M, Harms J. Hemivertebra resection by a posterior approach: innovative operative technique and first results. Spine 2002; 27(10):1116–1123
23. Campbell RM Jr, Hell-Vocke AK. Growth of the thoracic spine in congenital scoliosis after expansion thoracoplasty. J Bone Joint Surg Am 2003;85(3):409–420
24. Campbell RM Jr, Smith MD, Mayes TC, et al. The effect of opening wedge thoracostomy on thoracic insufficiency syndrome associated with fused ribs and congenital scoliosis. J Bone Joint Surg Am 2004;86(8):1659–1674
25. Lin Y, Tan H, Rong T, et al. Impact of thoracic cage dimension and geometry on cardiopulmonary function in patients with congenital scoliosis: a prospective study. Spine 2019;44(20):1441–1448
26. Campbell RM Jr. VEPTR: past experience and the future of VEPTR principles. Eur Spine J 2013; 22(2, Suppl 2):S106–S117
27. Thompson GH, Akbarnia BA, Campbell RM Jr. Growing rod techniques in early-onset scoliosis. J Pediatr Orthop 2007;27(3):354–361
28. Jenks M, Craig J, Higgins J, et al. The MAGEC system for spinal lengthening in children with scoliosis: a NICE medical technology guidance. Appl Health Econ Health Policy 2014;12(6):587–599

8 Neuromuscular Scoliosis in Adults

Alexandra J. White, Tyler J. Calton, and Jacob Hoffmann

Introduction

Neuromuscular scoliosis refers to spinal deformity due to neuromuscular pathway abnormalities. These disorders are due to a dysfunction in the pathway from brain, spinal cord, peripheral nerves, neuromuscular junction, and muscle. The abnormal sequence manifests in flaccidity, spasticity, or dyskinetic dysfunction of the muscle groups leading to an aberration of the entire spinal column. These patients often have poor head and trunk balance. Neuromuscular scoliosis often causes a more severe spinal deformity with a more progressive course compared to idiopathic scoliosis, and the risk of progression is high even after skeletal maturity.[1,2] Although extensive literature is devoted to neuromuscular scoliosis in children and, thus, on deformity in the immature skeleton, there are few reports about adult-onset neuromuscular scoliosis. The aim of this chapter is to compile available information on the etiologies, evaluation, prognosis, and operative and nonoperative management of adult-onset neuromuscular scoliosis and spinal deformity. In addition, this chapter aims to outline two common causes of adult-onset neuromuscular scoliosis from Parkinson disease (PD) and spinal cord injuries.

Neuromuscular scoliosis can lead to both coronal and sagittal misalignment.[3] It causes lateral curvature in the frontal plane, axial rotation in the horizontal plane, and disturbs the normal curvature in the sagittal plane.[4] The degree of physiological disability is directly related to the location and severity of the curve, potentially impacting mobility of the shoulder girdle and cervical spine, cardiopulmonary function (in the case of thoracic deformity), pelvic imbalance, and leg length discrepancy when in the lumbar spine.[3] Pelvic obliquity in lumbar scoliosis may impair patients' ability to sit without using their arms for balance, limiting their mobility and independence.[3] Very severe deformities, especially those leading to sagittal imbalance, can affect upright head balance, further limiting function. This limitation of mobility also impacts caregivers, complicating patient care, transport, and hygiene. The mechanical vector along which paraspinal muscles generate force is compromised in deformity, resulting in back pain along the curvature.[3] The costopelvic junction can become impinged, leading to pain on the concave side of the spinal curve.[3] Finally, spinal deformity can lead to cosmetic concerns, although these concerns appear less frequently in the adult population compared to children with neuromuscular scoliosis.[5]

Coronal or sagittal curvature may develop as a result of asymmetric tone in the paraspinal muscles.[3] The progression of deformity is exacerbated by osteoporosis in adults, especially in postmenopausal women.[5] Facet joints, joint capsules, discs, and ligaments may degenerate and ultimately lead to segmental instability, spinal stenosis, radiculopathy, claudication, and neurological symptoms.[5] Pelvic incidence is a major regulator of both lumbar lordosis and pelvic tilt, so spinopelvic balance also has an impact on the progression of adult scoliosis.[4,6]

Pearl

Neuromuscular scoliosis can lead to both coronal and sagittal misalignment causing physiologic disability.

Classification

Neuromuscular scoliosis can be classified based on the etiology and onset of the neurologic disease that leads to spinal deformity (**Box 8.1**).[3,7] Congenital upper motor neuron pathologies leading to neuromuscular scoliosis (in this case associated with spasticity) include cerebral palsy, Friedreich ataxia, and syringomyelia. Congenital lower motor and sensory neuron pathologies include spinal muscular atrophy (Werdnig-Hoffmann and Kugelberg-Welander disease), familial dysautonomia (Riley-Day syndrome), Charcot-Marie-Tooth disease, and Roussy-Lévy disease. Myelomeningocele is a mixed upper and lower motor neuron pathology that results in neuromuscular scoliosis. Congenital myopathies such as muscular dystrophies, arthrogryposis, and congenital hypotonia can lead to deformity. Acquired causes of neuromuscular scoliosis include structural lesions such as spinal cord tumors and trauma, as well as degenerative pathologies such as PD, transverse myelitis, and multiple sclerosis. Finally, viruses such as poliomyelitis can also progress to neuromuscular scoliosis.

Box 8.1 Classification of neuromuscular scoliosis

Primary neuropathies

- Upper motor neuron pathologies
  - Cerebral palsy
  - Spinocerebellar degeneration
    - Friedreich ataxia
  - Syringomyelia
  - Spinal cord tumor
  - Spinal cord trauma
- Lower motor neuron pathologies
  - Poliomyelitis
  - Other viral myelitides
  - Traumatic
  - Spinal muscular atrophy
    - Werdnig-Hoffmann disease
    - Kugelberg-Welander disease
  - Dysautonomia
    - Riley-Day syndrome
  - Combined upper and lower pathologies
    - Myelomeningocele
  - Charcot-Marie-Tooth disease
  - Roussy-Lévy disease

Primary myopathies

- Muscular dystrophy
    - Duchenne muscular dystrophy
    - Limb-girdle dystrophy
    - Facioscapulohumeral dystrophy
  - Arthrogryposis
  - Fiber-type disproportion
  - Congenital hypotonia
  - Myotonia dystrophica

Neuromuscular Scoliosis due to Parkinson Disease

The association between PD and spinal deformity has been widely described. One third of PD patients have abnormal posture.[8] The prevalence of scoliosis in PD has been estimated from 7 to 90% compared to 6 to 30% in the general population.[4] In fact, spinal deformity together with hand and gait symptoms can be a presenting symptom of PD.[9] In one 2016 study of 503 patients with PD in China, there was a 10.34% prevalence of coronal imbalance, a 7.75% prevalence of scoliosis, and a 16.5% prevalence of Pisa syndrome.[4] Pisa syndrome (PS) is a reversible lateral bending of the trunk by greater than 10 degrees in the standing position.[9] In this study, patients with PS had significantly greater severity of PD, worse chronic dorsal or lumbar pain, and longer duration of both disease and treatment.[10] These findings are corroborated by a 2015 study that demonstrated a significant association between magnitude of coronal Cobb angle and UPDRS score (a measure of PD symptom severity) in a cohort of PD patients.[11] However, a 2016 study of PD patients in Finland with a scoliosis prevalence of 50% found no difference in disease severity between subjects with scoliosis and those without.[4]

Animal studies have suggested an association between disease severity and degree of scoliosis, as well as an association between laterality of symptoms and laterality of curvature, but these findings are not consistently replicated in human studies. Therefore, the true etiology of scoliosis in PD remains unknown. Hemiparkinsonism induced in rats by injecting 6-hydroxydopamine into the left ventral tegmentum leads to ipsilateral deviation and ultimately to the development of scoliosis.[12] Dystonia may be one of the initiators of abnormal posture in scoliosis in PD, but ultimately soft tissue, muscle, and spinal changes will drive the progression of deformity.[9] This observation is in keeping with the higher incidence of scoliosis in women with PD, as women with PD tend to have dystonia more frequently.[11,13] Abnormal proprioception may also impair axial motor control, but further study is needed.[9] Rigidity and reduced spinal range of motion perpetuate the development of deformity. Preexisting spinal conditions or a history of spinal surgery can also compound the progression of deformity in PD, as does the use of L-dopa. One theory is that the neuromuscular changes caused by L-dopa have a negative impact on spinal structure.[14] This complex interplay between adult-onset pathology and preexisting comorbidities is a unique aspect of neuromuscular scoliosis in adults.[15]

As mentioned above, there is controversy as to whether there is a correlation between PD symptom laterality and scoliosis.[10,13] Most studies find that patients tend to lean away from their most affected side, but some found no difference.[9,11] For example, a 2009 prospective cohort study in Korea comparing PD patients with spinal asymmetry to PD patients with true scoliosis found no correlation between laterality of PD symptoms and scoliosis, and that the incidence of scoliosis did not differ based on L-dopa treatment status.[13] This study did find that the average age of PD patients with scoliosis was significantly greater, suggesting that duration of PD and preexisting age-related spinal deformity may contribute to the progression of scoliosis in PD, or that scoliosis is associated with a later age of PD onset.[13] PD patients with scoliosis may also have a greater duration of disease.[16]

Pearl

Soft tissue and muscular changes in Parkinson disease likely contributes to the associated spinal deformities, but the specific etiology of scoliosis in patients with Parkinson disease is currently unknown.

Neuromuscular Scoliosis after Spinal Cord Injury

Neuromuscular scoliosis occurs in the setting of asymmetric paraspinal and lateral trunk muscular tone in spinal cord injury (SCI).[17] Scoliosis can result from lateral compression or burst injuries.[18] Sometimes, inadequate initial treatment or immobilization can predispose to the development of deformity in the context of physiologic demands.[18] Compromise of spinal cord function can compound this process or lead to spinal deformity in and of itself.[7] Additional causes of postoperative spinal cord deformity include nonunion, failure of implants, Charcot spine, and iatrogenic causes.[18] Lack of motor function in the lower extremities also predisposes to the development of deformity.[7] One adult study reported a 21% incidence of spinal deformity in a retrospective cohort of 214 adult patients with SCI.[19] Higher American Spinal Injury Association (ASIA) grade and surgery after injury have been identified as risk factors for spinal deformity.[19] Spasticity and younger age at onset of injury may also contribute to the development of deformity.[19] Syringomyelia as a result of secondary spinal cord destruction is another contributory factor.[7] Operative intervention after trauma can also result in flat back syndrome.[18]

A flexion-compression injury to the anterior column of the thoracic spine may produce a focal kyphosis at that level, causing adjacent spinal regions to hyperextend, leading to instability and accelerated degenerative changes.[18] Although appropriate immobilization or surgical treatment will prevent progression of deformity, deformity may occur if there is not appropriate initial treatment.[18] Rib head dislocation and intrusion into the spinal canal at the convex apex of the scoliotic curve has been reported in posttraumatic scoliosis in an adult.[20] Spinal deformity may perpetuate disability after SCI by interfering with the ability to sit and limiting independence, and by limiting residual walking.[7]

Charcot spine, a degenerative spinal arthropathy, was initially described in individuals with tabes dorsalis, illustrating the importance of sensory feedback to maintaining spinal alignment.[3,21] Diabetic neuropathy, traumatic paraplegia, spinal cord trauma, uremic neuropathy, and leprosy can all lead to neuropathic arthropathy.[3] Spinal fusion at the time of or subsequently after SCI is a risk factor for Charcot arthropathy.[7] In the SCI population, repetitive microtrauma leading to increased stretch of neighboring ligaments without compensatory muscle contraction is thought to contribute to joint degeneration.[21] This is compounded by changes in bone homeostasis, changes in loading forces during daily activities such as transfers, and increased intervertebral joint forces secondary to long spinal fusions (>5 levels).[18,21] In a review of 166 cases of Charcot spine associated with SCI, 48% presented with spinal deformity.[21] Most cases occurred in the lumbar region, most commonly at L4–L5.[21] A review of 92 radiologic cases found spinal instability in 45%.[21] Notably, no difference in clinical presentation was seen between traumatic and nontraumatic (ischemia, transverse myelitis, neoplasm) causes of SCI, and most cases were in paraplegic and not tetraplegic patients.[21] Nonetheless, the prevalence of Charcot spine is low in SCI at approximately one in 220.[22]

Pearl

Appropriate initial treatment with stabilization and surgical intervention, if indicated, is crucial to prevent future progression of spinal deformity in patients with traumatic spine injuries.

Neuromuscular Scoliosis due to Other Causes

Adult neuromuscular scoliosis has been described in multiple sclerosis, neuropathy, and neurofibromatosis as well.[2] The progression of scoliosis has been reported in Stiff Person syndrome, an autoimmune disorder that leads to progressive, fluctuating muscular rigidity and spasms.[23] This progression of preexisting scoliosis occurred in a patient with an intrathecal baclofen pump: this complication is known in pediatric patients with cerebral palsy who undergo baclofen pump implantation.[23] Previous authors hypothesize that the baclofen further relaxed axial musculature in an asymmetric manner leading to deformity.[23]

Clinical Presentation

Back pain is a common presenting symptom as the curve convexities place abnormal strain on paraspinal muscles.[1,8] Patients may experience axial back pain at the apex of the convexity or radiculopathy and neurogenic claudication from compression of the spinal cord and roots.[7] Evaluation of back pain is complicated by common comorbidities of prior degenerative spinal disease, back pain, or spinal surgeries.[6] A localized kyphotic deformity of 30 degrees or greater predisposes to pain.[18] In PD, PS may be a precursor to development of scoliosis, and many patients with a clinical diagnosis of PS have scoliosis with a Cobb angle of 10 degrees or greater.[5]

Functional impairment is typically more frequent and severe in individuals with neuromuscular scoliosis compared to adolescent idiopathic scoliosis.[3] Patients may present with worsening gait instability and pelvic misalignment as the center of gravity is displaced from the base of stance.[1] This instability may impair sitting and standing balance, requiring the patient to use a hand for support and further limiting function.[1] Patients may report difficulty lying in bed due to the deformity. Sitting balance can lead to pressure sores, especially in wheelchair-bound patients.

Thoracic deformity can limit functional vital capacity and lead to restrictive lung disease, ultimately resulting in alveolar hyperventilation, carbon dioxide retention, pulmonary hypertension, and even cor pulmonale, as well as increasing the risk of pulmonary infections.[1] Patients with neuromuscular disease may have increased incidence of sleep disordered breathing.[1] Spasticity leads to increased nutritional requirements, predisposing to poor nutrition, which can further increase the risk of skin breakdown and impair ulcer healing.[1]

Evaluation

A thorough history is important to ascertain the progression of disease. Anteroposterior and lateral view X-rays are essential in demonstrating the progression of deformity: while standing, films are ideal, in that they demonstrate deformity in a weight-bearing state but may not be feasible in this patient population. In addition, flexion, extension, and lateral bending radiographs can provide information about the flexibility of deformity.[18] It is recommended to obtain full-length standing spine radiographs as early as possible in the progression of PD because of the known risk of scoliosis.[9] In PD, it is important to distinguish scoliosis from reversible postural abnormalities such as camptocormia and PS: the latter two improve by passive movement or supine position. In scoliosis, the structural curve with axial vertebral rotation will persist on supine imaging.[9] No matter the etiology of scoliosis, regular radiographs can help track the progression of deformity over time.[18] Computed tomography (CT) and magnetic resonance imaging (MRI) can be hopeful in the cause of neurologic deficits or in identifying injury to the paraspinal musculature and soft tissue.[18]

Physical exam should reveal the extent of deformity and may demonstrate shoulder asymmetry, rib prominence, pelvic obliquity, trunk imbalance, and hip deformity.[1] Examination of reflexes and elicitation of pathologic reflexes can help distinguish between upper and lower motor neuron pathology.[1] Limb-length discrepancy, contractures, and pressure ulcers or skin breakdown should also be identified.[1] It is important to assess the degree of functional impairment, (i.e., use of a wheelchair or walker).

Pulmonary function testing is important, given the risk of restrictive lung pathology, especially if surgical intervention is planned in large curvatures. Assessment of malnutrition and swallowing capacity may be indicated.

The Scoliosis Research Society published the Schwab Adult Spinal Deformity Classification in 2012. This classification correlates health-related quality of life outcomes and radiographic findings. First, the curve type is identified, then the difference between the angle of the pelvic incidence and the angle of the lumbar lordosis, followed by the sagittal vertical axis. Finally, pelvic tilt is important as it can compensate for the degree of sagittal misalignment.[24] However, this classification scheme has not been validated within the neuromuscular population.

Pearl

Due to adult progression of curvature in neuromuscular scoliosis, detailed physical examinations and two-view scoliosis radiographs are necessary at each appointment to determine the appropriate treatment plan.

Prognosis

The underlying neuromuscular pathology is the most important driver in the progression of neuromuscular scoliosis.[3] Pulmonary compromise leads to reduced forced vital capacity and restrictive lung pathology, which can ultimately progress to right-sided heart failure (cor pulmonale). In general, neuromuscular scoliosis will continue to progress without operative treatment.[7]

Nonoperative Treatment

Pain can be managed through oral medications such as NSAIDs and muscle relaxants. Sitting supports, spinal orthoses, and functional strengthening programs are all nonoperative interventions that can produce greater balance, independence, and function.[3] Wheelchair seating changes can also correct flexible curvature and accommodate inflexible deformity. These supports consist of wedging, lateral support, hip blocking, and seat cushion changes.[17] These interventions are helpful in preventing neuromuscular scoliosis in the SCI population by stopping the progression of functional scoliosis.[17,25] If scoliosis in PD is not accompanied by radiculopathy or severe coronal imbalance, close observation and physical therapy are appropriate.[15] Exercises that improve cardiovascular function may counterbalance the progressive pulmonary compromise.[3] The benefit of exercise to the axial musculature may be limited by neuromuscular dysfunction. Weight control is also important for preserving mobility.

Low-load prolonged stretching (LLPS) through night splinting and serial casting has been reported to improve muscle length and reduce spasticity and has been used to conservatively manage neuromuscular scoliosis after SCI.[17] LLPS can be augmented with botulinum toxin injections to reduce spasticity.[26] Similarly, baclofen pumps can be used to ameliorate spasticity. Facet, epidural, or nerve blocks can help localize the source of pain caused by degenerative spinal changes.[5]

Operative Treatment

It is important to emphasize that correction should be undertaken with the goal of improving quality of life, and that surgical intervention will not reverse the disorder that led to the deformity.[27] As scoliosis may impair lung function as it progresses, it is essential to undergo surgery before the restrictive lung pathology becomes so severe as to be a contraindication to surgical intervention. The goals of operative treatment in neuromuscular scoliosis include preventing progression and correcting the deformity, improving sitting and standing balance and preventing cardiopulmonary compromise.[2] Treatment can consist of decompression, stabilization, correction, and/or fusion.[5] Impaired sitting or standing balance, cardiopulmonary compromise, skin breakdown, progression of deformity, new-onset myelopathy or radiculopathy, and intractable pain are all indications for surgical intervention in neuromuscular scoliosis.[3]

Pearl

It is critical to spend time discussing goals and limitations of operative management with patients during the consent process so that expectations are shared between the surgeon and patient.

Complications in Operative Management of Neuromuscular Scoliosis

In the pediatric population, surgical treatment of neuromuscular scoliosis carries a much higher complication rate than surgery for adolescent idiopathic scoliosis.[2] Complications include neurologic injury (this can be due to spinal cord tethering), infection, and chylothorax in anterior approaches.[18]

In one retrospective review of 50 cases of posterior spinal fusion with segmental spinal instrumentation and pedicle screw fixation for neuromuscular scoliosis, which included children and adults up to age 43, 68% patients experienced perioperative complications and 2 (4%) patients died.[2] Major complications in this series included hemothorax or pneumothorax, pulmonary edema, pleural effusion, wound infection, and SCI, while minor perioperative complications included pneumonia, atelectasis, radicular symptoms, urinary tract infection, ileus, gastritis, vomiting, and wound dehiscence.[2] Postoperative complications included screw head prominence, decubitus ulcers, and implant loosening.[2]

Operative Intervention in Neuromuscular Scoliosis due to Parkinson Disease

Surgical decision-making for PD patients is complicated because while the decision to pursue surgery is usually led by pain and disability, these very patients are often those with the least optimal postoperative prognosis.[15] Previous authors have recommended that surgery is indicated in individuals with clinical and imaging evidence of myelopathy or radiculopathy,[15,28] which is in keeping with prior recommendations for surgery in this population.[9] Additional indications for surgery include deformity unresponsive to L-dopa, disability that has failed conservative management, and good functional performance.[15]

While general indications for correction of deformity are similar in PD patients and patients without PD, PD necessitates special considerations, given increased morbidity and mortality in this population.[15] A multidisciplinary approach can improve outcomes in spinal surgery in PD patients.[15] **Flowchart 8.1** demonstrates a guideline for indications and operative techniques in these patients. Upadhyaya et al recommend that short-segment decompression and fusion should be considered in the event of symptomatic deformity with stenosis.[28] Meanwhile, long-segment deformity correction should only be undertaken in patients who are motivated to walk, given its reported >50% complication rate.[28] Correction of spinopelvic alignment in PD patients is crucial, as incomplete correction can lead to further sagittal imbalance due to the forward displacement of the trunk and gravity line in PD.[15] Pedicle subtraction osteotomy may be necessary for achievement of sagittal alignment in patients with significant lumbar lordosis and pelvic incidence mismatch.[15] Because posterior muscles tend to be weak in PD and there is a flexor muscle predominance, additional sacral fixation points or iliac screw fixation are necessary for longer spinal instrumentation constructs.[15] L5–S1 interbody grafting can also enhance fusion rates at the lumbosacral junction.[15] A 2012 retrospective study of 12 PD patients who underwent posterior T2-sacral fusion found that good correction of sagittal and frontal balance allows for optimal clinical and radiological results even in the face of complications.[29] However, this study still reported proximal junctional kyphosis (PJK) and a revision rate of 50%.[30] Even so, the patient population was overall satisfied with the functional and cosmetic results of surgery.[30] In this study, postoperative or follow-up C7-SVL >10 cm, (i.e., a substantial sagittal imbalance), was associated with increased rates of scheduling or completion of revision surgery.[30] They recommend ICU care for 48 hours postop and TLSO use for 3 months to prevent instrumentation failure in poor bone quality.[30]

Deep brain stimulation of the subthalamic nucleus led to improvement of posture, Cobb angle, and C7 sagittal vertical axis in 2 out of 16 PD patients with scoliosis.[16] These patients were also both male and younger at the age of PD onset.[16]

PD may negatively impact spinal surgery outcomes in the elderly, and complication rates are high (33–86%) in this population.[29,31] Recurrent kyphosis is especially common, as mentioned in the Bourghli et al study discussed above.[30] Patients with dyskinesia have increased rates of rod fracture, compression fracture, and pseudoarthrosis after spinal fusion.[29] PD increases the risk for both osteoporosis and osteoporosis-related fractures.[15] This is compounded in women, who are typically postmenopausal once they develop scoliosis.[29,30] For example, severe postural instability can continue to predispose patients to catastrophic falls despite surgically corrected spinal alignment.[15] Greater postural instability in more severe disease increases the risk of imbalance.[15]

Operative Intervention in Neuromuscular Scoliosis due to Spinal Cord Injury

Surgery in the case of SCI is indicated if the deformity is progressive over time, or if there is a new or worsening neurologic deficit.[18] The goal of surgical intervention is to reestablish the integrity of all spinal columns and thus promote postural stability.[18]

Restoration of sagittal and coronal balance is the overall operative goal and may be achieved through posteriorly based osteotomies in severe deformities.[18] These deformities are best treated with surgical correction within 12 months of injury.[32]

Minimally Invasive Spine Surgery and Neuromuscular Scoliosis

The use of minimally invasive spine surgery has been reported in pediatric patients with neuromuscular scoliosis, with the goal of reducing hospital stay, pain, narcotic use, and blood loss.[33] The authors use a single narrow midline incision along the muscle plane through which they are able to insert

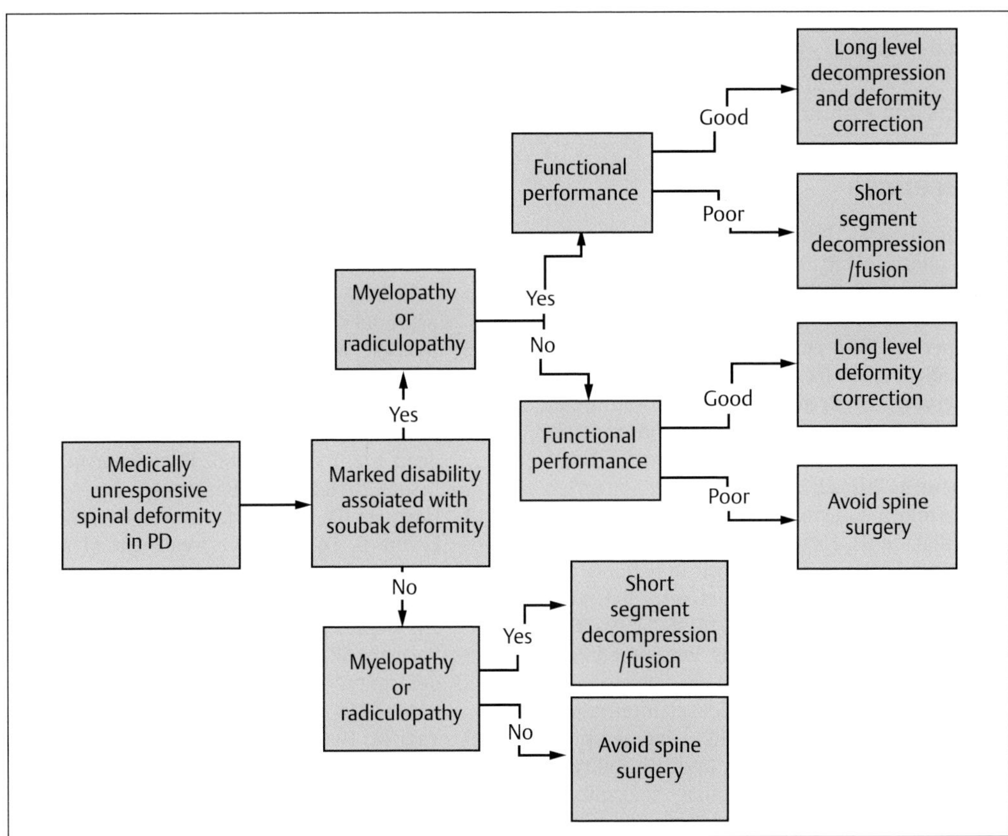

Flowchart 8.1 Suggested surgical decision algorithm for spinal deformities in patients with Parkinson disease.

pedicle screws, pass curved rods, partially or completely resect facet joints, and perform a variety of reduction maneuvers.[34] The technique reduces blood loss, risk of transfusion, and operative time.[33]

Conclusion

The pathophysiology of adult neuromuscular scoliosis is unique and complex, given the compounding influence of preexisting degenerative spinal changes and osteoporosis. Neuromuscular scoliosis can lead to marked functional impairment and limited independence, as well as severe cardiopulmonary compromise, and its course is progressive and severe. Operative intervention is the only definitive intervention to stop the progression of deformity. However, this population is highly prone to severe complications and adverse outcomes, so optimal surgical decision-making necessitates a careful appraisal of the risks and benefits and a multidisciplinary approach.

References

1. Allam AM, Schwabe AL. Neuromuscular scoliosis. PM R 2013;5(11):957–963
2. Modi HN, Suh S-W, Yang J-H, et al. Surgical complications in neuromuscular scoliosis operated with posterior-only approach using pedicle screw fixation. Scoliosis 2009;4:11
3. Berven S, Bradford DS. Neuromuscular scoliosis: causes of deformity and principles for evaluation and management. Semin Neurol 2002;22(2):167–178
4. Bissolotti L, Donzelli S, Gobbo M, Zaina F, Villafañe JH, Negrini S. Association between sagittal balance and scoliosis in patients with Parkinson disease: a cross-sectional study. Am J Phys Med Rehabil 2016;95(1):39–46
5. Aebi M. The adult scoliosis. Eur Spine J 2005; 14(10):925–948
6. Schwab FJ, Blondel B, Bess S, et al; International Spine Study Group (ISSG). Radiographical spinopelvic parameters and disability in the setting of adult spinal deformity: a prospective multicenter analysis. Spine 2013; 38(13):E803–E812
7. Heary RF, Albert TJ. Spinal deformities. The essentials [Internet]. 2nd ed. Thieme; 2014 [cited 2020 Oct 21]. https://medone-neurosurgery-thieme-com.ccmain.ohionet.org/ebooks/1343489#/ebook_1343489_SL57502381
8. Ashour R, Jankovic J. Joint and skeletal deformities in Parkinson's disease, multiple system atrophy, and progressive supranuclear palsy. Mov Disord 2006;21(11):1856–1863
9. Doherty KM, van de Warrenburg BP, Peralta MC, et al. Postural deformities in Parkinson's disease. Lancet Neurol 2011;10(6):538–549
10. Ye X, Lou D, Ding X, et al. A clinical study of the coronal plane deformity in Parkinson disease. Eur Spine J 2017;26(7):1862–1870
11. Choi HJ, Smith JS, Shaffrey CI, et al. Coronal plane spinal malalignment and Parkinson's disease: prevalence and associations with disease severity. Spine J 2015;15(1):115–121
12. Herrera-Marschitz M, Utsumi H, Ungerstedt U. Scoliosis in rats with experimentally-induced hemiparkinsonism: dependence upon striatal dopamine denervation. J Neurol Neurosurg Psychiatry 1990;53(1):39–43
13. Baik JS, Kim JY, Park JH, Han SW, Park JH, Lee MS. Scoliosis in patients with Parkinson's disease. J Clin Neurol 2009;5(2):91–94
14. Oh JK, Smith JS, Shaffrey CI, et al. Sagittal spinopelvic malalignment in Parkinson disease: prevalence and associations with disease severity. Spine 2014;39(14):E833–E841
15. Ha Y, Oh JK, Smith JS, et al. Impact of movement disorders on management of spinal deformity in the elderly. Neurosurgery 2015; 77(Suppl 4):S173–S185
16. Okazaki M, Sasaki T, Yasuhara T, et al. Characteristics and prognostic factors of Parkinson's disease patients with abnormal postures subjected to subthalamic nucleus deep brain stimulation. Parkinsonism Relat Disord 2018;57:44–49
17. Hastings JD, Dickson J, Tracy L, Baniewich C, Levine C. Conservative treatment of neuromuscular scoliosis in adult tetraplegia: a case report. Arch Phys Med Rehabil 2014;95(12): 2491–2495
18. Vaccaro AR, Silber JS. Post-traumatic spinal deformity. Spine 2001; 26(24, Suppl): S111–S118
19. Yagi M, Hasegawa A, Takemitsu M, Yato Y, Machida M, Asazuma T. Incidence and the risk factors of spinal deformity in adult patient after spinal cord injury: a single center cohort study. Eur Spine J 2015;24(1):203–208

20. Kishen TJ, Mohapatra B, Diwan AD, Etherington G. Post-traumatic thoracic scoliosis with rib head dislocation and intrusion into the spinal canal: a case report and review of literature. Eur Spine J 2010; 19(2, Suppl 2): S183–S186
21. Solinsky R, Donovan JM, Kirshblum SC. Charcot spine following chronic spinal cord injury: an analysis of 201 published cases. Spinal Cord 2019;57(2):85–90
22. Krebs J, Grasmücke D, Pötzel T, Pannek J. Charcot arthropathy of the spine in spinal cord injured individuals with sacral deafferentation and anterior root stimulator implantation. Neurourol Urodyn 2016;35(2): 241–245
23. Oh DC-S, Rakesh N, LaGrant B, Sein M. Advanced progression of scoliosis after intrathecal baclofen in an adult with Stiff Person syndrome: a case report. A A Pract 2020;14(6):e01204
24. Schwab F, Ungar B, Blondel B, et al. Scoliosis Research Society-Schwab adult spinal deformity classification: a validation study. Spine 2012;37(12):1077–1082
25. Hastings JD, Fanucchi ER, Burns SP. Wheelchair configuration and postural alignment in persons with spinal cord injury. Arch Phys Med Rehabil 2003;84(4):528–534
26. Marciniak C, Rader L, Gagnon C. The use of botulinum toxin for spasticity after spinal cord injury. Am J Phys Med Rehabil 2008; 87(4):312–317, quiz 318–320, 329
27. Heary RF, Albert TJ. Spinal deformities. The essentials [Internet]. [cited 2020 Oct 9]. Available from: https://medone-neurosurgery-thieme-com.ccmain.ohionet.org/ebooks/1343489#/ebook_1343489_SL57506128
28. Upadhyaya CD, Starr PA, Mummaneni PV. Spinal deformity and Parkinson disease: a treatment algorithm. Neurosurg Focus 2010;28(3):E5
29. Babat LB, McLain RF, Bingaman W, Kalfas I, Young P, Rufo-Smith C. Spinal surgery in patients with Parkinson's disease: construct failure and progressive deformity. Spine 2004;29(18):2006–2012
30. Bourghli A, Guérin P, Vital J-M, et al. Posterior spinal fusion from T2 to the sacrum for the management of major deformities in patients with Parkinson disease: a retrospective review with analysis of complications. J Spinal Disord Tech 2012;25(3):E53–E60
31. Moon S-H, Lee H-M, Chun H-J, et al. Surgical outcome of lumbar fusion surgery in patients with Parkinson disease. J Spinal Disord Tech 2012;25(7):351–355
32. Gertzbein SD. Scoliosis Research Society. Multicenter spine fracture study. Spine 1992; 17(5):528–540
33. Sarwahi V, Amaral T, Wendolowski S, et al. Minimally invasive scoliosis surgery: a novel technique in patients with neuromuscular scoliosis. BioMed Res Int 2015;2015:481945

9 Adolescent Idiopathic Scoliosis

Eric Schmidt, Kyle McGrath, Vikram Chakravarthy, and Jason Savage

Introduction

Adolescent idiopathic scoliosis (AIS) is an abnormal structural curvature of the spine that occurs in approximately 1 to 3% of otherwise healthy individuals between the ages of 10 and 16. AIS is only diagnosed in the absence of other causes of scoliosis such as neuromuscular disorders and congenital vertebral malformations. Adolescents are commonly screened for AIS with the Adams forward bend test using a scoliometer; however, a Cobb angle measurement on an upright coronal radiograph is necessary to confirm the diagnosis. AIS is characterized by a coronal Cobb angle of at least 10 degrees and can be managed conservatively with physical therapy and bracing. Surgery may be warranted depending on the progression and severity of the curve and the patient's associated functional impairment.[1] In this chapter, the natural history of AIS as well as current guidelines for screening and treating individuals with this deformity will be discussed.

Pearl

Adolescent idiopathic scoliosis (AIS) is an abnormal structural curvature of the spine occurring in otherwise healthy individuals between the ages of 10 and 16.

Epidemiology

Adolescent idiopathic scoliosis, as the name implies, is idiopathic with no confirmed cause. It is a diagnosis of exclusion that is made in otherwise healthy adolescents. While 2 to 3% of adolescents experience AIS, a significantly lower percentage of these patients ultimately require surgical intervention.[2] The prevalence of mild AIS (Cobb angle approximately 10 degrees) is similar among males and females; however, AIS is more common in females overall, and females are about 10 times as likely to progress to more severe AIS (Cobb angle >30 degrees).[3] AIS typically does not present with functional impairment, while trunk asymmetry and associated cosmetic complaints are among the most common presenting symptoms to surgeons and primary care physicians.[4]

Etiology

The pathogenesis of AIS remains largely unknown; however, a systematic review of current hypotheses by Sèze and Cugy has described a variety of hormonal, biomechanical, and genetic causes that have been linked to AIS.[5] Literature since 2000 has drawn correlations between AIS and abnormalities in spinal growth rates,[6] as well as melatonin,[7] leptin,[8] and calmodulin levels,[9] and many other factors without arriving at any clear conclusions.

The genetic influence of AIS is among the most widely researched links today. AIS has been observed in multiple members of the same family, with a variety of reported inheritance patterns.[1] Numerous studies have been done to help better understand the genetic component of this deformity; however, no single genetic locus has been found and agreed upon in the literature.[10–14] One meta-analysis studying the incidence of AIS in twins showed concordance for AIS in 73% of monozygotic twins and 36% of dizygotic twins.[15] Axenovich et al analyzed pedigrees of 101 families, 778 individuals in total, suggesting that pronounced forms of AIS (Cobb angle ≥10 degrees) demonstrated inheritance patterns consistent with an autosomal-dominant diallele model with incomplete penetrance. This study suggested that while no specific locus has been found, more clinically significant forms of AIS are likely due to a mutant allele with a predictable inheritance pattern.[16]

Biomechanical and histological models have also been used to help explain the development and progression of AIS. Due to the clinical relationship between adolescent growth spurts and curve progression, it has long been suspected that asymmetric vertebral growth has played a key role in pathogenesis of AIS. Wang et al collected intraoperative samples of vertebral growth plates in AIS patients undergoing anterior release and fusion and assessed them for histological grade and growth activity. When examining the growth plate of the apex vertebra on the concave side, they found not only a lower histological grade, but a significantly lower proliferative potential index and apoptosis index compared to the convex side at the same location. This suggests that there may be significant differences in chondrocyte kinetics and a reduction in growth activity on the concave side of the curve.[17] These findings then raise the question of whether or not the discrepancies in growth plate activity are a primary cause of asymmetric spinal curvature or a result of biomechanical differences incited by an alternative cause. The spines of scoliosis patients experience excessive loading on the concave side of the major curve due to a shifting of the load-bearing axis toward the facets of the concavity.[18] This would explain the aforementioned histological differences, as stated by the Hueter-Volkmann law, that skeletal growth can be significantly restricted by increased mechanical compression of the growth plate, as well as accelerated by reduced loading relative to normal values.[19] Without more conclusive data at present time, this discussion presents a "chicken or the egg" dilemma as the biomechanical loading discrepancies may incite these histological changes entirely, or only further perpetuate a curve initiated by an underlying genetic and molecular cause.

Pearl

The etiology of AIS is not well defined; however, numerous genetic and biomechanical factors are thought to contribute to the development of AIS.

Natural History

The natural history of AIS has been covered extensively by Weinstein and associates. Untreated AIS can progress with extreme variability due to several known (the patient's curve pattern) and unknown factors (e.g., genetic predisposition). Much of today's reliable natural history data has come out of a group of cohort studies from the University of Iowa beginning in 1950,[20-26] through which it was first determined that prognosis can largely be predicted by a patient's curve pattern and age of onset.[20]

Untreated AIS has primarily been studied in terms of curve progression, including the most significant long-term associated sequelae, such as cardiopulmonary compromise, back pain, and psychosocial concerns.[1] Several factors are taken into account when assessing a patient's risk of major curve progression, including skeletal maturity (as determined by age, onset of menses, and closure of triradiate cartilage), curve magnitude (Cobb angle), curve apex location, as described in Risser Sign and Sanders Score. Weinstein's longitudinal follow-up of AIS patients into adulthood demonstrated that 68% of major curves progressed.[1,26] Nachemson et al composed a chart to screen for skeletally immature patient's risk of progression based only on the patient's Cobb angle and age at detection. For curves <20 degrees, patients presenting earlier than 13 years of age had only a 25%

chance of progressing, and only a 10% chance if presenting between 13 and 15 years. By comparison, patients with a more significant curve (>40 degrees) presenting earlier than 13 years of age had a documented 100% chance of progressing, and a 90% chance if presenting between ages 13 and 15, further emphasizing the importance of early detection and proper management.[2] Position of the apex has also shown significant correlation to risk of curve progression, with the highest rate of progression being observed in patients with a thoracic level apex.[27] Furthermore, while major thoracic curves have a high risk of progression, those of 50 to 75 degrees magnitude place patients at the highest risk of progression among any curve magnitude or location, regardless of skeletal maturity.[26]

Skeletal maturity is a vital component of curve assessment on presentation because the timing of adolescent growth can give physicians a great deal of insight into the patient's prognosis. Having an accurate assessment of prognosis at a young age can alter the course of treatment and prevent significant curve progression. Adolescent curve progression can occur at a significant rate during the rapid adolescent growth phase (up to 2 degrees per month), with the rate of growth progression correlating positively to the height of the patient.[28] Throughout adulthood, however, progression slows but can still occur at a clinically significant rate. Upon reaching skeletal maturity, thoracic curves >50 degrees and lumbar curves >30 degrees can still progress up to 1 degree per year, while thoracic curves <30 degrees are not likely to progress.[23,26] This in turn reiterates the importance of properly managing adolescent curves at a young age as the deformity they present with can have major long-term implications on curve progression.

The relationship between curve progression and the associated long-term sequelae has been extensively studied. Among the sequelae, only pulmonary symptoms have been directly associated with curve magnitude.[23,26] Major thoracic curves >80 degrees have shown significant effects on reducing pulmonary vital capacity. Thoracic curves of this magnitude are also associated with shortness of breath as reported by patients, while major lumbar curves (>50 degrees) are not.[25,26] Having a thoracic Cobb angle of ≥50 degrees at skeletal maturity is also a strong predictor of decreased pulmonary function later in life, but it is only attributed to curve progression.[23,26] This signifies that someone presenting with a curve ≥50 degrees at skeletal maturity is likely to have their curve progress later in life, significantly impacting pulmonary function. Although correlations between curve progression and a decline in pulmonary function have been identified, it is important to note that Weinstein and Dolan found no difference in 50-year all-cause mortality or mortality related to pulmonary or cardiac complications due to curvature between untreated AIS and controls.[25]

While curve magnitude and progression can allow physicians to predict changes in pulmonary functions, clinically important correlations such as back pain and psychosocial concerns have not yet been well defined. Most patients with severe AIS will develop clinically significant radiographic osteoarthritic changes throughout their life; however, the patient's reported level of back pain does not seem to be correlated to the severity of these changes or the severity of the curve. Back pain is reported more frequently in adult patients with untreated AIS (77%) compared with age-matched controls (37%), but this seems to be unrelated to curve type or severity.[25] The only exception of note is that lateral listhesis of the thoracolumbar curves in AIS is associated with a higher frequency of back pain than other curve patterns.[22] When comparing untreated AIS patients to unmatched controls, only minimal differences in functional and physical disability have been identified.[25] From a psychosocial aspect, significant disturbances have been seen in 19% of AIS patients, 94% of whom had a curve >40 degrees.[29] Beyond that, there seems to be no significant difference in clinical depression in AIS patients overall compared to age- and sex-matched controls; however, about one-third of AIS patients have reported reduced physical ability, difficulty purchasing clothes, and self-consciousness.[30]

Evaluation of AIS Patients and Determining Curve Subtype

Adolescents with significant curves typically present to their clinician with cosmetic asymmetry or are referred for further testing upon a positive screening test. Adolescents are commonly screened with the Adams' forward bend test and a scoliometer, assessing shoulder height discrepancy and trunk rotation. It has been shown that current screening tests are very successful (93.8% sensitivity and 99.2% specificity) at detecting AIS when three separate screening tests are utilized together (e.g., the forward bend test, scoliometer measurement, and Moiré topography).[3] Adolescents who receive a positive screen must be worked up further to receive a definitive diagnosis. This requires a coronal radiograph to determine the Cobb angle, likely accompanied by a lateral view radiograph as well as a lateral bending radiograph to assess for curve flexibility. Of note, a thorough neurological examination as well as an assessment for leg-length discrepancy should be done at the time of diagnosis to rule out malignant pathology.[31]

Evaluation of these patients should also include an assessment of overall spinal balance, accounting for the relationship between the major and minor curves. Minor curves, as will be discussed in more detail, may be compensatory and therefore have surgical implications. Pubertal stage of the patient also should be taken into account. As discussed above, the age at which a patient presents with any given curve type and magnitude can have serious implications on the patient's prognosis. Tools commonly used to assess skeletal maturity include the Risser stage and closure of the triradiate cartilage. The Risser stage is an evaluation of the ossification of the iliac apophysis. In the United States, ossification of the iliac apophysis is divided into quarters that tend to ossify sequentially from no ossification (stage 0) to when the apophysis commences fusion to the iliac wing (stage 4) and ultimately when the ossified apophysis fuses to the iliac wing (stage 5). This sequence is correlated to completion of vertebral growth and is a valuable tool in assessing skeletal maturity as it relates to AIS curve progression.[32] The triradiate cartilage can be used to assess skeletal maturity as well. This epiphyseal plate is a "Y"-shaped junction between the ischium, ilium, and pubis. Its ossification can be monitored via radiographs, and typically reaches complete closure between the ages of 12 and 15, with females closing 2 to 3 years prior to males on average.[33]

A detailed analysis of the deformity itself is vital for adequate understanding of the pathology and creation of an appropriate treatment plan. Conventionally, curve analysis begins with Cobb angle measurement as well as acquiring supine lateral bending radiographs to assess degree of curve flexibility.[34] Determining curve flexibility is important because it allows the physician to delineate structural and nonstructural curves. Nonstructural curves are more flexible than structural curves, and can be purely compensatory in order to retain spinal balance. If it is determined that these curves can be corrected with flexibility testing, then they should not be fused as they may spontaneously get corrected if the major curve is corrected. There are a variety of ways to assess curve flexibility, including traction radiographs under anesthesia (TUA), fulcrum radiographs, and supine-bending radiographs. It has been demonstrated (with limited statistical analysis) that when comparing these three methods, fulcrum radiographs demonstrated a great deal of flexibility for moderate thoracic curves (40–65 degrees) with no significant difference to TUA. Both fulcrum and supine-bending radiographs were superior to TUA in moderate lumbar curves as well; however, TUA was superior to fulcrum and supine-bending radiographs for severe (>65 degrees) thoracic and lumbar curves.[34] Multiple studies have also demonstrated differential curve measurements comparing Schroth position to normal position on X-ray. In a pilot study of 10 patients by Skaggs et al, when X-rays were taken in the Schroth position, there was a mean change in the major Cobb angle of 6 degrees compared to normal standing position.[35]

In addition to understanding curve flexibility, accurate classification of the curve is also vital. The most commonly seen curve in AIS is a right thoracic major curve with compensatory left minor lumbar curve.[4,36] However, AIS is commonly understood as a three-dimensional deformity, exhibiting abnormal motion in multiple planes. The coupling phenomenon describes how motion in one plane can influence motion in other planes, with the classic example being that lateral bending of vertebral segments induces rotation in those segments. This idea can help us understand why AIS is a three-dimensional deformity, often exhibiting abnormal curvature in coronal, sagittal, and rotational planes.[18] King et al described five types of thoracic curves in 1983,[37] and while this classification system was heavily used to guide treatment options for many years, it could not be used to describe scoliosis as a three-dimensional deformity.[38] In 2001, Lenke et al developed a more comprehensive classification system, taking into account lumbar curves and sagittal alignment[36] (**Fig. 9.1**).

Lenke classification system includes curve type (1 through 6) with a lumbar modifier (A, B, C) and sagittal plane modifier (−, N, +). The curve type is based on the location of the major (structural) curve and the structural properties of the minor curve(s). The lumbar modifier is determined based on the central sacral vertical line (CSVL) and its relationship to the apex vertebra in the lumbar curve. The sagittal plane modifier is unique, in that it addresses the degree of thoracic kyphosis. Bernhardt et al demonstrated that AIS patients can have decreased thoracic kyphosis or even lordosis compared to normal patients.[39] The thoracic sagittal profile indicates whether the patient's kyphosis is below normal (−), within normal range (N), or above normal (+).[36]

Conservative Management of AIS Patients

Determining the appropriate steps in managing AIS is dependent on a number of factors, with a significant amount of interplay. These include gender, age, curve type and magnitude, and pubertal stage, which includes timing of menarche in females, Risser stage, and other methods of measuring bone development/growth stage.[40,41] Progression is considered to be a curve advancement of >5 to 6 degrees on serial radiographs, especially in curves >20 degrees.[42]

In general, structural curves less than 20 to 25 degrees can be managed conservatively, with interval evaluation and repeat scoliosis radiographs every 3 to 6 months, depending on skeletal maturity at time of diagnosis.[31,42] If the curve demonstrates progression or is between 25 and 40 degrees at time of diagnosis in a skeletally immature patient, consideration should be given to bracing, especially in those patients at high risk for progression.[31,42–45] In patients with similar curve magnitudes who are nearing skeletal maturity or are of older age, observation may be employed initially, given the lower probability of curve progression, supported by Nachemson, Lonstein, and Weinstein research on the natural history of AIS.[26,40–42] Those with curves of 45 degrees with remaining growth potential or 50 degrees at skeletal maturity can be considered surgical candidates.

Bracing for AIS has long been a topic of debate with discrepancy of results in the literature. The main goal of bracing (typically, a thoracolumbosacral orthosis, or TLSO) is to prevent further curve progression during skeletal immaturity, which could necessitate

Type	Proximal thoracic	Main thoracic	Thoracolumbar/ lumbar	Curve type
1	Nonstructural	Structural (major*)	Nonstructural	Main thoracic (MT)
2	Structural	Structural (major*)	Nonstructural	Double thoracic (DT)
3	Nonstructural	Structural (major*)	Structural	Double major (DM)
4	Structural	Structural (major*)	Structural	Triple major (TM)
5	Nonstructural	Nonstructural	Structural (major*)	Thoracolumbar/Lumbar (TL/L)
6	Nonstructural	Structural	Structural (major*)	Thoracolumbar/Lumbar-main Thoracic (TL/L–MT)

*Major = largest cobb measurement (always structural)

Structural criteria (Minor curves)

Proximal thoracic	• Side-bending Cobb ≥25° • T2–T5 kyphosis ≥ +20°
Main thoracic	• Side-bending Cobb ≥25° • T12–L2 kyphosis ≥ + 20°
Thoracolumbar/ lumbar	• Side-bending Cobb ≥25° • T12–L2 kyphosis ≥ + 20°

Minor = all other curves with structural criteria applied.

Location of Apex (SRS definition)

Curve	Apex
Thoracic	T2 body–T11/12 disc
thoracolumbar	T12 body–L1 body
lumbar	L1/2 disc–L4 body

Modifiers

Lumbar spine modifier	CSVL to lumbar apex
A	CSVL between Pedicles
B	CSVL touches Apical body(ies)
C	CSVL completely medial

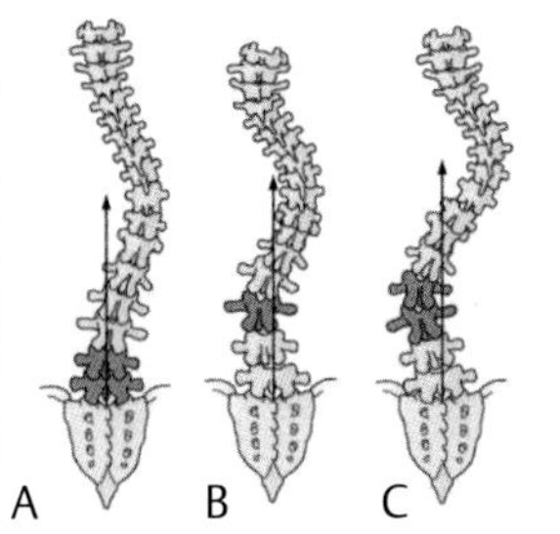

A B C

Thoracic sagittal profile (T5–T12)		CSVL to lumbar apex
–	Hypo	<10°
N	Normal	10°–40°
+	Hyper	>40°

Classification: Curve type (1–6) + Lumbar modifier (A, B, C) + Thoracic sagittal modifier (–, N, +) (i.e., 2A+)
SRS = Scoliosis Research Society; CSVL = Center Saeral Vertical Line

Fig. 9.1 Lenke classification of curve type.

surgery. Evidence both in support and against bracing are primarily retrospective or of low-grade evidence in nature, limiting interpretation of its results.[46–48] In recent years, the Bracing in Adolescent Idiopathic Scoliosis Trial (BrAIST) performed at the University of Iowa demonstrated reliable evidence in support of bracing in AIS patients, measured by preventing progression to a curve of 50 degrees. This was a multicenter prospective randomized study evaluating 242 patients divided into a randomized cohort and a preference-based cohort (bracing vs. observation), with those wearing the brace required to wear it for at least 18 hours a day. Similar to the guidelines set forth by the Scoliosis Research Society (SRS) Committee on Bracing and Nonoperative Management in 2006, patients were required to be 10 to 15 years of age, with Risser grades of 0 to 2, and largest curve measuring 20 to 40 degrees. In both the randomized and preference-based cohorts, bracing was deemed significantly impactful in preventing curve progression, with those randomly assigned to bracing achieving a success rate of 75% as compared to the 42% success rate in those being observed. In addition, this study established a dose-effect correlation related to the amount of hours the brace was worn during the day and prevention of curve progression.[49] Bracing is considered successful if curve progression is halted to a degree below which surgery would be considered by the time the patient achieves skeletal maturity.[50,51]

Hawary et al identified three factors that contributed to failure in bracing: poor brace compliance, skeletal immaturity, and a Cobb angle greater than 30 degrees at initiation of treatment.[43] Further studies are required to delineate the exact patient population that may benefit most from bracing, especially to avoid bracing patients who despite fitting radiological parameters may still experience curve progression. This is especially notable in skeletally immature patients with curves ranging from 30 to 40 degrees, with literature demonstrating the likelihood of progression to range from 56 to 100%.[52] In addition, high-quality studies that clarify the exact amount of in-brace time need to be performed, to better improve patient perception and compliance. This is especially important in light of the psychosocial impact that wearing a brace may have on an adolescent.[53]

The Schroth exercise method is another nonoperative treatment for the management of AIS that may be employed. It is composed of a unique set of individualized exercises addressing spinal alignment in all three anatomical planes with the primary goal to improve body mechanics and spinal stabilization. A meta-analysis by Park et al evaluating 15 studies across the literature concluded that Schroth exercises may be more beneficial for scoliosis patients with a Cobb angle of 10 to 30 degrees.[54] Schreiber et al presented results from their intention to treat trial evaluating the effect of 6-month Schroth intervention added to standard of care compared to standard of care alone, finding the addition of Schroth exercise decreased the curve severity in AIS.[55] Further controlled studies must be performed to ultimately determine spinal manipulative therapy's efficacy, as summarized by Théroux et al's meta-analysis in 2017 which assessed all prospective studies in the literature, concluding that they were at "substantial risk of bias."[56]

Surgical Management of AIS Patients

Patient selection and choosing the "appropriate" upper and lower instrumented vertebra are important aspects of AIS surgery. Natural history studies have demonstrated that patients with curves greater than 45 to 50 degrees are at high likelihood to demonstrate progressive deformity, which could potentially result in pain and/or pulmonary dysfunction.[25] As described previously, part of the initial work-up of patients should include full-length scoliosis X-rays in standing and lateral bending positions, at a minimum. This is invaluable for surgical planning, as it provides information about the patient's curve magnitude, type, and overall spinal balance. Lateral bending X-rays are also of importance as they may further define the nature of the patient's curve(s). Determining the major curve (structural curve), or the curve of largest magnitude, is critical. Minor curves (i.e., curves of lesser magnitude), may or may not be structural, and lateral bending films should demonstrate correction of nonstructural curves. This information is utilized to determine an individualized surgical plan to best treat the patient's deformity while minimizing unnecessary fusion of additional levels. Preoperative work-up may also include acquisition of a computed tomography (CT) of the spine to rule out structural anomalies, such as hemivertebrae, and a magnetic resonance imaging (MRI) to rule out spinal cord or spinal canal abnormalities such as neoplasm and syringomyelia, especially in patient's presenting with a neurological deficit. The ultimate goal of surgical intervention is preventing curve progression through arthrodesis and attempting to correct the curve(s) through as limited of a fusion as possible, all while ensuring the maintenance of global spinal balance.[57–59]

Once the decision to perform surgical intervention has been agreed upon, numerous options exist including standard posterior pedicle screw fixation with derotation and reduction, utilization of tether technology for realignment, thoracoscopic approaches, and growing-rod constructs. Often based on today's surgical methods the role for rib resection in realignment is rarely required, and arguably, the need for vertebral column resections is diminishing as well. In light of modern posterior instrumentation systems (i.e., pedicle screw and rod constructs), anterior approach utilization has fallen out of favor, especially in the setting of mild and moderate cases. A prospective study by Wang et al demonstrated no difference in efficacy of treating moderate lumbar and thoracolumbar patients when comparing anterior and posterior approaches.[60] This was further supported in a systematic review and meta-analysis performed by Lin et al, concluding that anterior and posterior approaches provided similarly satisfactory outcomes overall. For coronal deformity, anterior and posterior techniques resulted in similar correction. Posterior instrumentation was found to be superior in correcting sagittal deformity in thoracolumbar and lumbar cases. The degree of thoracic kyphosis created in anterior approaches, however, was found to be superior to that of posterior approaches,[61] indicating that certain patients could still benefit from an anterior approach.

Surgical decision-making in AIS is complex and dependent on a multitude of variables, including curve subtype and flexibility, shoulder balance and T1 tilt, and degree of thoracic or thoracolumbar kyphosis, to suggest a few.[58] Much consideration has been given to performing selective fusions to treat AIS, specifically fusing the structural curves while leaving the nonstructural components unfused, thereby limiting operative time, blood loss, and sparing motion, especially in the lumbar region.[58,62] This is especially important given that spontaneous curve corrections up to 70% in lumbar curves and 41% in thoracic curves has been reported,[58] indicating that in certain cases longer segment fusion may be unnecessary and can place the patient at undue risk. Puno et al retrospectively compared patients treated according to Lenke criteria to patients who were treated outside of these guidelines, concluding that better radiological outcomes were seen in those treated via Lenke methodology.[63]

In 2007, Lenke published an overview of general principles for selection of fusion levels in each curve subtype, with a focus on selecting proximal and distal fusion levels in order to level the shoulders and prevent an "adding-on" effect distally, whereby the patient's lumbar curve can worsen, leading to decompensation.[58,62] Despite these general principles, there are no formal guidelines dictating management, as such there has been robust debate around these topics with a wide variance in opinions and results.[58,59,64–66] Ultimately, each patient's surgical plan requires a thorough analysis of the preoperative imaging, precisely defining the nature of each curve (i.e., structural vs. nonstructural and global coronal/sagittal imbalance) and specific subfactors (e.g., T1 tilt, clavicle angle, degree of hypokyphosis, rotary components, etc.). Surgeons treating this pathology should make an effort to review the currently available body of literature before committing to a surgical plan to treat this complex pathology.

Pearl

Management of AIS depends on several factors, with curve magnitude and patient age being key determining factors. Conservative management often includes physical therapy, exercise, and bracing, while surgical management is reserved for more severe cases.

Conclusion

AIS is one of the most common structural deformities seen in the adolescent population. It often occurs in otherwise healthy individuals, and despite significant research, the pathogenesis is not yet well understood. There remains a great deal of mystery surrounding the development of this disease from the genetic level to the biomechanical level, leading to treatment plans that are intended to limit progression rather than prevent the onset of this disease. For skeletally immature patients with curves up to 40 degrees, conservative measures—especially bracing—have demonstrated considerable value in preventing significant long-term progression. Surgical decision-making for AIS patients is complex and multifactorial, with consistently evolving techniques and recommendations. Further study in all areas of this disease is warranted to optimize patient outcomes.

References

1. Weinstein SL, Dolan LA, Cheng JC, Danielsson A, Morcuende JA. Adolescent idiopathic scoliosis. Lancet 2008;371(9623):1527–1537
2. Nachemson AL, Lonstein JE, Weinstein SL. Report of the Prevalence and Natural History Committee of the Scoliosis Research Society. Denver: Scoliosis Research Society; 1982
3. Grossman DC, Curry SJ, Owens DK, et al; US Preventive Services Task Force. Screening for adolescent idiopathic scoliosis. JAMA 2018;319(2):165–172
4. Benzel EC, Steinmetz MP. Pediatric spinal deformities and deformity correction. In: Benzel's spine surgery: Techniques, complication avoidance, and management. Philadelphia, PA: Elsevier; 2017:1374–1390
5. de Sèze M, Cugy E. Pathogenesis of idiopathic scoliosis: a review. Ann Phys Rehabil Med 2012;55(2):128–138
6. Caballero A, Barrios C, Burgos J, Hevia E, Correa C. Vertebral growth modulation by hemicircumferential electrocoagulation: an experimental study in pigs. Eur Spine J 2011; 20(Suppl 3):367–375
7. Machida M, Dubousset J, Yamada T, Kimura J. Serum melatonin levels in adolescent idiopathic scoliosis prediction and prevention for curve progression: a prospective study. J Pineal Res 2009;46(3):344–348
8. Burwell RG, Aujla RK, Grevitt MP, et al. Pathogenesis of adolescent idiopathic scoliosis in girls: a double neuro-osseous theory involving disharmony between two nervous systems, somatic and autonomic expressed in the spine and trunk: possible dependency on sympathetic nervous system and hormones with implications for medical therapy. Scoliosis 2009;4:24
9. Lowe TG, Edgar M, Margulies JY, et al. Etiology of idiopathic scoliosis: current trends in research. J Bone Joint Surg Am 2000; 82(8):1157–1168
10. Wise CA, Barnes R, Gillum J, Herring JA, Bowcock AM, Lovett M. Localization of susceptibility to familial idiopathic scoliosis. Spine 2000;25(18):2372–2380
11. Salehi LB, Mangino M, De Serio S, et al. Assignment of a locus for autosomal dominant idiopathic scoliosis (IS) to human chromosome 17p11. Hum Genet 2002; 111(4-5):401–404
12. Miller NH, Justice CM, Marosy B, Zhang J, Wilson AF. Familial idiopathic scoliosis: evidence of autosomal susceptibility loci. Paper presented at the 38th Annual meeting of the Scoliosis Research Society Sept 10–13, 2003; Quebec, Canada
13. Justice CM, Miller NH, Marosy B, Zhang J, Wilson AF. Familial idiopathic scoliosis: evidence of an X-linked susceptibility locus. Spine 2003;28(6):589–594
14. Chan V, Fong GC, Luk KD, et al. A genetic locus for adolescent idiopathic scoliosis linked to chromosome 19p13.3. Am J Hum Genet 2002;71(2):401–406
15. Kesling KL, Reinker KA. Scoliosis in twins. A meta-analysis of the literature and report of six cases. Spine 1997;22(17):2009–2014, discussion 2015

16. Axenovich TI, Zaidman AM, Zorkoltseva IV, Tregubova IL, Borodin PM. Segregation analysis of idiopathic scoliosis: demonstration of a major gene effect. Am J Med Genet 1999;86(4):389–394
17. Wang S, Qiu Y, Zhu Z, Ma Z, Xia C, Zhu F. Histomorphological study of the spinal growth plates from the convex side and the concave side in adolescent idiopathic scoliosis. J Orthop Surg Res 2007;2(1):19
18. Benzel EC. Deformity prevention and correction: complex clinical strategies. In: *Biomechanics of spine stabilization*. New York: Thieme; 2015:354–395
19. Stokes IA. Mechanical effects on skeletal growth. J Musculoskelet Neuronal Interact 2002;2(3):277–280
20. Ponseti IV, Friedman B. Prognosis in idiopathic scoliosis. J Bone Joint Surg Am 1950;32A(2):381–395
21. Collis DK, Ponseti IV. Long-term follow-up of patients with idiopathic scoliosis not treated surgically. J Bone Joint Surg Am 1969;51(3):425–445
22. Weinstein SL, Zavala DC, Ponseti IV. Idiopathic scoliosis: long-term follow-up and prognosis in untreated patients. J Bone Joint Surg Am 1981;63(5):702–712
23. Weinstein SL, Ponseti IV. Curve progression in idiopathic scoliosis. J Bone Joint Surg Am 1983;65(4):447–455
24. Weinstein SL. Idiopathic scoliosis. Natural history. Spine 1986;11(8):780–783
25. Weinstein SL, Dolan LA, Spratt KF, Peterson KK, Spoonamore MJ, Ponseti IV. Health and function of patients with untreated idiopathic scoliosis: a 50-year natural history study. JAMA 2003;289(5):559–567
26. Weinstein SL. The natural history of adolescent idiopathic scoliosis. J Pediatr Orthop 2019; 39(6, Suppl 1):S44–S46
27. Bunnell WP. The natural history of idiopathic scoliosis before skeletal maturity. Spine 1986;11(8):773–776
28. Sanders JO. Maturity indicators in spinal deformity. J Bone Joint Surg Am 2007; 89(Suppl 1):14–20
29. Ascani E, Bartolozzi P, Logroscino CA, et al. Natural history of untreated idiopathic scoliosis after skeletal maturity. Spine 1986;11(8):784–789
30. Mayo NE, Goldberg MS, Poitras B, Scott S, Hanley J. The ste-justine Adolescent Idiopathic Scoliosis cohort study. Spine 1994; 19(14, Supplement):1573–1581
31. Jada A, Mackel CE, Hwang SW, et al. Evaluation and management of adolescent idiopathic scoliosis: a review. Neurosurg Focus 2017;43(4):E2
32. Hacquebord JH, Leopold SS. In brief: The Risser classification: a classic tool for the clinician treating adolescent idiopathic scoliosis. Clin Orthop Relat Res 2012;470(8):2335–2338
33. Parvaresh KC, Pennock AT, Bomar JD, Wenger DR, Upasani VV. Analysis of acetabular ossification from the triradiate cartilage and secondary centers. J Pediatr Orthop 2018; 38(3):e145–e150
34. Hamzaoglu A, Talu U, Tezer M, Mirzanli C, Domanic U, Goksan SB. Assessment of curve flexibility in adolescent idiopathic scoliosis. Spine 2005;30(14):1637–1642
35. Skaggs K, Lin AJ, Andras LM, Illingworth KD, Skaggs DL. Standing in Schroth trained position significantly changes Cobb angle and leg length discrepancy: a pilot study. [published online ahead of print, 2020 Jun 26] Spine Deform 2020;8(6):1185–1192
36. Lenke LG, Betz RR, Harms J, et al. Adolescent idiopathic scoliosis: a new classification to determine extent of spinal arthrodesis. J Bone Joint Surg Am 2001;83(8):1169–1181
37. King HA, Moe JH, Bradford DS, Winter RB. The selection of fusion levels in thoracic idiopathic scoliosis. J Bone Joint Surg Am 1983;65(9):1302–1313
38. Cummings RJ, Loveless EA, Campbell J, Samelson S, Mazur JM. Interobserver reliability and intraobserver reproducibility of the system of King et al., for the classification of adolescent idiopathic scoliosis. J Bone Joint Surg Am 1998;80(8):1107–1111
39. Bernhardt M, Bridwell KH. Segmental analysis of the sagittal plane alignment of the normal thoracic and lumbar spines and thoracolumbar junction. Spine 1989;14(7):717–721
40. Lonstein JE, Carlson JM. The prediction of curve progression in untreated idiopathic scoliosis during growth. J Bone Joint Surg Am 1984;66(7):1061–1071
41. Nachemson AL, Peterson LE. Effectiveness of treatment with a brace in girls who have adolescent idiopathic scoliosis. A prospective, controlled study based on data from the Brace Study of the Scoliosis Research Society. J Bone Joint Surg Am 1995;77(6):815–822
42. Lonstein JE. Scoliosis: surgical versus non-surgical treatment. Clin Orthop Relat Res 2006;443(443):248–259
43. Hawary RE, Zaaroor-Regev D, Floman Y, Lonner BS, Alkhalife YI, Betz RR. Brace

treatment in adolescent idiopathic scoliosis: risk factors for failure-a literature review. Spine J 2019;19(12):1917–1925
44. Weiss HR, Negrini S, Rigo M, et al; SOSORT guideline committee. Indications for conservative management of scoliosis (guidelines). Scoliosis 2006;1:5. Published 2006 May 8
45. Richards BS, Bernstein RM, D'Amato CR, Thompson GH. Standardization of criteria for adolescent idiopathic scoliosis brace studies: SRS Committee on Bracing and Nonoperative Management. Spine 2005;30(18):2068–2075, discussion 2076–2077
46. Schiller JR, Thakur NA, Eberson CP. Brace management in adolescent idiopathic scoliosis. Clin Orthop Relat Res 2010;468(3): 670–678
47. Stokes OM, Luk KD. The current status of bracing for patients with adolescent idiopathic scoliosis. Bone Joint J 2013;95-B(10): 1308–1316
48. Karavidas N. Bracing in the treatment of adolescent idiopathic scoliosis: evidence to date. Adolesc Health Med Ther 2019;10:153–172. Published 2019 Oct 8
49. Weinstein SL, Dolan LA, Wright JG, Dobbs MB. Effects of bracing in adolescents with idiopathic scoliosis. N Engl J Med 2013; 369(16):1512–1521
50. Dolan LA, Weinstein SL. Surgical rates after observation and bracing for adolescent idiopathic scoliosis: an evidence-based review. Spine 2007; 32(19, Suppl):S91–S100
51. El-Hawary R, Chukwunyerenwa C. Update on evaluation and treatment of scoliosis. Pediatr Clin North Am 2014;61(6):1223–1241
52. Karol LA, Virostek D, Felton K, Jo C, Butler L. The effect of the Risser stage on bracing outcome in adolescent idiopathic scoliosis. J Bone Joint Surg Am 2016;98(15):1253–1259
53. Piantoni L, Tello CA, Remondino RG, et al. Quality of life and patient satisfaction in bracing treatment of adolescent idiopathic scoliosis. Scoliosis Spinal Disord 2018;13:26
54. Park JH, Jeon HS, Park HW. Effects of the Schroth exercise on idiopathic scoliosis: a meta-analysis. Eur J Phys Rehabil Med 2018; 54(3):440–449
55. Schreiber S, Parent EC, Khodayari Moez E, et al. Schroth physiotherapeutic scoliosis-specific exercises added to the standard of care lead to better Cobb angle outcomes in adolescents with idiopathic scoliosis: an assessor and statistician blinded randomized controlled trial. PLoS One 2016;11(12):e0168746
56. Théroux J, Stomski N, Losco CD, Khadra C, Labelle H, Le May S. Spinal manipulative therapy for adolescent idiopathic scoliosis: a systematic review. J Manipulative Physiol Ther 2017;40(6):452–458
57. Moe JH. Modern concepts of treatment of spinal deformities in children and adults. Clin Orthop Relat Res 1980; (150):137–153
58. Trobisch PD, Ducoffe AR, Lonner BS, Errico TJ. Choosing fusion levels in adolescent idiopathic scoliosis. J Am Acad Orthop Surg 2013; 21(9):519–528
59. Tambe AD, Panikkar SJ, Millner PA, Tsirikos AI. Current concepts in the surgical management of adolescent idiopathic scoliosis. Bone Joint J 2018;100-B(4):415–424
60. Wang Y, Fei Q, Qiu G, et al. Anterior spinal fusion versus posterior spinal fusion for moderate lumbar/thoracolumbar adolescent idiopathic scoliosis: a prospective study. Spine 2008;33(20):2166–2172
61. Lin Y, Chen W, Chen A, Li F, Xiong W. Anterior versus posterior selective fusion in treating adolescent idiopathic scoliosis: a systematic review and meta-analysis of radiologic parameters. World Neurosurg 2018;111: e830–e844
62. Lenke LG. The Lenke classification system of operative adolescent idiopathic scoliosis. Neurosurg Clin N Am 2007;18(2):199–206
63. Puno RM, An KC, Puno RL, Jacob A, Chung SS. Treatment recommendations for idiopathic scoliosis: an assessment of the Lenke classification. Spine 2003;28(18):2102–2114, discussion 2114–2115
64. Lee CS, Hwang CJ, Lee DH, Cho JH. Five major controversial issues about fusion level selection in corrective surgery for adolescent idiopathic scoliosis: a narrative review. Spine J 2017;17(7):1033–1044
65. Kuklo TR, Lenke LG, Graham EJ, et al. Correlation of radiographic, clinical, and patient assessment of shoulder balance following fusion versus nonfusion of the proximal thoracic curve in adolescent idiopathic scoliosis. Spine 2002;27(18):2013–2020
66. Themes U. (2016, July 16). Pediatric and adult scoliosis. Retrieved August 31, 2020, from https://neupsykey.com/pediatric-and-adult-scoliosis/

10 Iatrogenic Cervical Spine Deformity

Taofiq D. Sanusi, Michael McLarnon, and Nikolay Peev

Introduction

All spinal surgeries have the intention to either prevent or correct spinal deformity, but the possibility of causing spinal deformity through surgery also exists. Iatrogenic spinal deformity is defined as an entity occurring as a result of a surgical procedure not appropriately tailored to the specific problem and patient.

Epidemiology of Iatrogenic Deformity

Iatrogenic cervical spine deformity occurs secondary to sagittal and/or coronal imbalance, resulting from a surgical or radiotherapy treatment of cervical pathology.[1] It is one of the commonest causes of deformity in the cervical spine.

The cervical spine is prone to deformity. This is due mainly to its wide range of mobility, the coronal orientation of facet joints, and curvilinear end plates. There is also no external bracing, as the rib cage, which supports the thoracic spine. Concomitantly, there is a heavy reliance on surrounding musculature, ligamentous, and soft tissue support. This results in a trade-off, namely a superior range of motion in the cervical spine at the expense of reduced structural stability. Surgery of the cervical spine may invariably disrupt these supporting tissues.

The majority of deformity occurs in the sagittal plane—the commonest observed deformity is cervical kyphosis,[1] which may result in pain, physical deformity, and neurological symptoms.

Risk Factors in the Development of Iatrogenic Deformity

Patient Age

Cervical kyphosis can occur in any age group, but it is more prevalent in older patients due to degenerative disease. Pediatric deformities are commonly reported following trauma, spine surgery, Chiari malformations, syringomyelia, connective tissue disorders, and tumor resection.[2]

Radiation and Postoperative Radiotherapy

Radiation reduces bone density, resulting in a weakened spine. This increases the risk of anterior and lateral wedging, as well as damaging the extensor muscles and surrounding soft tissues that help to support the spine.[3]

Hypermobility States

An increased range of movements seen in certain connective tissue disorders like Marfan syndrome, Ehlers-Danlos syndrome, and Down syndrome increases the risk of cervical spine deformity. Hyperflexion and hyperextension are associated with the development of postoperative kyphosis.[4]

Osteoporosis

Osteoporosis is a structural weakening of the bone secondary to an imbalance between osteogenic and osteoclastic activities, thus resulting in a predisposition to fracture and deformity.

Preexisting Cervical Kyphosis

A preexisting loss of normal cervical lordosis is a risk factor, as the weakening of posterior muscular-ligamentous support from surgery may lead to a further abnormal anterior shifting of weight distribution.[5,6]

Spine Tumor

Extradural and intradural tumors can lead to cervical kyphosis. However, malignant lesions are more prone to instability and hence kyphosis due to the tendency for invasion and subsequent destruction of the bones and supporting muscles and ligaments.[1]

Causes of Iatrogenic Deformity

These include surgical technique and anatomical areas involved, the direction of approach, positioning issues, improper distractor placement, type and extent of instrumentation, and inadequate postoperative immobilization.[5]

Multilevel Procedures

Multilevel cervical spine surgery is strongly associated with an increased risk of postoperative deformity, especially posterior approaches without fixation. C2–C3 involvement is known as having high potential for kyphosing postoperatively, due to the unique role of C2 in the sagittal balancing via the longissimus capitis and longissimus cervicis muscles.

Anatomical Disruption

Disrupting the anatomical integrity is a major factor in promoting the iatrogenic deformity, for example, when comparing laminectomy to laminoplasty—lower levels of deformity are observed when laminoplasty is chosen as opposed to laminectomy. Laminoplasty may help prevent postoperative kyphosis, especially in patients with loss of normal cervical lordosis and in pediatric groups.[5]

Excessive facetectomy also could lead to structural instability—as a rule, no more than 50% of the facet should be removed when performing decompressions to prevent structural instability and resulting deformity.

Disruption of extensor muscles in the neck, in particular semispinalis cervicis, is known to be associated with cervical spine kyphosis. Resection of the C2 process/lamina or muscles attached to C2–C3 is now a well-recognized factor promoting cervical spine kyphotic deformity.

Pearls

- Avoid more than 50% facet joint resection when performing laminectomy.
- Laminoplasty is preferable to laminectomy when possible.
- Avoid resection of muscles and ligaments when possible.
- C2–C3 is crucial for the maintenance of the cervical lordotic configuration.

Surgeries Commonly Associated with Iatrogenic Deformity

Multiple level cervical spine procedures—especially if posterior elements are disrupted without fixation—will increase the risks of postoperative deformity.[7] Anterior cervical spine procedures can also predispose to iatrogenic deformities, albeit to a lesser extent.

Anterior Cervical Surgery

The following anterior surgeries are associated with iatrogenic deformity[4]:

- Anterior cervical discectomy without fusion (ACF).
- Anterior cervical discectomy with fusion (ACDF) +/− plating.
- Multilevel ACDF with stand-alone cages.
- Dynamic cervical plates.
- Cervical disc replacement.
- Corpectomy.

Plating provides additional anterior buttressing and thus appears to result in significantly less kyphotic deformity compared to patients not receiving plating[8]; however, the clinical relevance of this is unknown.

Corpectomy is believed to predispose to kyphosis due to the replacement of a normal lordotic spinal segment with a more neutrally aligned graft. For multilevel procedures, circumferential management (360-degree fixation) should be considered.[5]

Posterior Cervical Surgery

The following posterior surgeries are associated with iatrogenic deformity[5]:

- Facetectomy.
- Laminectomy.
- Laminoplasty.

Due to the relatively high prevalence of deformity secondary to these procedures, if any risk factors coexist (such as osteoporosis, multilevel surgery, preexisting kyphosis), fixation should be considered.[1]

For multilevel laminectomy, Fu[4] suggests performing laminectomy and fusion with multiple lateral mass screws and rods to prevent kyphosis in some select cases. There is, however, associated morbidity, in the form of reduced range of motion with extensive fixation.[4]

Pearls

- Anterior cervical discectomy with fusion (ACDF) is seen as a good surgical solution for single- or multilevel disc degeneration. If performed satisfactorily, it can preserve lordosis, and even can create lordosis in patients with loss of lordosis across multiple levels.
- Anterior cervical surgery is the preferable option when the patient is at risk of cervical kyphotic deformity.

Biomechanics of Deformity

The center of gravity in the head directly overlies the occipital condyle, roughly 1 cm above and anterior to the external auditory canal. Any deviation from normal head alignment results in increased leverage and load on the spine, which can lead to muscle strain and pain.[9,10]

This is well illustrated by Duboussett[11] in his cone of economy, whereby balance is conceptualized by drawing a line through the body and feet (**Fig. 10.1**). The model allows for equal movement in all directions and demonstrates that within a small range of motion from the center, minimum leverage is applied, and minimum effort is required to maintain posturing. In normal subjects, their spinal curvatures are maintained within this range to facilitate ease of movement and pain-free walking.

Outside of this range, one enters the conus of maximum work, where there is a large lever arm and a mismatch between muscular works required to simply maintain posturing. Too much energy is expended for small movements and both functional deformity and pain occur.[12]

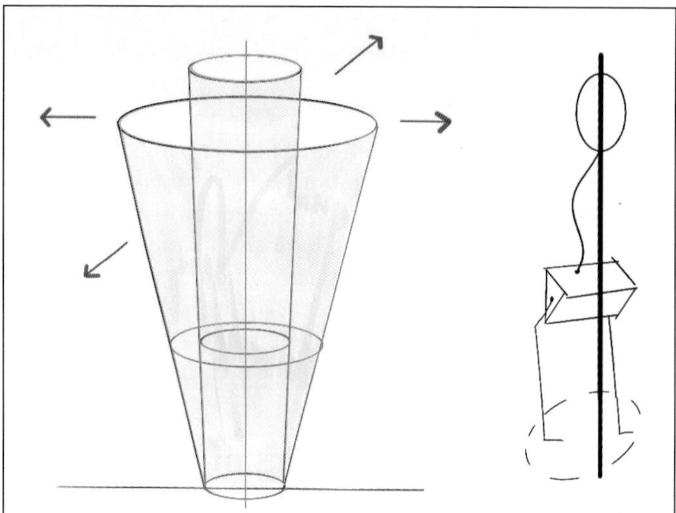

Fig. 10.1 Conus of economy and maximum work.

Clinical Picture/Important Signs and Symptoms

Symptoms of cervical spine deformity can be broadly categorized into pain, neurological symptoms, physical impairment, and functional impairment.[12]

Pain is the commonest reported symptom.[1] Pain occurs due to muscular fatigue from strain, and this can be identified as a mechanical type of pain because it usually improves with rest and/or immobilization.

Neurological symptoms, radiculopathy and myelopathy, are also common.[12] Myelopathy is deemed as the main indication for intervention,[12] over and above pain relief. Myelopathy is thought to result in the kyphotic segment, either as a new phenomenon or postsurgical recurrence, due to direct compression or stretch myelopathy. Radicular symptoms may result from any impingement upon nerve roots due to mechanical instability causing foraminal narrowing or deformation.

Functionally and cosmetically, the most severe form of cervical kyphosis may be described as "chin-on-chest" or "swan-neck" deformity.[1]

Clinical Examination

- Full neurological examination of limbs.
- Assessment of abdominal and sphincter reflexes.
- Spine examination.
- Functional assessment of gait, gaze, and mobility.

Classification of Deformity

Cervical deformity is assessed radiologically, with functional and myelopathy assessments furthering the clinical significance and consequences of the deformity.

The cervical deformity can be classified into five primary groups (**Flowchart 10.1**)[4]:

- Primary sagittal with deformity in the cervical spine.
- Primary sagittal with deformity at the cervicothoracic junction (at C7/T1 or T2).
- Primary sagittal deformity in the apex of the thoracic spine.
- Primary coronal deformity, (i.e., cervical scoliosis) (C2–C7, Cobb angle >15 degrees).
- Primary craniovertebral junctional deformity.

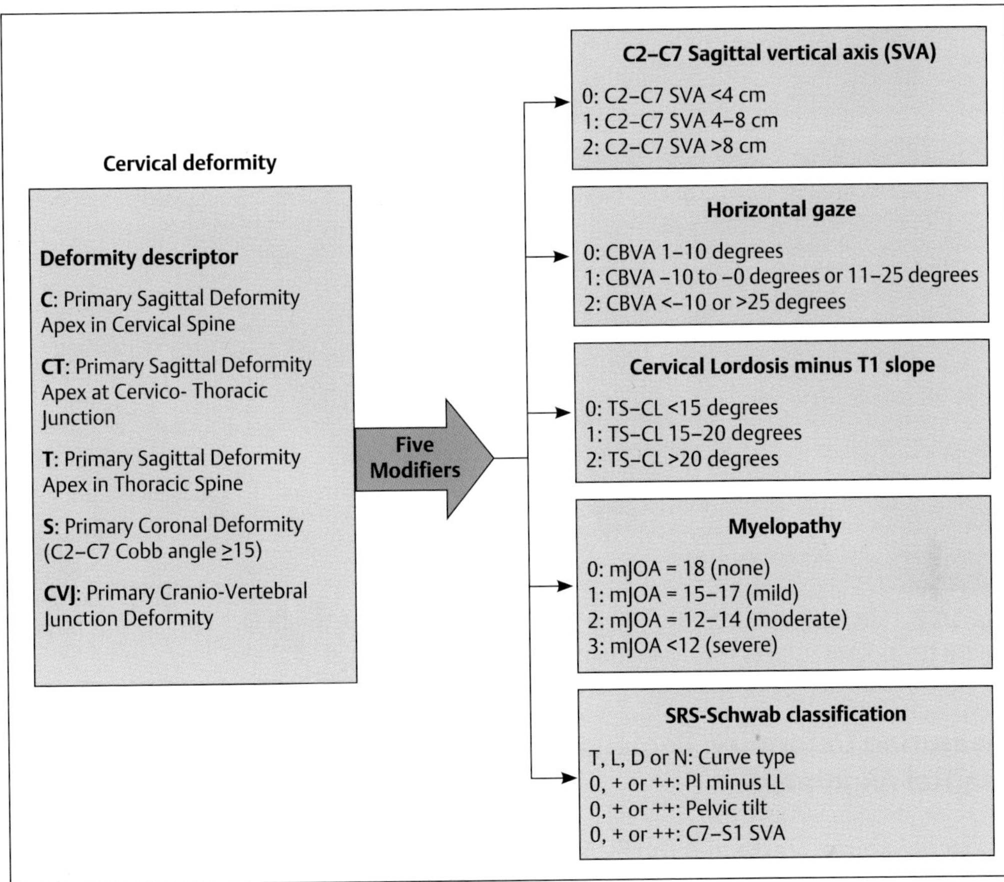

Flowchart 10.1 Classification of cervical deformity. Adapted from Rhee.[5]

Imaging and Measuring Cervical Deformity

Measuring Deformity: Cervical Lordosis

The three primary methods to assess cervical lordosis include Cobb angles, Jackson physiological stress lines, and the Harrison posterior tangent method,[5,9] the most common of which is the Cobb angle typically measured from C1 to C7 or C2 to C7.

The Cobb angle is calculated by drawing four lines on the radiograph: two lines are drawn along the C2–C7 end plates, and then two perpendicular lines are drawn to these. The angle subtended by the perpendicular lines is used to represent cervical lordosis[5] (**Fig. 10.2a**).

The Jackson physiological stress line method requires drawing two lines, both parallel to the posterior surface of the C7 and C2 vertebral bodies, and measuring the angle between them[9] (**Fig. 10.2b**).

The Harrison posterior tangent method involves drawing lines parallel to the posterior surfaces of all cervical vertebral bodies from C2 to C7 and then summing the segmental angles for an overall cervical curvature angle.[9]

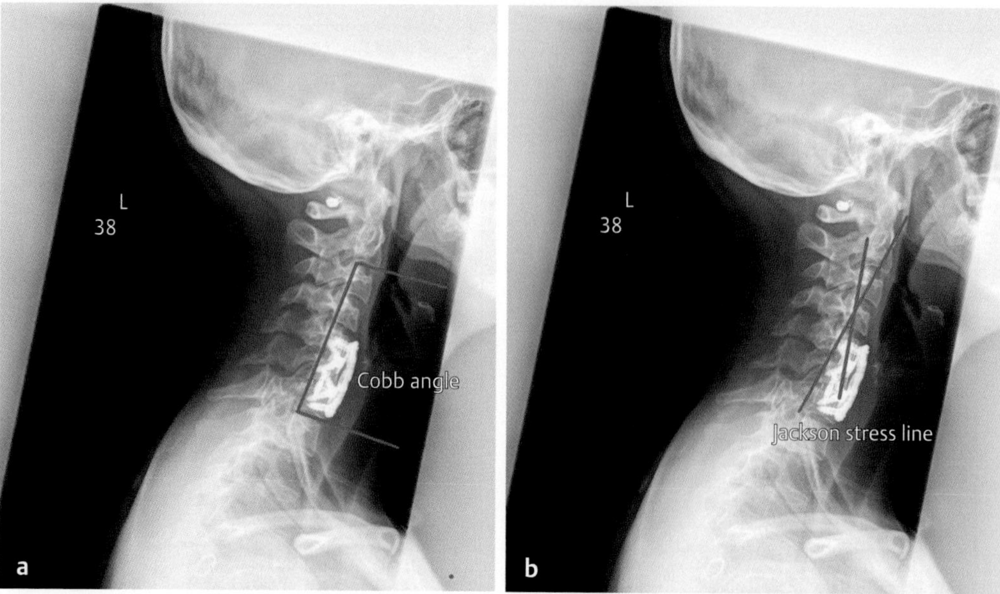

Fig. 10.2 Measuring deformity. These illustrate the **(a)** Cobb angle and **(b)** Jackson physiological stress lines used in the evaluation of cervical lordosis.

Measuring Deformity: Regional Sagittal Alignment

Cervical Sagittal Vertical Axis (SVA) (Fig. 10.3)

SVA, the C2–C7 sagittal vertical axis, is the biggest coronal cervical parameter[1] and assesses the balance of the head in relation to the spine. The angle should ideally be between 0 and 4 cm in healthy individuals. It is considered moderate deformity if the angle is between 4 and 8 cm and significant deformity if >8 cm.[1] Regionally, the cervical SVA can be defined using the distance between a plumb line dropped from the dens of C2 and the posterosuperior aspect of C7.[9] The cervical SVA is closely related to the Cobb angle.[5,9]

Cervical Lordosis Minus T1 Slope (Fig. 10.4)

On cervical X-ray, this looks at the relationship between the cervical slope and its balance to the upper thoracic slope. Take the T1 slope (TS), sloped to parallel (e.g., the floor), and subtract the normal cervical lordosis (in degrees). Normal is <15 degrees, and 0 is perfectly normal. Anything greater than 15 is abnormal. A greater degree of cervical lordosis is required for a bigger thoracic kyphosis and vice versa.

Measuring Deformity: Global Assessment

The Scoliosis Research Society (SRS)-Schwab Classification looks at thoracolumbar pathology in combination with cervical pathology to assess overall deformity when considering a surgical approach.

Pelvic incidence is also an important measurement when assessing global spinal alignment.

The C2 and C7 SVA (**Fig. 10.5**) have both been used to define sagittal alignment globally by measuring the distance between the C2 and C7 plumb lines, respectively, from the posterior superior corner of the sacrum.[9] SVA has a significant correlation with the

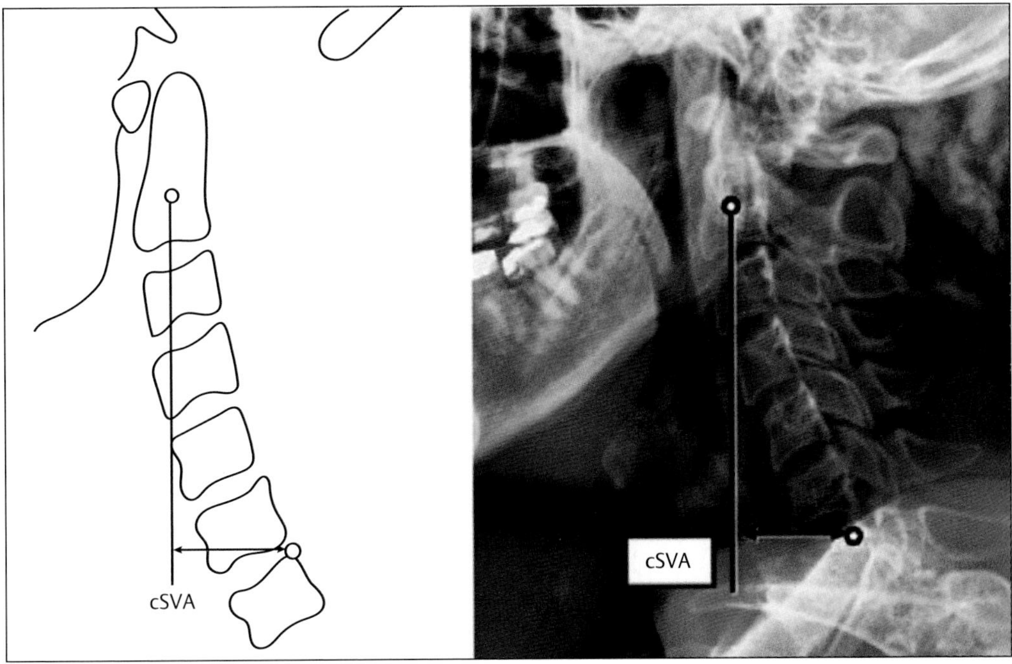

Fig. 10.3 Cervical sagittal vertical axis (cSVA).

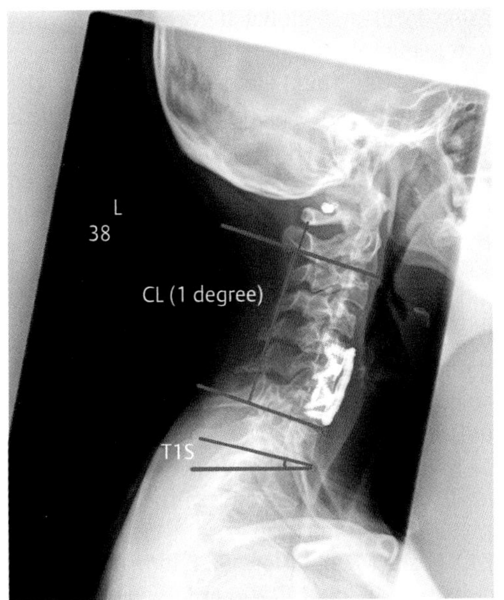

Fig. 10.4 Cervical lordosis minus T1 slope.

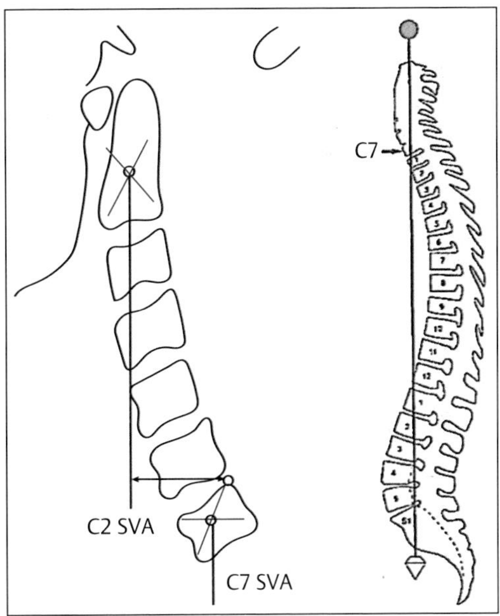

Fig. 10.5 The C2 and C7 sagittal vertical axis (SVA).

social responsiveness scale (SRS), Oswestry Disability Index (ODI), and 12-Item Short Form Survey (SF-12).[1] The pelvis is intimately associated with SVA; pelvic retroversion can compensate for a larger SVA and help to bring the body back into the conus of economy.[12]

By combining the cervical measurements and the global measurements of the pelvic incidence–lumbar lordosis (PI-LL) mismatch, C7–S1 SVA and pelvic tilt, the surgeon can have a complete picture for surgical planning.[1]

Functional Measurements and Myelopathy Assessment

Horizontal Gaze: CBVA (Fig. 10.6)

The chin-brow vertical angle (CBVA) is a measurement of horizontal gaze.[1,5,9,13] It is defined as the angle subtended between a line drawn from the patient's chin to their brow and a vertical line. A normal CBVA is within 1 and 10 degrees. The angle is measured by a photograph with the patient standing straight with the neck in a neutral position.[5,9] Horizontal gaze is reportedly a good measure of patient health-related quality of life (HRQOL).[9]

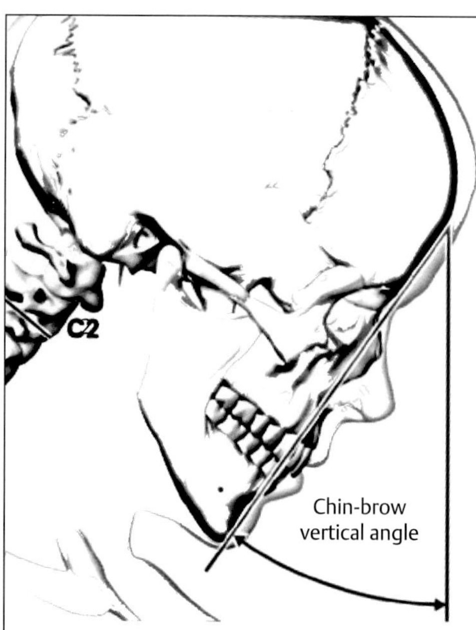

Fig. 10.6 Horizontal gaze: chin-brow vertical angle (CBVA).

Myelopathy Assessment

It is important to look at the patient's neurological status, and the most commonly observed tool in the literature is the modified Japanese Orthopaedic Association (JOA) scale.[1] The scale accounts for many aspects of myelopathy including functional measurements.

Investigations for Surgery

Lateral X-ray, swimmer's X-ray, and spinal X-ray with flexion and extension in the cervical spine should be performed to determine local and global deformity, including extension into the upper thoracic spine.

Next, one must determine whether the deformity is rigid or flexible/reducible. This is usually related to ankylosis. Dynamic plain lateral radiographs and thin-cut computed tomography (CT) scans are required to assess this.[1]

If either anterior or posterior fusion is observed, the deformity is termed *rigid*. If no fusion is observed or if the patient's deformity is reducible on cervical extension, as observed on lateral radiograph, the deformity is deemed *flexible*.

Magnetic resonance (MR) cervical spine is useful in determining the degree of myelopathy/radiculopathy. A cervical spine DEXA scan would provide information on density. CT or MR angiogram is recommended in surgical preassessment to look at the location of vertebral artery.[14]

Modified Delphi Cervical Spine Deformity Classification

Ames et al have proposed a combined approach for classifying and assessing cervical spine deformity with multipliers relating to severity[15,16] (**Flowchart 10.1**).

Preoperative Planning

The following needs to be considered before attempting corrective surgery:

- The extent of the regional and global deformity.
- Presence/absence of myelopathy or radiculopathy.
- Functional status.
- Patient risk factors and morbidity.
- Previous surgeries.
- A measure of benefit from potential surgery.
- Rigid versus fixed deformity.
- Whether fusion is present at any level.

Pearls

- Sagittal balance parameters should be considered when planning cervical spine surgery in order to prevent or correct cervical spine deformity.
- Iatrogenic cervical spine deformity could be prevented in many cases if the cervical spine sagittal balance parameters are appropriately incorporated in the preoperative surgical plan and the surgery is executed according to the calculated desirable angles.

Strategies for Deformity Correction

The principles of revision surgery generally come under one of three categories.[6] These involve correction of the deformity by:

- Lengthening of the anterior column.
- Shortening of the posterior column.
- Decompression of the spinal segment and prevention of myelopathy.

Deformity Morphology and Surgical Approach

Flexible Deformity

Flexible deformities are those that may be reduced.

They can be treated by preoperative traction and then surgical release/fusion, either from an anterior or posterior approach.[5] The relative advantages and disadvantages of each approach are outlined in **Table 10.1**.

Flexible deformities can usually be managed with a single-stage procedure.[9]

Rigid Deformity

Patients with a rigid deformity can be managed with anterior, posterior, or circumferential (combined) approach.[1] The approach chosen is related to the presence of fusion, location of joint fusion, and patient bone quality.

Fixed Without Fusion

An anterior only or circumferential approach with anterior release followed by posterior fusion may be considered.[5,6] This can be decided based on the severity of the deformity, and the extent of revision surgery (multilevel, corpectomy, etc.).

Fixed and Fused

Osteotomies may be required in the context of ankylosis to restore satisfactory lordosis.[5,6] The approach should be decided based upon the location of fusion (anterior, posterior, or both).

Circumferential approaches will generally result in greater correction of deformity.[9]

The specific procedures with regard to different approaches are outlined in **Table 10.2**.

Table 10.1 Anterior surgery

Surgical approach	Advantages	Disadvantages
Anterior surgery	• Less associated morbidity • As initial surgery is likely posterior, avoidance of additional posterior surgeries • Preservation of remaining extensor musculature (located posteriorly) • Restoration of height to anterior column and normal lordosis	• Poorer fixation with anterior approach • No correction of posterior tension band
Posterior surgery	• Superior fixation • Mechanical advantage: acts on the posterior tension band	• May not achieve satisfactory cord decompression in neurological patients if there is anterior compression or OPLL • Limited graft surface area • Revision approach through scar is difficult • Increased pain and infection rate • Further damage to soft tissues
Circumferential	• Provides greater stability, especially if the patient had corpectomy and laminectomy at a vertebral level	• Time-consuming • Higher chance for postoperative and intraoperative morbidity

Table 10.2 Surgical options in deformity correction

Anterior	• Osteotomy for fused anterior column • Anterior cervical discectomy with fusion (ACDF) +/– plating
Posterior	• Posterior instrumentation/fusion ± decompression for the flexible deformity • Smith-Peterson osteotomy ± decompression for the semirigid deformity • Pedicle subtraction osteotomy or vertebral column resection for ankylosed cervicothoracic junction kyphosis
Circumferential	• Anterior-posterior approach • Anterior-posterior-anterior approach • Posterior-anterior-posterior approach

Outcomes: Surgical and Radiological Assessment

Treatment goals of the deformity surgery are to correct and fuse the deformity, remove reasons for myelopathy, and provide pain relief. The normalization of the sagittal axis should also be a desirable result.[5]

The same functional and radiological assessments should be performed postoperatively to assess the success of the surgery.

Patient-related quality-of-life scores are often useful in portraying patient[14,17] impression of the success of reintervention.

Conclusion

In conclusion, iatrogenic cervical spine deformity is a common occurrence. The best form of treatment should be prevention, which involves careful planning to determine the most appropriate surgical technique for each patient. Reference should be made to patient risk factors and surgeries with a higher rate of deformity as a complication. The symptomatic patient or asymptomatic patient with likely progression should receive intervention. This can initially be conservative but usually involves surgical reintervention, intending to correct the deformity, alleviate pain, and re-establish good functionality in the cervical spine.

References

1. Joaquim AF, Riew KD. Management of cervical spine deformity after intradural tumor resection. Neurosurg Focus 2015;39(2):E13
2. Bell DF, Walker JL, O'Connor G, Tibshirani R. Spinal deformity after multiple-level cervical laminectomy in children. Spine 1994;19(4):406–411
3. Kunieda E, Nishimura G, Kaneko T, Hirobe S, Masaki H, Kamagata S. Spinal deformity after intra-operative radiotherapy for paediatric patients. Br J Radiol 2010;83(985):59–66
4. Fu K-M. Seminar: cervical deformity. Video lecture. 2018
5. Rhee JM, ed. Iatrogenic cervical deformity. Seminars in Spine Surgery. Elsevier; 2011
6. Lee D-H. Iatrogenic cervical sagittal plane deformity following surgery.
7. Deformiteler İS. Iatrogenic spinal deformities. Turk Neurosurg 2014;24(1):75–83
8. Steinmetz MP, Kager CD, Benzel EC. Ventral correction of postsurgical cervical kyphosis. J Neurosurg 2003; 98(1, Suppl)1–7
9. Chi JH, Tay B, Stahl D, Lee R. Complex deformities of the cervical spine. Neurosurg Clin N Am 2007;18(2):295–304
10. Kim HJ, Lafage V. Seminar: spinal deformity principles. Video lecture. 2018
11. Dubousset J. Three-dimensional analysis of the scoliotic deformity. In: Weinstein SL, ed. Pediatric Spine: Principles and Practice. New York, NY: Raven Press; 1994.
12. Etame AB, Wang AC, Than KD, La Marca F, Park P. Outcomes after surgery for cervical spine deformity: review of the literature. Neurosurg Focus 2010;28(3):E14
13. Pesenti S, Lafage R, Lafage V, Panuel M, Blondel B, Jouve J-L. Cervical facet orientation varies with age in children: an MRI study. J Bone Joint Surg Am 2018;100(9):e57
14. Moustafa IM, Diab AA, Taha S, Harrison DE. Addition of a sagittal cervical posture corrective orthotic device to a multimodal rehabilitation program improves short- and long-term outcomes in patients with discogenic cervical radiculopathy. Arch Phys Med Rehabil 2016;97(12):2034–2044
15. Tan LA, Riew KD, Traynelis VC. Cervical spine deformity—part 1: biomechanics, radiographic parameters, and classification. Neurosurgery 2017;81(2):197–203
16. Ames CP, Blondel B, Scheer JK, et al. Cervical radiographical alignment: comprehensive assessment techniques and potential importance in cervical myelopathy. Spine 2013; 38(22, Suppl 1)S149–S160
17. Takeshita K, Seichi A, Akune T, Kawamura N, Kawaguchi H, Nakamura K. Can laminoplasty maintain the cervical alignment even when the C2 lamina is contained? Spine 2005; 30(11):1294–1298

11 Adult Degenerative Scoliosis

Aftab Younus and Adrian Kelly

Introduction

From a conceptual viewpoint understanding the term *degenerative scoliosis* begins by understanding that it is just one form of a disease that exists under the umbrella term of *adult scoliosis*. Adult degenerative scoliosis refers to a structural curve that develops after skeletal maturity in a previously normal spine.[1] Adult scoliosis is however an umbrella term that, while including adult degenerative scoliosis, refers to all forms of scoliosis occurring in skeletally mature individuals irrespective of whether the deformity began before skeletal maturity or thereafter.[2] On a global scale, advances in medical care are translating into longer life spans and when coupled with accelerated age-related spinal degeneration the prevalence of adult degenerative scoliosis is increasing at an alarming rate and so are patient expectations for deformity correction for both cosmetic and functional reasons, as well as to alleviate pain.[3] In terms of quantifying the magnitude of the problem, two retrospective cohort systematic reviews considered elderly subjects with previously normal spinal curvature and reported a prevalence of 30 to 60%.[4,5] In terms of understanding adult degenerative scoliosis, the attending spinal surgeon must appreciate the intimate association between the coronal deformity itself and the accompanying issues of central and lateral recess spinal stenosis and positive sagittal imbalance, all three of which form the corners of a conceptual triangle of understanding.[6]

Pathogenesis

Defining adult degenerative scoliosis has at its starting point the same broader definition of adult scoliosis which is defined as a Cobb angle of greater than 10 degrees measured in the coronal plane. Refining this to refer specifically to adult degenerative scoliosis means including the same definition but further including the point of the deformity commencing in adulthood and occurring in a previously normal spine.[1,7] The pathogenesis of adult degenerative scoliosis has at its foundation the same starting point of degenerative spine disease, namely, age-related desiccation of the intervertebral disc. Understanding why only a subset of aging adults develop adult degenerative scoliosis is afforded by the concept that relatively symmetrical spinal degeneration, as occurs in the general population, will not lead to the deformity. In those patients that develop adult degenerative scoliosis a crucial pathophysiological concept to appreciate is the asymmetry of disc and facet joint degeneration which leads to progressive imbalance of axial loading and the subsequent deformity.[8] Synonyms of the term *adult degenerative scoliosis* include lateral rotatory subluxation, lateral subluxation, lateral listhesis, lateral spondylolisthesis, and rotatory listhesis.[9] These terms must however be specifically contextualized as occurring in an adult with a previously straight spine to fulfill the definition of adult degenerative scoliosis.[1,7] In patients who develop adult degenerative scoliosis, asymmetrical desiccation of multiple intervertebral discs leads to asymmetrical disc space collapse. This, in turn, leads to asymmetrical facet joint degeneration usually at multisegmental levels. The subsequent asymmetrical facet strain leads to accelerated degenerative changes which include narrowing of the facet joint space, osteophyte formation of both the facet and limbus of the vertebral end plate, subchondral sclerosis, and subchondral cyst formation. Further abnormalities in the pathophysiology of adult degenerative scoliosis include hypertrophy of the ligamentum flavum, laxity of the interspinous ligament, and, as an end result, spinal instability. This explains the multisegmental and importantly multidirectional instability which by the very nature of the intervertebral disc and facet joint degeneration being asymmetrical, the milieu for adult degenerative scoliosis to develop is created.[3,8] Asymmetrical axial loading accelerates asymmetrical spinal degeneration which in turn accelerates progression of the deformity by three degrees or more annually.[10] Besides the deformity itself, osteophyte formation and the ligamentous flavum hypertrophy lead to narrowing of the central canal, lateral recesses, and foramina of the bony spine. One retrospective cohort comprehensive study found that the most common complication of degenerative scoliosis is spinal stenosis; however, this research found that patients are more likely to present with symptoms of central stenosis and radiculopathy than with either symptom alone.[11]

Besides the fundamental coronal deformity used in the diagnosis of adult degenerative scoliosis, another cornerstone of the disease, which is invariably present to some degree, is sagittal imbalance. The importance of this parameter is supported by the same retrospective cohort systematic review and another prospective cohort systematic review where sagittal malalignment directly correlated with both quality of life and the amount of axial back pain.[12,13] Measured globally on full-length weight-bearing sagittal spine films by a plum line, dropped vertically from the center of the body of C7 which should pass through the posterosuperior corner of the sacrum in ideally sagittal-balanced individuals, a line falling up to 4 cm anterior to this sacral landmark is regarded as a physiological variation that is unlikely to result in symptoms.[7] Truly understanding sagittal balance must however start with the realization that it is in fact determined by three parameters: lumbar lordosis, thoracic kyphosis, and pelvic incidence.[14] Of these three parameters, in terms of their importance in the development of adult degenerative scoliosis, lumbar lordosis or more specifically asymmetrical degenerative lumbar rotatory scoliosis is the most important consideration. The two retrospective cohort systematic reviews propose that it is the predominance of asymmetrical lower lumbar curvature that underpins the development and progression of adult degenerative scoliosis.[3,15]

Pearls

- Progression of the deformity and degeneration of the disc lead to decrease in size of the spinal canal due to the osteoarthritis of disc and facet joint.
- Less space available for the neural elements.
- Osteophyte growth and ligamentous flavum hypertrophy contribute to constriction of the bony spine's central canal, lateral recesses, and foramina and degenerative deformity.

Clinical Evaluation

Patients with adult degenerative scoliosis most commonly present with axial back pain as their primary complaint. Three retrospective cohort studies reported the frequency of this in up to 90% of cases".[3,16,17] It is important to take a thorough history of the exact nature of the axial backache as subtle nuances provide valuable information regarding management and expected outcome. Axial backache caused by the spinal deformity itself is commonly localized only to the convexity of the curve and is poorly localized. This form of axial back pain responds to rest as the pain trigger is predominantly paraspinal muscle fatigue. The existence of lumbar kyphosis together with adult degenerative scoliosis, in fact the two are part of the same disease process, leads to a flat back syndrome and here the axial back pain is quite particular, in that in the presence of a significant positive sagittal balance the patient will complain of axial lower lumbar back pain localized to the central part of the lower lumbar spine, iliac crests, and sacrum with identifiable and well-localized trigger points radiating rostrally. Spinal instability is another cause of axial back pain in adult degenerative scoliosis and this may be subtle or overt often needing dynamic imaging to diagnose.[3] Lenke et al provides a different perspective of the above. In their retrospective cohort systematic review they reported an important distinction between two types of adult degenerative scoliosis related to axial back pain. In this paper, pure axial backache of a tolerable nature, not relieved leaning forward, is predominantly the result of sagittal imbalance while an increase in the severity of the axial pain to an intolerable level that is relieved by leaning forward usually indicates the cause of the axial pain to be spinal stenosis and neurogenic claudication.[18] Determining the pain trigger in patients presenting with purely axial back pain in adult degenerative scoliosis is challenging. One prospective cohort clinical trial, which considered purely radiographical parameters, demonstrated significance between the severity of the axial back pain and thoracolumbar kyphosis, lateral listhesis, and the obliquity of specifically the L3 and L4 end plates. In this same paper, patient age, Cobb angle, the amount of sagittal imbalance, and listhesis failed to demonstrate significance.[19]

Classical unilateral leg pain occurs in the context of foraminal nerve root compression which can occur either from single- or multilevel foraminal disc herniations or from facet joint degeneration with foraminal osteophytic projections, specifically from the superior articular process of the inferior vertebrae which constitutes the posterior wall of the intervertebral foramen, causing nerve root impingement. Classical bilateral leg pain, albeit not always symmetrical in nature, occurs in the context of central spinal stenosis.[20] Applying these classical explanations to completely explain the radicular pain experienced by patients with adult degenerative scoliosis would however be an oversimplification. Without including central spinal stenosis and the subsequent leg pain from neurogenic claudication, the etiology of the radiculopathy experienced by patients with adult degenerative scoliosis is quite specific. Across the convex side of the curve, the radiculopathy is better explained by dynamic traction on the nerve roots which may occur with absolutely no compression being seen on imaging. On the concave side of the curve, the radiculopathy occurs as a result of foraminal stenosis in keeping with the classical understanding. Hence, in adult degenerative scoliosis, a retrospective cohort systematic review reported that bilateral leg pain should not be misdiagnosed as central spinal stenosis and neurogenic claudication and that this may be a bilateral radiculopathy should always be borne in mind.[21]

The clinical course of patients with adult degenerative scoliosis is usually a progressively increasing deformity with increasing symptomatology and worsening axial backache over many years. Superimposed leg pain and eventually gradual leg weakness occurs in the advanced stages of the disease.[10] Predictors of curve progression that have demonstrated statistical significance in a prospective cohort study of adult degenerative scoliosis included curves with a Cobb angle greater than 30 degrees; lateral listhesis of 6 mm or more; L5 depth measured from an imaginary horizontal intercrestal line and curves with an increased apical rotational component.[22] Acute neurological deterioration and sphincter involvement infrequently occur, and on reimaging, acute curve progression from, for example, an osteoporotic lumbar compression fracture or a significant disc herniation may be seen.[3]

Comprehensive patient evaluation must consider more than just the science of adult degenerative scoliosis and must consider all aspects of each patient. Each patient comes with his or her own agenda framed from their social and environmental context and their expectations form a critical part of their evaluation. Medical comorbidities such as a significant tobacco history, ischemic heart disease, previous cerebrovascular accident, diabetes mellitus, psychiatric history, and dietary habits are paramount considerations that need to be taken into account. The exact details of previous conservative treatments employed as well as any previous spinal surgery are further variables that directly impact patient evaluation and subsequent management.

Finally, the attending spinal surgeon performing a patient evaluation in the context of adult degenerative scoliosis must always have in the back of their mind a working differential diagnosis before arbitrarily attributing all symptomatology to the presenting spinal deformity. Local diseases such as pelvic malignancies, aneurysms of the abdominal aorta, osteoarthritis of the hip joint, abdominal wall hernias, and sacroiliitis must all be entertained and excluded. Other diseases distant from the lumbar spine such as cervical spondylotic myelopathy, acute cholecystitis, and pancreatic carcinoma are mimickers of the axial backache of adult degenerative scoliosis.[3]

Signs and Symptoms

Signs

- Paucity of neurologic deficit despite profound symptoms.
- May have positive femoral nerve stretch test or straight-leg raise with disc herniation.
- Adult degenerative scoliosis is usually a progressively increasing deformity with worsening of neurology.
- Cervical and lumber spinal stenosis can coexist; therefore, a detailed examination of both areas and the upper and lower extremities is essential.

Symptoms

- Lower backache (95%), claudication (91%), leg pain (71%), leg weakness (33%).
- Exacerbated by walking, relieved by sitting or leaning forward.
- May have radicular pain with lumber disc herniation.
- Cosmesis concerns.

Diagnostic Imaging

Lumbar symptoms dictate lumbar radiographic imaging be done as a first-line investigation. Once significant deformity is present, full-length, standing, posteroanterior radiographs to assess coronal balance and lateral, spinal radiographs to assess sagittal balance are mandatory. Flexion and extension views are routinely requested not only to assess the flexibility of the curves but also to rule out instability and its contribution to axial pain. Computed tomographic spine imaging is valuable to better define bony anatomy in patients being considered for surgery.[10] In the presence of radiculopathy, magnetic resonance imaging (MRI) as a preoperative surgical planning tool is commonly done; however, due to the complexity of the deformity, these images have been reported in a retrospective cohort systematic review to be difficult to assess.[3]

The specifics of how the initial, full-length, spinal radiographic images are performed contribute significantly to their value. No shoes should be worn and any lower limb length discrepancies should be measured and recorded. Radiography that includes rostrally the occiput and caudally the hip joints in a single posteroanterior and lateral spinal view is essential to assess the Cobb angle and pelvic parameters. Lateral radiography of the hips and knees is included to assess the flexibility of a patient's maximum correction of compensatory hip and knee flexion. A goniometer utilizes the Cobb method to measure the Cobb angle on the coronal curve. Here, the angle between the most deviated end plates at the superior and inferior ends of the primary curve is measured between intersecting perpendicular lines. Sagittal balance is measured on the sagittal full-length radiographic views by a plum line dropped vertically from the center of the body of C7 which should transverse the posterior third of the S1 superior end plate, though up to 4 cm anterior to this is considered an acceptable physiological variation.[10,23] The Cobb angle on both the posteroanterior view and lateral view and the sagittal balance on the lateral view are used as initial evaluation methods to not only dictate management but also measure curve progression in patients being managed conservatively under surveillance.

Further imaging modalities include computed tomographic scans augmented by myelography, which is useful because it concurrently assesses bony and neurological anatomy. This is offered as an alternative to MRI images; however, now-a-days it is less frequently used except where clear contraindications to MRI exist such as the presence of an MRI incompatible cardiac pacemaker. One prospective cohort study proposes discography as an imaging modality useful for specifically assessing each lumbar disc space individually to determine its specific contribution as a pain trigger and thereby its need to be incorporated into any fusion surgery being planned. Anasetti et al's recommendation is controversial.[24] EOS™ (Electro Optical System) imaging is a novel technique that utilizes low-dose biplanar radiography to reconstruct a three-dimensional assessment of the entire skeletal system in a standing position and thereby defines the degenerative lumbar scoliosis, thoracic kyphosis, and the compensatory hip and knee flexion qualitatively in a single view. The two-dimensional dedicated views described to specifically measure the Cobb angles, pelvic parameters, and sagittal alignment needed to define clinical decision-making in degenerative lumbar scoliosis are all simultaneously performed with the EOS system. An additional advantage of the three-dimensional qualitative skeletal view is ease of patient understanding.[25]

- Plain radiograph:
  - Remains essential to survey bone quality, spinal alignment, and arthritic conditions and may reveal destructive lesions.
  - Disc space collapse, osteophyte formation, and loss of lordosis are common features.
  - Full radiograph of the cervical, thoracic, and lumbar spine can be done on a single film.
  - Cobb angle measured on the anteroposterior view of the X-rays.
- MRI scan:
  - The technique of choice, if the patient has neurology.
  - It helps in evaluating the patency of the spinal canal.
  - Very sensitive and noninvasive.
- CAT scan—Myelography:
  - Next best option, if MRI scan is not available.
  - Cross-sectional area of less than 100 mm^2 suggests spinal stenosis.

Management

Nonsurgical Treatment

Conservative measures commonly employed by primary care physicians who by and large incidentally discover the degenerative scoliosis on routine radiological investigations performed for other reasons include out-patient medication and lumbosacral and thoracolumbosacral braces. These are not only poorly tolerated in the elderly but are ineffective in the context of the transverse instability that dictates curve progression in degenerative scoliosis. The muscle deconditioning that occurs with chronic bracing results in worsening curve progression rather than stabilization of the deformity and several retrospective cohort systematic reviews reported no beneficial effect.[3,4] Other conservative ineffective treatment modalities prescribed include exercise, swimming, yoga, and chiropractic spinal manipulation.[3]

The significance of the medical comorbidities in patients presenting with degenerative scoliosis is well recognized, and in poor surgical candidates, many spinal surgeons often advocate a trial of conservative measures incorporating physical therapy and nonsteroidal anti-inflammatory medication. Two retrospective cohort systematic reviews noted facet joint blocks, epidural blocks, nerve root blocks, and trigger point injections to be adjunctive short-term conservative treatment modalities.[3,10] One retrospective cohort systematic review and one retrospective cohort study reported the ineffectiveness of these as long-term treatment modalities in degenerative scoliosis.[13,26]

Common pharmacological agents prescribed by both primary care physicians and spinal surgeons include nonsteroidal anti-inflammatory medications, opioid analgesics, and muscle relaxants. The benefit of these is limited by considerable side effects which include gastrointestinal and renal concerns with regard to nonsteroidal anti-inflammatory medications, and dependence and an accelerated development of chronic pain syndrome with regard to opioid-based medications. Other useful pharmacological agents are gabapentin which effectively manages neuropathic pain as well as tricyclic antidepressants taken at night due to their sedating effects.[8]

Pearls

- Bracing is poorly tolerated in elderly patient with degenerative scoliosis.
- Nonoperative patients had no significant change in Owestry Disability Index (ODI) or leg pain.
- Surgically treated patients had significant improvement in mean score for leg pain (5.4 vs. 2.2, $p < 0.001$) and ODI (41 vs. 24, $p < 0.001$).[27]

Surgical Treatment

Degenerative scoliosis is a surgical disease best managed surgically and the conservative measures should at best be regarded as palliative in nonsurgical candidates secondary to significant medical comorbidities. One retrospective systematic review reported the goals of scoliosis corrective surgery to be (1) sagittal balance restoration, (2) symptomatic neural element decompression, (3) complication avoidance, and (4) improved quality of life.[23] Applying these principles to patients with degenerative scoliosis who are in the advanced years of life with significant medical comorbidities is difficult and requires patient-specific surgical treatment goals.

Correction surgery incorporating long-segment fusion has been reported to provide the best chance of achieving a satisfactory outcome.[22,28] Lenke in a retrospective cohort systematic review advised minimal surgical intervention to solve a patient's symptoms as the optimal strategy in degenerative scoliosis.[18]

Minimally invasive techniques have been adapted to degenerative scoliosis; however, no clear benefit has been reported in advanced degenerative scoliosis due to the complex multisegment nature of the disease process requiring multiple multilevel interventions be performed to correct the deformity.[29,30] One prospective and one retrospective cohort study note that advances in minimally invasive techniques continue to be developed as spinal surgeons increasingly recognize the direct association between complications, especially surgical site infection, and the extensiveness of any surgical procedure including, as an independent variable, the number of levels fused.[31,32]

The indications for surgery in adult degenerative scoliosis are progressive neurological deficit, disabling axial back pain nonresponsive to conservative measures, disabling pain and fatigue secondary to documented curve progression with sagittal and/or coronal imbalance, and cosmesis in those that request and can physiologically tolerate the corrective surgery.[3,33]

Pearls

- Surgical indications:
  - Progressive neurologic symptoms, which is rare.
  - Failure of nonoperative treatment:
    - Lower back pain.
    - Radicular pain.
- Selection of operative versus nonoperative treatment of adult degenerative scoliosis is dependent on the surgeon decision, which is based on:
  - Larger curves.
  - More frequent leg and lower back pain.
  - More episodes of severe lower back pain in the last 6 months.

Posterior Decompression Alone

One retrospective cohort systematic review noted that decompression alone is only suitable in one very specific instance, namely, symptomatic central spinal stenosis presenting as neurogenic claudication or lateral recess spinal stenosis presenting as a radiculopathy, no associated instability, a mild deformity, namely, a Cobb angle of or below 20 degrees, and maintained sagittal balance.[3] Decompression in the presence of deformity should be, however, approached with caution as the deformity itself may in fact be causing the compression and in this situation the compression is better alleviated by correcting the deformity itself. A second consideration is an iatrogenic destabilization of the deformity by performing the decompression causing accelerated curve progression.[23] For this reason two retrospective cohort systematic reviews reported that decompression should not be performed at either the proximal or distal ends of the curve or the curve apex.[16,34] Regarding the risk of iatrogenic destabilization by decompression alone, further factors that should be considered are the degree of disc collapse and extent of surrounding end-plate osteophytes which buffer the risk for curve progression as opposed to less disc space collapse and a relative scarcity of osteophytes where more anticipated curve progression may be expected to occur.[7] Limiting the extent of decompression to one or two levels and employing minimally invasive techniques with less paraspinal musculature dissection were proposed in a retrospective cohort study and a retrospective cohort systematic review as further means to limit curve progression, if decompression only is being considered.[29,35]

The procedures included under the decompression umbrella are laminectomy, laminotomy, foraminotomy, and extraforaminal decompression. These procedures, as long as they are done with due diligence and respect to the surrounding soft tissues, have little to no effect on preventing or causing deformity progression. They furthermore do nothing to address instability and importantly the most commonly reported disabling symptom in patients with degenerative scoliosis, namely, axial back pain.[3] In these patients, close postoperative surveillance at regular intervals should be routinely employed to exclude the development of instability and rapid curve progression presenting clinically as worsening axial back pain.

Pearls

- Posterior decompression alone is mainly done for symptomatic central spinal stenosis, with mild degenerative scoliosis.
- It does not address instability or scoliosis.
- If aggressive laminectomy is performed, then there is danger of future progression of the curve.

Posterior Decompression and Posterior Fusion Alone

The relentless nature of degenerative scoliosis is characterized by progressive deformity and worsening instability. For this reason, decompression alone is usually reserved for mild curves or as a palliative procedure in poor surgical candidates. The mainstay of surgical treatment for degenerative scoliosis is curve correction augmented by posterior fusion which not only addresses the axial back pain but also indirectly relieves neuropathic pain and radiculopathy caused by traction of neural elements on the convex side of the curve and compression of neural elements on the concave sides of the curve. Adjunctive direct decompression of symptomatic radiographically confirmed sites on neural compression may be undertaken in the same setting.

Fusion may be obtained without posterior instrumentation but in these cases the deformity is fused in situ utilizing bone graft which does nothing to correct the deformity or the degree of axial back pain already present. Some degree of curve correction can be achieved through the use of posterior instrumentation alone which offers segmental fixation anchor points through pedicle screw placement and when combined with an adequate release of the posterior elements, including the facet joints, some triplanar correction can be achieved. The amount of correction that can be achieved is, however, limited to mild-to-moderate curves and is unsuitable for rigid curves where an anterior release becomes mandatory, especially important in the presence of significant coronal imbalance. In a retrospective cohort systematic review, the decision to augment a decompression procedure with posterior instrumented fusion is recommended when one or more of the recognized factors for curve progression are present, namely, lateral listhesis greater than 6 mm, rotation, and spondylolisthesis.[3]

While coronal imbalance has enjoyed greater attention in older series, sagittal imbalance is now recognized to be equally important. Pelvic incidence is an additional parameter of paramount importance that becomes fixed once skeletal maturity has been achieved. This angle is defined by the angle between a perpendicular line drawn from the midpoint of the sacral end plate and a line drawn from the femoral head axis of rotation to the midpoint of the sacral end plate.[36] Correcting lumbar lordosis to be as equal as possible to pelvic incidence reduces hip and knee flexion as compensatory mechanisms, and thereby the energy of ambulation.[37] Corrected lumbar lordosis translates into corrected sagittal balance in degenerative scoliosis and this in turn has translated into increased patient satisfaction in several large surgical series.[36–38]

Pearls

- Posterior spinal fusion with fusion in situ will not correct the whole deformity.
- Fusion in situ can provide stability and good clinical outcomes without the risk of neurologic injury from reduction techniques.
- Posterior only correction is a useful surgical strategy to treat most type of spinal deformity and often it provides small degree of correction as anterior/posterior fusion.

Decompression with Posterior Fusion and Augmented Interbody Support

Due to the fundamental pathophysiology of degenerative scoliosis being asymmetrical disc space collapse, it follows logically that asymmetrical augmented interbody correction through interbody support would offer significant beneficial deformity correction which is not afforded by decompression and posterior instrumented fusion alone. While the anterior retroperitoneal approaches to the lumbar spine allow direct visualization, direct anterior release, direct correction of disc space height and a higher fusion rate, they are unfortunately fraught with significant morbidity. Besides the avoidable complications of vascular and visceral injuries which occur even in experience hands, the complications of postoperative paralytic ileus and retrograde ejaculation in males are according to two retrospective cohort studies far less predictable and difficult to avoid.[39,40] Advancements in minimally invasive technology provided spinal surgeons with a direct approach to the anterior lumbar disc space through the development of the lateral lumbar interbody fusion. Through a stab incision to the flank and serial dilatation via a trans-psoas approach, the morbidity of the anterior approaches was avoided; however, a new set of complications arose and persisted despite the incorporation of intraoperative neurophysiological monitoring with recurring injuries to the lumbar plexus. One prospective nonrandomized trial noted the procedure to be unsuitable to the L5–S1 disc space which is the predominant level needing correction to correct sagittal imbalance.[30]

The posterior lumbar interbody fusion (PLIF) technique allowed spinal surgeons to correct coronal imbalance and completely avoid the complications of the anterior and lateral approaches. The disadvantage of the approach is that significant nerve root retraction is needed to place the implant and contributes to a significant percentage of patients complaining of postoperative neuropathic pain and weakness. A further disadvantage is that if the implant is not placed anteriorly enough it becomes a pivot for inducing kyphosis.[38,39] The transforaminal interbody fusion device incorporates a facetectomy and thereby avoids the nerve root retraction needed to place the posterior lumbar interbody device. The disadvantage is that the necessary facetectomy induces instability and therefore pedicle screws and rods must be placed on the ipsilateral side to maintain stability. The compression across these ipsilateral rods to correct sagittal imbalance by pivoting the correction across the implant may in turn cause contralateral nerve root compression, and therefore, a prophylactic contralateral foraminotomy is commonly performed as contralateral pedicle screws and rods. A further complication of the transforaminal lumbar interbody device is that it must be rotated inside the disc space to lie parallel with the anterior limbus of the end plate and during this rotation breach of the anterior annulus can occur with subsequent vascular injury.[41,42] Although long-term outcomes are lacking regarding these procedures, purely due to their recent development and slow implementation, a retrospective cohort study noted them to be of benefit through immediate scoliosis correction on postoperative imaging, reduced hospital stay, and a lower complication rate as compared to the traditional open approaches.[29]

Pearls

- Transforaminal lumbar interbody fusion (TLIF) may achieve the goals with a posterior only approach.
- To assist in correction of deformity, the cage may be biased to the concavity of the scoliosis to address the coronal plane.
- After the facetectomy and posterior compression, lordosis can be restored.
- In general, a posterior interbody technique is less effective than an anterior lumbar interbody technique with a cage but anterior lumber interbody cage technique has more complication.
- TLIF has less neurological complication than the PLIF.

Staged Procedures

Prolonged surgical procedures place severe physiological strain on elderly patients taken to the operating room for correction of degenerative scoliosis. Intraoperative patient repositioning is difficult and complications such as airway dislodgement can occur. Fatigue of the surgical team is a further reality contributing to suboptimal results and an increased complication rate. Two studies, one a retrospective cohort and the other a clinical control trial, reported benefit from staging the anterior and posterior procedures in the context of separate surgical approaches to the anterior and posterior lumbar spine. These benefits are seen not only in terms of a shorter postoperative recovery period, reduced blood loss, and reduced complications but also in complex deformities, as they got further translated into better deformity correction.[43,44]

The patient's condition dictates the actual interval period between surgeries and the second stage is performed as early as possible to facilitate mobilization. Additional opportunity to correct hematological values to normal in the interoperative period is of value as well as the ability to exclude complications such as surgical site infection.[45]

Posterior Osteotomies

Both kyphosis and hypolordosis are amenable to correction by relative anterior column lengthening by posterior column shortening. These techniques not only restore sagittal balance but through asymmetrical removal of bone can correct coronal imbalance and rotation.

Spinal curve flexibility is an important consideration in adult degenerative scoliosis. This is defined as a curve that does not correct by 50% or more preoperatively on bending forward or intraoperatively on traction fluoroscopy. While the lumbar curve in adult degenerative scoliosis is almost invariably rigid, the secondary thoracic curve commonly corrects to some degree, but not enough to be regarded as truly flexible. In most cases, thoroughly releasing the posterior elements is required and performing osteotomies augments the spinal surgeon's ability to obtain an acceptable correction.[16] Consideration for the degree of correction required as well as the relative flexibility of the curve are the two cornerstones dictating the choice of osteotomy to be performed.

Smith-Peterson osteotomies were originally described for already fused spines which relied on the mobility of a disc space for correction. Here the spinous processes, lamina, and facet joints are removed, and a wedge is made into the anterior column either with an osteotome and mallet or an ultrasonic bone knife. The remaining superior and inferior posterior columns are then forcedly closed and held as such with pedicle screws and rods. A landmark retrospective cohort study reported that 10 degrees of sagittal correction can be obtained per level and the resultant bone-on-bone closure between the inferior surface of the remaining superior vertebral body and the superior surface of the remaining inferior vertebral body facilitates the anterior column fusion.[46] The disadvantages of the Smith-Peterson osteotomy are that (1) the considerable blood loss during each osteotomy is not warranted by the small degree of correction, which in reality is only a little more than 5 degrees per level; and (2) in the context of adult degenerative scoliosis, the forced closure of the posterior column effectively "snaps" the remaining anterior degenerated disc space which may cause a vascular injury directly anterior to this. A case series reported that a safer option in milder but requiring more flexible deformities is Ponte osteotomy which involves resecting the spinous processes, lamina, and facets at multiple levels and achieving a more gradual correction of approximately 3 to 5 degrees per level. The blood loss in the Smith-Péterson osteotomy is avoided as is the trauma incurred by the traumatic "snap" of the anterior disc space. The disadvantage of the Ponte osteotomy is that it requires flexibility of the curve to be achieved and in fact the procedure was first described for the treatment of Scheuermann disease in adolescents and young adults.[47]

Pedicle subtraction osteotomies (PSOs) are reserved for fixed sagittal imbalance deformities where more marked correction is needed. By performing a spinous process resection and bilateral lamina resection, access is gained to the pedicles of a single vertebral body. The pedicles are then wholly or partially resected and thereafter by working either from within the boundaries of partially resected pedicles, or directly on the vertebral body itself through the pedicular openings, but importantly staying within the boundaries of a single vertebral body, the cancellous bone is removed anteriorly and laterally with curettes. The remaining superior and inferior end plates, with a variable amount of remaining cancellous bone attached to each depending on the amount of desired correction needed, are then opposed and held closed with pedicle screws and rods in superior and inferior vertebrae. A retrospective cohort study reported that up to 30 degrees correction can be achieved per procedure. PSOs are often undertaken as a single intervention and afforded the same amount of correction as three Smith-Peterson osteotomies. This procedure should not be undertaken by novice surgeons and has a steep learning curve in unexperienced hands.[48]

By asymmetrically resecting more from one side of the vertebral body, coronal imbalance can also be corrected. This is done by performing a longer wedge on the opposite side of the coronal imbalance and a shorter wedge on the side of the coronal imbalance, and hence, during closing of the wedge the coronal imbalance is simultaneously addressed at the same time as the sagittal imbalance.[49] Another adaptation of the classical PSO, which lowers the blood loss considerably, is to incorporate either the superior or inferior disc space into the resection, and hence, only wedge either the superior vertebra if the inferior disc space is being incorporated or the inferior vertebra if the superior disc space is being incorporated. The former is more commonly performed than the latter. It is important if the disc space is being incorporated that the disc material and annulus are removed completely and a burr is used to decorticate the underlying end plate to facilitate fusion of the cancellous bone onto the end plate from which the disc was resected. By differentially wedging the vertebral body, coronal imbalance can be simultaneously corrected during closure of the wedge onto the exposed subcortical bone from the decorticated end plate.

Pearls

- Smith-Peterson osteotomy should be performed for only small deformity that require 10 to 20 degrees of deformity correction with possibility of requiring anterior column support.
- PSOs are reserved for fixed sagittal imbalance deformities where more marked correction is needed.
- For larger deformity that require angle greater than 30 degrees of correction a PSO may be the right choice.

Length of Fusion Construct

Classical teaching in scoliosis surgery is underpinned by three fundamental premises on the subject of length of fusion. The first of these is that decompressed areas should be incorporated into the fusion construct. The second premise is that constructs should not be stopped at the apex of curves, as this serves as a point for the development of adjacent level disease, which often progresses to the development of an acute kyphotic deformity. The final premise is regarding junctional areas, in almost all cases of degenerative scoliosis the thoracolumbar junction, which should not be the point of terminus in fusion constructs for the same fear regarding the development of junctional kyphosis.

A controversial point regarding length of fusion is regarding constructs terminating at L5 versus the need to include S1. A retrospective cohort study noted that stopping a fusion at L5 is problematic and reportedly results at best in worsening axial back pain from the L5–S1 motion segment and at worse secondary L5–S1 spondylolisthesis with worsening axial back pain and radiculopathy.[50]

Further controversy involves additional measures needed when involving the L5–S1 disc space in the fusion construct. It is recommended that incorporation of the L5–S1 disc space will require either, but in L5–S1 hypolordosis commonly both sacral screws and anterior column offer support to prevent flat back syndrome and/or spondylolisthesis. The debate here arises from well-known secondary sacroiliac joint pain, as a cause of late-onset worsening axial back pain, in fusion constructs extending to S1 but ignoring the incurred excessive sacroiliac joint axial and rotational loading. Here, spinal surgeons debate regarding the need to incorporate one or two sacroiliac screws, with or without arthrodesis of the sacroiliac joint, to prevent excessive loading onto this fibrous joint. Two studies, one a prospective cohort and the other a retrospective cohort systematic review, noted that sacroiliac screws are rarely placed as part of the primary intervention in adult degenerative scoliosis and are reserved for the development of this complication.[51,52]

Pearls

- Fusion should not be stopped at the apex of the curve.
- The severe lateral subluxation is included in the fusion.
- The spondylolisthesis and retrolisthesis are included in the fusion.
- The upper instrumented vertebra is better to be horizontal than tilted.
- It is debatable whether the proximal fusion level should be extended to T10 or stop at the lumbar spine.

Complications

The complication rates reported in adult degenerative scoliosis surgery must be understood as dependent on the physiological age of the patient, the specifics of the surgical corridor utilized, and the number of interventions.[53] Across several series, complications listed can be grouped as (1) skeletal, incorporating pseudoarthrosis, hardware failure, compression fractures, and junctional kyphosis; (2) neurological, incorporating radiculopathy, paresthesias, paraparesis, and paraplegia; (3) systemic, incorporating respiratory distress syndrome, deep vein thrombosis and secondary thromboembolic disease, urinary tract infection, and myocardial infarction; and (4) surgical site infection.[3,10,54]

The complication rates were higher as compared to other surgical subspecialties, as reported in the 1970s, and ranged between 20 and 40 percent.[8] Significant advances in preoperative patient optimization, anesthesia, instrumentation, and resuscitation afforded a marked drop in the complication rate which three decades later, but still two decades ago, was reported to be 13.4% in a landmark study from the Scoliosis Research foundation database which considered 4,980 surgical cases of adult scoliosis.[54] A more recent meta-analysis published less than a decade ago reported less optimistic results. In this study which considered 49 articles and 3,299 subjects, the incidence of adverse events in the perioperative period was reported to be 40%.[55]

The extent of the surgical intervention is correlated with a higher complication rate and posterior osteotomies are at the forefront in terms of not only skeletal complications but also neurological complications.[54–56] Intraoperative neurophysiological monitoring has become mandatory in these cases to ensure benefit outweighs risk as deformity correction while incurring a neurological injury is unacceptable in modern spinal surgery practice.[57] Overall infection rates in scoliosis surgery are 1 to 2%; however, in adult degenerative surgery this value is 3 to 5%.[58] The rate of pseudarthroses is similarly higher in adult degenerative scoliosis than in scoliosis surgery in younger patients and in degenerative scoliosis where patients have long fusion constructs; this is reported to occur in up to 24% of cases.[59]

Proximal junctional kyphosis is defined as an increase in kyphosis of greater than 10 degrees at the proximal end of a fusion construct and is a well-recognized complication of adult degenerative scoliosis surgery occurring in 20 to 39% of cases.[60,61] Proximal junction failure is a specific subtype of proximal junction kyphosis and is defined as kyphosis occurring together with structural failure of the vertebra immediately cephalad to the most superior instrumented level or failure of the most cephalad instrumented vertebra itself. Proximal junctional failure has been significantly associated with worsening axial pain, junctional instability, new-onset neurological deficit, and importantly the need for revision surgery. Hence while proximal junctional kyphosis is diagnosed more frequently than proximal junctional failure the implications of being diagnosed with proximal junctional kyphosis are not as marked as the latter and the risks as well as the revision surgery rate is significantly less.[62]

Pearls

- Excessive blood loss can occur during the operation.
- Early postoperative complication includes epidural hematoma, pulmonary embolism, and respiratory failure.
- Late complications include adjacent segment disease, pseudarthrosis and instrumentation failure, and proximal junctional kyphosis.
- Pseudarthrosis most commonly occurs at L5–S1 level, when it fuses to sacrum.
- High pelvis incidence and larger pelvic tilt may be associated with sagittal decompensation due to insufficient correction. In these patients, a high degree of correction lumber lordosis is needed.

Outcome

While the above paints a seemingly ominous picture of surgery performed for adult degenerative scoliosis, studies confirmed a quality-of-life improvement in over 94% of cases.[53,63] Patients with marked deformity have the worst disability and these same patients commonly need the most extensive surgical procedures for correction, specifically those with the highest complication rates. It is, however, this same group that benefits the most from surgery for degenerative scoliosis correction and shows the most marked improvement in quality of life.[53] Red flags studied and proven to predict a worse outcome irrespective of the type of surgery performed included a psychiatric history and tobacco use.[64]

In terms of quantifying outcome a recent multicenter randomized North American clinical control trial compared operative versus nonoperative treatment for symptomatic adult degenerative lumbar scoliosis and used as its outcome measures the Scoliosis Research Society Score-22 (SRS-22) and the Owestry Disability Index (ODI). In this study, the follow-up period was 2 years. Sixty-three patients were enrolled in the randomized cohort, 30 in the operative group and 33 in the observational group. Two hundred and twenty-three patients comprised the observational group of which 112 were ultimately managed operatively and 111 nonoperatively. In this study it is reported that, in both the randomized cohort and the observational cohort, the operative group demonstrated statistically significant advantages in 2 year outcome in both the SRS-22 and the ODI. The overall conclusion of this study was that patients who are symptomatically controlled medically should be left alone while symptomatic patients who fail a trial of medical therapy are best managed operatively.[64] In the authors' opinion, a criticism of these studies is the relatively short follow-up period. Several studies do however support adult degenerative scoliosis as a disease best managed surgically.[18,22,28,65]

A further factor alluded to in a recent study that contributes to outcome is the amount of fatty infiltration in the paravertebral muscles which by offering poor muscular support is at least in part contributory to poor outcome and persistent pain due to increased bony stresses. The amount of fatty infiltration in the multifidus muscle on the concave side of the curve was measured on MRI and correlated positively with outcome.[66] This emphasizes the importance of paraspinal muscle strengthening in both preventing curve progression and maintaining postsurgical curve correction and thereby outcome. Another study noted the failure of spinal deformity classification systems to include body mass index despite it being a significant influencer of outcome.[67] Other studies echo this thinking and note that despite being poorly explored, body mass index is a significant factor in determining outcome.[68–70]

Conclusion

In contrast to other spinal deformities, adult degenerative scoliosis is increasing in prevalence. Its natural course is slow progression over decades and overall it is largely a benign disease. While the pathophysiology is uniform, the expression of this is extremely varied and each patient needs individualistic treatment based on their specific needs, tailored to their resilience to undergo an operative intervention. From palliative interventions such as regional blocks and spinal cord stimulators to extensive corrections with their inherent surgical risk but substantial benefit, the surgery for adult degenerative scoliosis requires the attending spinal surgeon to have a deep understanding of the complexity, not only of spinal anatomy and spinal radiology, but of the benefits and risks of the surgical procedures themselves. The Cobb angle in adult degenerative scoliosis is not as much of a dominant role player as it is in idiopathic curves, and other factors such as lateral listhesis, spondylolisthesis, spinal stenosis, and sagittal imbalance, all play an equal, if not more important, role. Minimally invasive techniques are here to stay and offer minimalistic interventions at considerably less risk. The role of the larger procedures is however steadfast when larger corrections are needed, and both are required in modern spinal practice in a patient-specific manner. Understanding patient expectations and balancing these with realistic surgical outcomes through thorough informed consent forms a pillar in ensuring postoperative patient satisfaction.

References

1. Grubb SA, Lipscomb HJ, Coonrad RW. Degenerative adult onset scoliosis. Spine 1988;13(3):241–245
2. Vanderpool DW, James JI, Wynne-Davies R. Scoliosis in the elderly. J Bone Joint Surg Am 1969;51(3):446–455
3. Ploumis A, Transfledt EE, Denis F. Degenerative lumbar scoliosis associated with spinal stenosis. Spine J 2007;7(4):428–436
4. van Dam BE. Nonoperative treatment of adult scoliosis. Orthop Clin North Am 1988; 19(2):347–351
5. Aebi M. The adult scoliosis. Eur Spine J 2005; 14(10):925–948
6. Zeng Y, White AP, Albert TJ, Chen Z. Surgical strategy in adult lumbar scoliosis: the utility of categorization into 2 groups based on primary symptom, each with 2-year minimum follow-up. Spine 2012;37(9):E556–E561
7. Gupta MC. Degenerative scoliosis. Options for surgical management. Orthop Clin North Am 2003;34(2):269–279
8. Benner B, Ehni G. Degenerative lumbar scoliosis. Spine 1979;4(6):548–552
9. Toyone T, Tanaka T, Kato D, Kaneyama R, Otsuka M. Anatomic changes in lateral spondylolisthesis associated with adult lumbar scoliosis. Spine 2005;30(22):E671–E675
10. Ascani E, Bartolozzi P, Logroscino CA, et al. Natural history of untreated idiopathic scoliosis after skeletal maturity. Spine 1986; 11(8):784–789
11. Sengupta DK, Herkowitz HN. Lumbar spinal stenosis. Treatment strategies and indications for surgery. Orthop Clin North Am 2003;34(2):281–295

12. Jackson RP, McManus AC. Radiographic analysis of sagittal plane alignment and balance in standing volunteers and patients with low back pain matched for age, sex, and size. A prospective controlled clinical study. Spine 1994;19(14):1611–1618
13. Schwab F, Patel A, Ungar B, Farcy JP, Lafage V. Adult spinal deformity-postoperative standing imbalance: how much can you tolerate? An overview of key parameters in assessing alignment and planning corrective surgery. Spine 2010;35(25):2224–2231
14. Heary HF, Albert TJ. Spinal deformities: the essentials. New York: Thieme Medical Publishers; 2007
15. Lowe T, Berven SH, Schwab FJ, Bridwell KH. The SRS classification for adult spinal deformity: building on the King/Moe and Lenke classification systems. Spine 2006; 31(19, Suppl)S119–S125
16. Berven SH, Deviren V, Mitchell B, Wahba G, Hu SS, Bradford DS. Operative management of degenerative scoliosis: an evidence-based approach to surgical strategies based on clinical and radiographic outcomes. Neurosurg Clin N Am 2007;18(2):261–272
17. Nasca RJ. Surgical management of lumbar spinal stenosis. Spine 1987;12(8):809–816
18. Silva FE, Lenke LG. Adult degenerative scoliosis: evaluation and management. Neurosurg Focus 2010;28(3):E1
19. Schwab FJ, Smith VA, Biserni M, Gamez L, Farcy JP, Pagala M. Adult scoliosis: a quantitative radiographic and clinical analysis. Spine 2002;27(4):387–392
20. Ascani E, Bartolozzi P, Logroscino CA, et al. Natural history of untreated idiopathic scoliosis after skeletal maturity. Spine 1986; 11(8):784–789
21. Foley KT, Holly LT, Schwender JD. Minimally invasive lumbar fusion. Spine 2003; 28(15, Suppl)S26–S35
22. Pritchett JW, Bortel DT. Degenerative symptomatic lumbar scoliosis. Spine 1993;18(6): 700–703
23. Oskouian RJ Jr, Shaffrey CI. Degenerative lumbar scoliosis. Neurosurg Clin N Am 2006; 17(3):299–315, vii
24. Anasetti F, Galbusera F, Aziz HN, et al. Spine stability after implantation of an interspinous device: an in vitro and finite element biomechanical study. J Neurosurg Spine 2010;| 13(5):568–575
25. Illés T, Somoskeöy S. The EOS™ imaging system and its uses in daily orthopaedic practice. Int Orthop 2012;36(7):1325–1331
26. Glassman SD, Bridwell K, Dimar JR, Horton W, Berven S, Schwab F. The impact of positive sagittal balance in adult spinal deformity. Spine 2005;30(18):2024–2029
27. Cho KJ, Suk SI, Park SR, et al. Short fusion versus long fusion for degenerative lumbar scoliosis. Eur Spine J 2008;17(5):650–656
28. Anand N, Baron EM, Khandehroo B, Kahwaty S. Long-term 2- to 5-year clinical and functional outcomes of minimally invasive surgery for adult scoliosis. Spine 2013;38(18):1566–1575
29. Isaacs RE, Hyde J, Goodrich JA, Rodgers WB, Phillips FM. A prospective, nonrandomized, multicenter evaluation of extreme lateral interbody fusion for the treatment of adult degenerative scoliosis: perioperative outcomes and complications. Spine 2010; 35(26, Suppl)S322–S330
30. Guigui P, Devyver B, Rillardon L, Ngounou P, Deburge A, Ghosez JP. Intraoperative and early postoperative complications of lumbar and lumbosacral fusion: prospective analysis of 872 patients. Rev Chir Orthop Repar Appar Mot 2004;90(1):5–15
31. Daubs MD, Lenke LG, Cheh G, Stobbs G, Bridwell KH. Adult spinal deformity surgery: complications and outcomes in patients over age 60. Spine 2007;32(20):2238–2244
32. Bradford DS, Tay BK, Hu SS. Adult scoliosis: surgical indications, operative management, complications, and outcomes. Spine 1999; 24(24):2617–2629
33. Birknes JK, White AP, Albert TJ, Shaffrey CI, Harrop JS. Adult degenerative scoliosis: a review. Neurosurgery 2008; 63(3, Suppl) 94–103
34. Lonstein JE. Scoliosis: surgical versus nonsurgical treatment. Clin Orthop Relat Res 2006;443(443):248–259
35. Lafage V, Schwab F, Patel A, Hawkinson N, Farcy JP. Pelvic tilt and truncal inclination: two key radiographic parameters in the setting of adults with spinal deformity. Spine 2009;34(17):E599–E606
36. Legaye J, Duval-Beaupère G, Hecquet J, Marty C. Pelvic incidence: a fundamental pelvic parameter for three-dimensional regulation of spinal sagittal curves. Eur Spine J 1998; 7(2):99–103
37. Schwab FJ, Blondel B, Bess S, et al; International Spine Study Group (ISSG). Radiographical spinopelvic parameters and disability in the setting of adult spinal deformity: a prospective multicenter analysis. Spine 2013; 38(13):E803–E812

38. Madan S, Boeree NR. Outcome of posterior lumbar interbody fusion versus posterolateral fusion for spondylolytic spondylolisthesis. Spine 2002;27(14):1536–1542
39. Cunningham BW, Polly DW Jr. The use of interbody cage devices for spinal deformity: a biomechanical perspective. Clin Orthop Relat Res 2002; (394):73–83
40. Potter BK, Freedman BA, Verwiebe EG, Hall JM, Polly DW Jr, Kuklo TR. Transforaminal lumbar interbody fusion: clinical and radiographic results and complications in 100 consecutive patients. J Spinal Disord Tech 2005;18(4):337–346
41. Kwon BK, Berta S, Daffner SD, et al. Radiographic analysis of transforaminal lumbar interbody fusion for the treatment of adult isthmic spondylolisthesis. J Spinal Disord Tech 2003;16(5):469–476
42. Viviani GR, Raducan V, Bednar DA, Grandwilewski W. Anterior and posterior spinal fusion: comparison of one-stage and two-stage procedures. Can J Surg 1993;36(5): 468–473
43. Shufflebarger HL, Grimm JO, Bui V, Thomson JD. Anterior and posterior spinal fusion. Staged versus same-day surgery. Spine 1991; 16(8):930–933
44. Bridwell KH, Edwards CC II, Lenke LG. The pros and cons to saving the L5-S1 motion segment in a long scoliosis fusion construct. Spine 2003;28(20):S234–S242
45. Smith Peterson MN, Larson CB, Aufranc EO. Osteotomy of the spine for correction of flexible deformity in rheumatoid arthritis. Clin Orthop Relat Res 1969; (66):6–9
46. Geck MJ, Macagno A, Ponte A, Shufflebarger HL. The Ponte procedure: posterior only treatment of Scheuermann's kyphosis using segmental posterior shortening and pedicle screw instrumentation. J Spinal Disord Tech 2007;20(8):586–593
47. Suk SI, Chung ER, Kim JH, Kim SS, Lee JS, Choi WK. Posterior vertebral column resection for severe rigid scoliosis. Spine 2005;30(14): 1682–1687
48. Cecchinato R, Berjano P, Aguirre MF, Lamartina C. Asymmetrical pedicle subtraction osteotomy in the lumbar spine in combined coronal and sagittal imbalance. Eur Spine J 2015;24(Suppl 1):S66–S71
49. Edwards CC II, Bridwell KH, Patel A, et al. Thoracolumbar deformity arthrodesis to L5 in adults: the fate of the L5-S1 disc. Spine 2003;28(18):2122–2131
50. Maigne JY, Planchon CA. Sacroiliac joint pain after lumbar fusion. A study with anesthetic blocks. Eur Spine J 2005;14(7):654–658
51. Yoshihara H. Sacroiliac joint pain after lumbar/ lumbosacral fusion: current knowledge. Eur Spine J 2012;21(9):1788–1796
52. Schwab FJ, Lafage V, Farcy JP, Bridwell KH, Glassman S, Shainline MR. Predicting outcome and complications in the surgical treatment of adult scoliosis. Spine 2008; 33(20):2243–2247
53. Sansur CA, Smith JS, Coe JD, et al. Scoliosis research society morbidity and mortality of adult scoliosis surgery. Spine 2011;36(9):E593–E597
54. Yadla S, Maltenfort MG, Ratliff JK, Harrop JS. Adult scoliosis surgery outcomes: a systematic review. Neurosurg Focus 2010;28(3):E3
55. Norton RP, Bianco K, Lafage V, Schwab FJ; International Spine Study Group Foundation. Complications and intercenter variability of three-column resection osteotomies for spinal deformity surgery: a retrospective review of 423 patients. Evid Based Spine Care J 2013;4(2):157–159
56. Fisher RS, Raudzens P, Nunemacher M. Efficacy of intraoperative neurophysiological monitoring. J Clin Neurophysiol 1995;12(1): 97–109
57. Murata Y, Takahashi K, Hanaoka E, Utsumi T, Yamagata M, Moriya H. Changes in scoliotic curvature and lordotic angle during the early phase of degenerative lumbar scoliosis. Spine 2002;27(20):2268–2273
58. Kim YJ, Bridwell KH, Lenke LG, Rhim S, Cheh G. Pseudarthrosis in long adult spinal deformity instrumentation and fusion to the sacrum: prevalence and risk factor analysis of 144 cases. Spine 2006;31(20):2329–2336
59. Li G, Passias P, Kozanek M, et al. Adult scoliosis in patients over sixty-five years of age: outcomes of operative versus nonoperative treatment at a minimum two-year follow-up. Spine 2009;34(20):2165–2170
60. Acosta FL Jr, McClendon J Jr, O'Shaughnessy BA, et al. Morbidity and mortality after spinal deformity surgery in patients 75 years and older: complications and predictive factors. J Neurosurg Spine 2011;15(6):667–674
61. Yagi M, Akilah KB, Boachie-Adjei O. Incidence, risk factors and classification of proximal junctional kyphosis: surgical outcomes review of adult idiopathic scoliosis. Spine 2011;36(1):E60–E68

62. Watanabe K, Lenke LG, Bridwell KH, Kim YJ, Koester L, Hensley M. Proximal junctional vertebral fracture in adults after spinal deformity surgery using pedicle screw constructs: analysis of morphological features. Spine 2010;35(2):138–145
63. Hostin R, McCarthy I, O'Brien M, et al; International Spine Study Group. Incidence, mode, and location of acute proximal junctional failures after surgical treatment of adult spinal deformity. Spine 2013; 38(12):1008–1015
64. Kelly MP, Lurie JD, Yanik EL, et al. Operative versus nonoperative treatment for adult symptomatic lumbar scoliosis. J Bone Joint Surg Am 2019;101(4):338–352
65. Xie D, Zhang J, Ding W, et al. Abnormal change of paravertebral muscle in adult degenerative scoliosis and its association with bony structural parameters. Eur Spine J 2019;28(7):1626–1637
66. Naresh-Babu J, Viswanadha AK, Ito M, Park JB. What should an ideal adult spinal deformity classification system consist of? Review of the factors affecting outcomes of adult spinal deformity management. Asian Spine J 2019;13(4):694–703
67. Xu L, Sun X, Huang S, et al. Degenerative lumbar scoliosis in Chinese Han population: prevalence and relationship to age, gender, bone mineral density, and body mass index. Eur Spine J 2013;22(6):1326–1331
68. Fu L, Chang MS, Crandall DG, Revella J. Does obesity affect surgical outcomes in degenerative scoliosis? Spine 2014;39(24): 2049–2055
69. Smith JS, Shaffrey CI, Glassman SD, et al; Spinal Deformity Study Group. Clinical and radiographic parameters that distinguish between the best and worst outcomes of scoliosis surgery for adults. Eur Spine J 2013; 22(2):402–410
70. Smith JS, Shaffrey CI, Berven S, et al; Spinal Deformity Study Group. Operative versus nonoperative treatment of leg pain in adults with scoliosis: a retrospective review of a prospective multicenter database with two-year follow-up. Spine 2009;34(16):1693–1698

12 Limited Surgical Intervention for Adult Spine Deformity: Philosophy and Techniques

Inyang Udo-Inyang, Jr., Assem Sultan, and R. Douglas Orr

Introduction

Spinal deformities including scoliosis has been classically described and initially studied among adolescent patients who suffered from idiopathic scoliosis.[1] The focus in these patients and approach to surgical correction have been largely directed toward addressing the absolute values of regional structural and compensatory curves predominantly in the thoracic region and mainly in the coronal plane.[2–6] Clinically, these patients may seek surgical evaluation for cosmetic concerns and rarely will have pain and/or significant functional disability unless very late in the course of the disease. In the world of adult spine, the morbidity of deformity is mainly due to the sagittal plane component and is predominantly a lumbar spine disease.[7–9] There is little to no correlation between the absolute values of lordosis, kyphosis, or coronal plane Cobb angle. Clinically, activity-related axial back pain is very common, and many patients present with symptoms of radiculopathy and/or neurogenic claudication.[10] "Global spine balance" is a far more important concept in adult spine deformity and is dependent on several global, regional, and spinopelvic parameters as discussed in multiple previous studies.[2–10]

Goals of Treatment

Defining the goals of treatment through shared decision making with patients and families is the first step for a favorable outcome and sound surgical planning. In general, goals of surgical treatment are to decompress central or foraminal stenosis, address segmental instability, and restore and maintain sagittal and coronal plane correction. When treating these complex patients, it is important to adopt a patient-specific risk-benefit approach that encompasses patient expectations, their medical comorbidities, and the anticipated postoperative time-to-recovery. Currently, there is a plethora of research on the surgical management of adult spine deformity. However, a broad range of surgical techniques exists, and the ideal surgical option remains controversial. Some authors advocate for an "all or none" approach where long-segment instrumentation, interbody spacers, and three-column osteotomies are utilized to achieve sagittal and coronal balance while also decompressing the neural elements at levels of stenosis. The risk of severe complications can be relatively high in these patients and estimated to be between 25 and 40% of patients in some reports.[7,11,12] In recent years, the concept of "limited surgery" has emerged and describes a highly focused approach that addresses segmental pathology while mitigating the risks of an all-open approach. This can be of particular importance in patients with limited number of degenerated segments that also maintain their global spine balance and have flexible deformity.[13] Recognizing patients who may benefit from limited surgery is the hallmark of this philosophy, as the risk of failure and even the need for more complex procedures is increased if limited surgery is utilized for the incorrect indications or suboptimally executed.

Pearls

- Preoperative discussion with patients should set very clear goal and expectations.
- There remains no ideal approach to adult spine deformity, and surgical decision making should address this complex problem on a case-by-case basis.
- Adult spine deformity correction surgery has a high morbidity with up to 40% complication rates in the literature.
- A more focused or limited approach may therefore achieve clinical goals while avoiding risks of massive deformity correction.

Limited Surgical Options

Decompression Alone

Patients who present with predominant symptoms of leg pain due to isolated nerve root radiculopathy in the presence of maintained and balanced spine may benefit from neurologic decompression alone.[14–16] These patients commonly present with rotatory subluxation with foraminal and nerve root impingement in the concavity of the curve. Considerable pain relief with selective nerve block administered at suspected levels is a strong predictor of subsequent successful decompression, regardless of the duration of this effect. Studies have shown that decompression alone may carry an increased risk of deformity progression in these patients due to inadvertent destabilization with exposure and bony resections especially with conventional open techniques.[11,14–16] Therefore, minimally invasive and minimal access decompression techniques augmented by microscopic visualization may be a better option in these patients.[14] In addition, it is important to note that decompression alone should be avoided in the presence of a rotatory subluxation or a slip at the apex of deformity, as these patients require fusion in addition to decompression. In summary, decompression alone can be a valuable option in elderly patients with low functional demands who present with radiculopathy predominant symptoms in a well or relatively balanced spine. There is a potential risk of deformity progression that can be avoided with careful patient selection and meticulous surgical techniques.

Pearls

- In adult spine deformity patients, if the majority of their symptoms come from nerve root entrapment, decompression alone may be a feasible and clinically relevant option in select patients.
- These patients will commonly present with rotatory subluxation with majority of symptoms from the concavity of their coronal curve. Extreme care should be taken as open decompression can destabilize these patients. Therefore, microscopic decompression is a better option.
- Identify patients who present with symptoms of compression from the apex of the curve. These patients will frequently require fusion and partial correction and would not do well long term with decompression alone.

Segment Fusion and Posterior Column Osteotomies

In many patients with adult spine deformity, symptoms can be isolated to a single or few levels of pathology, most commonly due to degenerative spondylolisthesis and/or rotatory subluxation, while they still maintain a reasonably balanced spine. In these patients, short-segment instrumented fusion focused on the problematic levels may be an option to relieve their symptoms while avoiding the morbidity of a full deformity correction surgery.[13] Direct central or foraminal decompression can also be performed if indicated.

In recent years, the incorporation of advanced navigation systems, newer generation interbody spacers, and versatile pedicle screws as well as meticulous surgical techniques has helped achieve better results in these patients.[13,17] A combination of reduction maneuvers such as direct vertebral derotation, rod translation, and approximation using persuader tools can be combined to correct focal deformity and achieve stability. In addition, interbody fusion seems to achieve higher fusion rates when compared to posterolateral fusion and can aid in achieving reduction of rotatory subluxation with transforaminal lumbar interbody fusion (TLIF).[18–20] In addition, restoration of disc space height with this technique can achieve indirect foraminal decompression. Choice of bone graft, substitutes, and expanders is critical for achieving successful fusion and avoiding reoperation for pseudoarthrosis. The use of bone morphogenetic protein (BMPs-2) is currently available and is used off-label in adult spine deformity patients and seems to lead to more solid and higher rates of fusion. However, they may have smaller role to play when short-segment fusion is indicated compared to full deformity correction surgery.

In a study by Kurra et al,[13] the authors compared long-term outcomes (minimum 5 y) of limited fusion using TLIFs in 41 patients with degenerative spondylolisthesis in the setting of degenerative scoliosis with neutral coronal and sagittal balance. The study evaluated patients who underwent TLIF for three levels or less. Revision rate was 41% in the cohort and was highest among patients who had one level TLIF (48%). There was no statistically significant correlation between preoperative coronal curve magnitudes and revision surgeries, though it should be noted that patients with curves that measured greater than 20 degrees had higher rates of revision surgeries (75%; $p = 0.343$) in the global lumbar curve deformity group. Despite the relatively high revision rate in the cohort, this technique remains a valuable option in patients with neutral sagittal and coronal alignment with far less perioperative risks and postoperative complications. Further research directly comparing outcomes and revision rates using this technique versus long-segment fusion is required to better understand the role and utility of each method.

Pearls

- Adult spine deformity patients with "balanced spine" may initially be addressed through short-segment decompression and instrumented fusion alone.
- New technologies and meticulous techniques have allowed improved correction and higher success rate in these patients compared to more historical results.
- Recent research has demonstrated that revision rates may still be high in these patients particularly in those who undergo one level TLIF versus higher levels (2 or 3) and in patients with coronal curves of 20 degrees or more.

Other Limited Options

Interspinous spacers such as the X-Stop have been used to treat mild-to-moderate spinal stenosis in patients without deformity with variable results.[21] Data from reports showing successful utilization is driven from lower quality, industry-funded studies. It may be used off-label as a salvage option in patients with deformity and concurrent mild-to-moderate stenosis. There is currently no reliable evidence and further studies are warranted.

Conclusion

Careful patient selection is essential when limited surgery is considered among adult spine deformity patients. In patients who present with severe degenerative scoliosis with sagittal and/or coronal imbalance, and who are healthier with fewer comorbidities, addressing the totality of disease and restoring global spin balance is warranted. Therefore, these patients are best treated with long-segment instrumented fusion, multilevel osteotomies, and interbodies. Limited surgery can be a safe and alternative option in patients who are older, have lower functional demands, are more prone to complications of major deformity correction, and most importantly, present with a balanced spine and a primarily focal problem. Decompression alone is an option for those presenting with predominantly radicular pain and is best done through minimal access approaches. Short-segment instrumented fusion is an option to provide regional stabilization in patients with balanced spine with good results and potentially lower risk for major complications compared to long-segment fusion.

References

1. Lenke LG, Betz RR, Harms J, et al. Adolescent idiopathic scoliosis: a new classification to determine extent of spinal arthrodesis. J Bone Joint Surg Am 2001;83(8):1169–1181
2. Ohrt-Nissen S, Shigematsu H, Cheung JPY, Luk KDK, Samartzis D. Predictability of coronal curve flexibility in postoperative curve correction in adolescent idiopathic scoliosis: the effect of the sagittal profile. Global Spine J 2020;10(3):303–311
3. Mohanty SP, Pai Kanhangad M, Gullia A. Curve severity and apical vertebral rotation and their association with curve flexibility in adolescent idiopathic scoliosis. Musculoskelet Surg 2020; (April): 10.1007/s12306-020-00660-0
4. Pesenti S, Prost S, Pomero V, et al. Does static trunk motion analysis reflect its true position during daily activities in adolescent with idiopathic scoliosis? Orthop Traumatol Surg Res 2020;106(7):1251–1256
5. Qadir I, Shah A, Alam SR, Hussain H, Akram R, Aziz A. Impact of metal density on deformity correction in posterior fusions for adolescent idiopathic scoliosis: a retrospective cohort study. Ann Med Surg (Lond) 2020;52:44–47
6. Ohrt-Nissen S, Luk KDK, Samartzis D, Cheung JPY. Selection of the lowest instrumented vertebra in main thoracic adolescent idiopathic scoliosis: is it safe to fuse shorter than the last touched vertebra? Eur Spine J 2020;29(8):2018–2024
7. Demirkiran G, Theologis AA, Pekmezci M, Ames C, Deviren V. Adult spinal deformity correction with multi-level anterior column releases description of a new surgical technique and literature review. Clin Spine Surg 2016;29(4):141–149
8. Haddas R, Satin A, Lieberman I. What is actually happening inside the “cone of economy”: compensatory mechanisms during a dynamic balance test. Eur Spine J 2020; 29(9):2319–2328
9. Merrill RK, Kim JS, McNeill IT, et al. Negative sagittal balance following adult spinal deformity surgery. Global Spine J 2018;8(2):149–155
10. Glassman SD, Bridwell K, Dimar JR, Horton W, Berven S, Schwab F. The impact of positive sagittal balance in adult spinal deformity. Spine 2005;30(18):2024–2029
11. Zanirato A, Damilano M, Formica M, et al. Complications in adult spine deformity surgery: a systematic review of the recent literature with reporting of aggregated incidences. Eur Spine J 2018;27(9):2272–2284
12. Samuel AM, Maza N, Vaishnav AS, et al. Medical optimization of modifiable risk factors before thoracolumbar three-column osteotomies: an analysis of 195 patients. Spine Deform 2020;8(5):1039–1047
13. Kurra S, Lavelle WF, Silverstein MP, Savage JW, Orr RD. Long-term outcomes of transforaminal lumbar interbody fusion in patients with spinal stenosis and degenerative scoliosis. Spine J 2018;18(6):1014–1021
14. Hansraj KK, Cammisa FP Jr, O’Leary PF, et al. Decompressive surgery for typical lumbar spinal stenosis. Clin Orthop Relat Res 2001; (384):10–17
15. San Martino A, D’Andria FM, San Martino C; MARTINO. The surgical treatment of nerve root compression caused by scoliosis of the lumbar spine. Spine 1983;8(3):261–265
16. Frazier DD, Lipson SJ, Fossel AH, Katz JN. Associations between spinal deformity and outcomes after decompression for spinal stenosis. Spine 1997;22(17):2025–2029
17. Kelleher MO, Timlin M, Persaud O, Rampersaud YR. Success and failure of minimally invasive decompression for focal lumbar spinal stenosis in patients with and without deformity. Spine 2010;35(19): E981–E987
18. Bae J, Theologis AA, Strom R, et al. Comparative analysis of 3 surgical strategies for adult spinal

deformity with mild to moderate sagittal imbalance. J Neurosurg Spine 2018;28(1): 40–49

19. Liow MHL, Goh GSH, Chua JL, et al. Sagittally balanced degenerative spondylolisthesis patients with increased sacral slope and greater lumbar lordosis experience less back pain after short-segment lumbar fusion surgery. Clin Spine Surg 2020;33(5):E231–E235
20. Park SW, Ko MJ, Kim YB, Le Huec JC. Correction of marked sagittal deformity with circumferential minimally invasive surgery using oblique lateral interbody fusion in adult spinal deformity. J Orthop Surg Res 2020;15(1):13
21. Mo Z, Li D, Zhang R, Chang M, Yang B, Tang S. Comparative effectiveness and safety of posterior lumbar interbody fusion, Coflex, Wallis, and X-stop for lumbar degenerative diseases: a systematic review and network meta-analysis. Clin Neurol Neurosurg 2018; 172:74–81

13 Coronal Balance and Its Importance in Spinal Surgery

Tansu Gürsoy, Kemal Paksoy, and Onur Yaman

Introduction

The frequency of deformity seen in adults varies by 32 to 60%.[1] The Scoliosis Research Society (SRS)-Schwab classification is an effective classification in adult deformity assessment. However, the coronal disorder, which is common in adult deformities, has not been considered.[2] The incidence of coronal imbalance in adult deformities varies between 19.3 and 34.8%.[3–5] It is often difficult to correct both the coronal plane and the sagittal plane, especially in curvatures that are rigid. The complication rate in adult deformity surgery is quite high. The incidence of major complications varies between 30 and 60% and the need for repeat surgery ranges from 10 to 42%.[6]

Coronal imbalance after surgery causes pain, loss of function, and decreased quality of life.[7,8] Daubs et al reported that having more than 4-cm central sacral vertical line (CSVL) before surgery changed the SRS-22 scores. Acaroğlu et al reported that one of the factors affecting health-related quality-of-life (HRQOL) values after surgery was coronal imbalance. Ploumis et al reported that coronal imbalance before surgery affected the surgical results more significantly than sagittal imbalance.[8–12] Koller et al reported that CSVL increased after surgery, affecting the postsurgical clinical condition in patients.[8]

Therefore, maintaining sagittal balance during surgery as well as maintaining coronal balance will increase the chances of success.

Pearl

Coronal balance is correlated with health-related quality-of-life (HRQOL).

How is Coronal Balance Assessed?

All spinal vertebrae should be seen on the standing scoliosis radiography. The distance between the vertical line down from T1 or C7 (C7PL-C7 Plumb Line) and the central vertical line (CSVL) shows the coronal balance distance (CBD) (**Fig. 13.1**).

If the vertical line down from C7 to the ground plane remains on the concave side of the main curvature in the lumbar region, the concave imbalance is mentioned, and if this line (C7 plumb line) remains on the convex side of the lumbar main curvature, the convex imbalance is mentioned. According to the publications of Bao and his colleagues, this distance is classified as Type A if below 3 cm on the concave side, Type B if more than 3 cm on the concave side, and Type C if more than 3 cm on the convex side[5] (**Table 13.1**).

An exact limit value has not been determined to be considered as coronal imbalance. Ploumis et al stated this value as 5 cm, while Daubs stated this value as 4 cm.[3,9,11,13] Obeid et al evaluated this value as 2 cm.[12]

Obeid et al evaluated the coronal imbalance in two groups:

Type 1. Concave coronal imbalance: In the anterior posterior scoliosis graph, if the

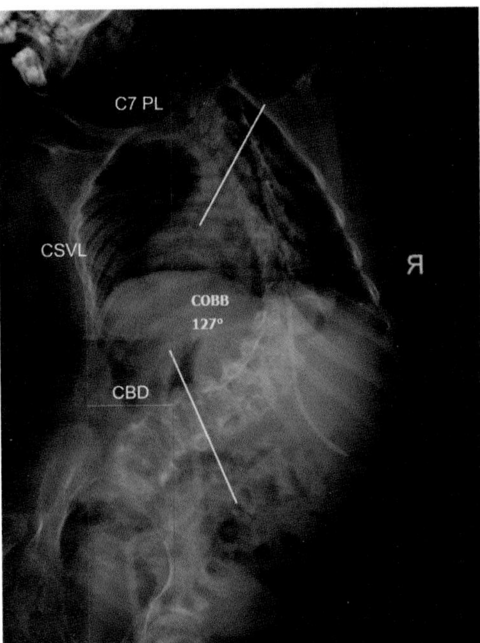

Fig. 13.1 Calculation of coronal balance: coronal balance distance (CBD) is the distance between C7PL (C7 plumb line) and central sacral vertical line (CSVL). CBD is shown by *white line*. C7PL (C7 plumb line) is shown by *red line*. CSVL is shown by *blue line*.

plumb line down from T1 remains on the concave side of the main coronal curvature (**Fig. 13.2**).

Type 2. Convex coronal imbalance: In the anterior posterior scoliosis graph, if the plumb line down from T1 remains on the convex side of the main coronal curvature (**Fig. 13.3**).

What are the Factors that Cause Coronal Imbalance?

The presence of L4 coronal tilt on the convex side before surgery, increased body mass index (BMI), wide coronal curvature, and osteoporosis are some factors that increase coronal imbalance after surgery.[14]

Table 13.1 Classification of coronal imbalance according to Bao et al.[5]

	Concave side	Convex side
Type A	<3 cm	
Type B	>3 cm	
Type C		>3 cm

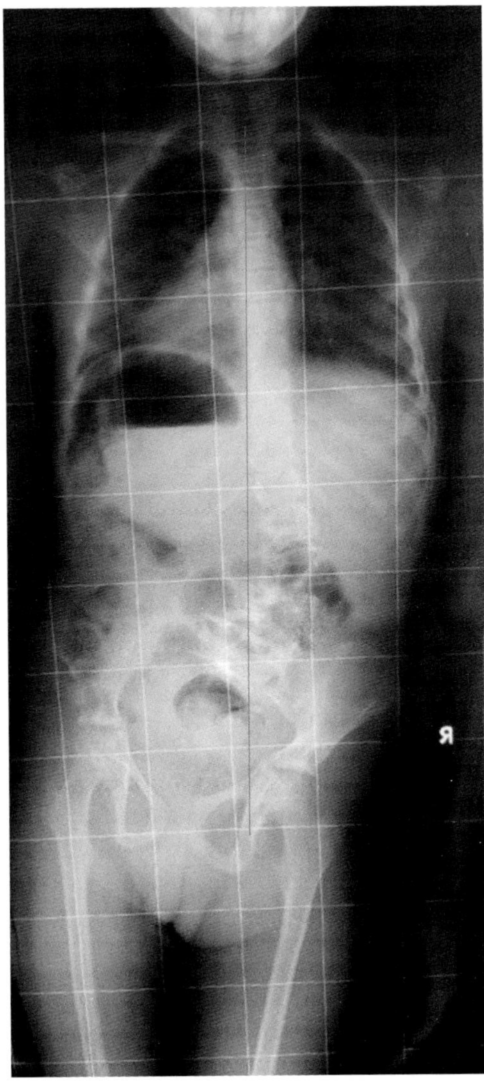

Fig. 13.2 T1 plumb line remains on the concave side of the main curvature (concave coronal curvature).

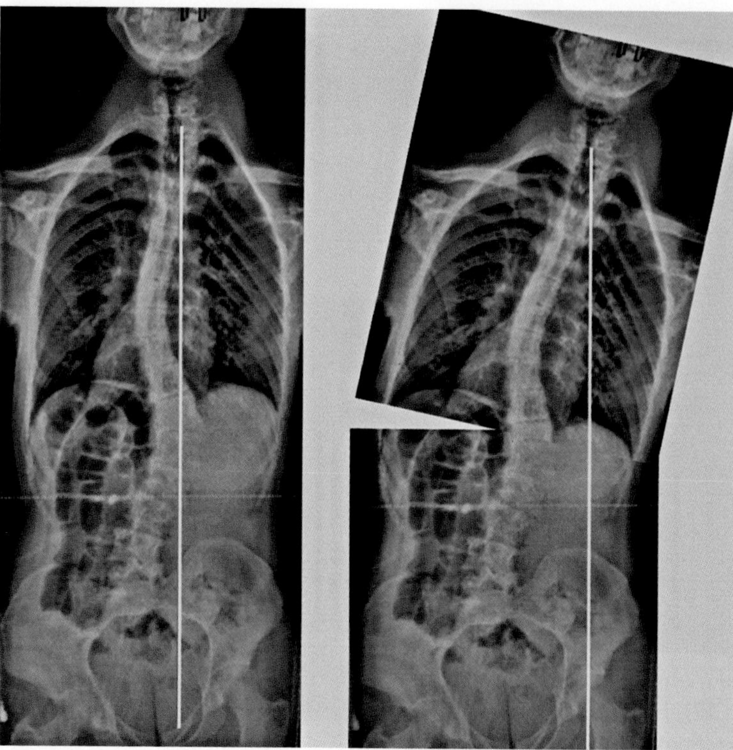

Fig. 13.3 T1 plumb line remains on the convex side of the main curvature (convex coronal curvature).

Correction of L4 and L5 tilts during surgery will correct the coronal imbalance that will occur after surgery. Lewis et al reported that 5-degree tilt at L4 level caused a coronal imbalance of approximately 3.5 cm at C7 level. Ensuring that the L4 and L5 pedicles are parallel in the Anterior Posterior (AP) fluoroscopic images during surgery will give the surgeon an idea of whether it corrects coronal balance or not.[14]

Also Sitte et al in his publications reported that residual in the lower instrument vertebra (LIV) caused degeneration in the adjacent segment and increased the rates of add-on and revision surgery.[15]

It is necessary to pay attention to the correction of the fractional curvature in the lumbosacral region, especially when correcting the curvature in the lumbar region. Distraction of the concave curvature, especially in the lumbosacral region, corrects the curvature in the coronal plane, but since it is a kyphotic maneuver in the sagittal plane, it causes the reduction in lumbar lordosis. The main cause of coronal imbalance that occurs after surgery is lumbosacral fractional curvature rather than lumbar main curvature.[14]

Pearls

- Increased BMI, L4 convex tilt increases coronal imbalance after surgery.
- Residual in the lower instrument vertebra causes degeneration in the adjacent segment.

Factors that Increase the Rate of Pseudoarthrosis[16–18]

- Preoperative lumbar lordosis (LL), sagittal vertical axis (SVA), high pelvic incidence (PI).
- Failure to provide lumbar lordosis after surgery.
- Postoperative SVA > 5 cm.
- High BMI.[3–5]

Distal Adjacent Segment Disease (ASD)

Standing in the distal movable lumbar vertebra while performing long-segment instrumentation increases the rate of distal ASD 9-33%.[19,20] High postsurgical SVA and lumbar hypolordosis are other factors that increase distal ASD. Another factor is the increased lordotic L5–S1 disc angle. High unfractionated curvature increases distal ASD after surgery.[20]

Proximal ASD and Proximal Junctional Kyphosis (PJK)

Patients with long-segment instrumentation have a 13 to 39%, average 20%, risk of developing proximal ASD.[19,21,22] Factors that increase the rate of proximal ASD include elderly patients, overcorrection of the lobar lordosis, and overcorrection of the SVA.[23]

Factors that increase proximal PJK include major corrections in lumbar lordosis and SVA, elderly patients, low BMD, thoracic kyphosis >30 degrees, ligament injury, lack of sagittal balance, and instrumentation to the sacrum.[21,23,24]

How is Coronal Imbalance Corrected?

Obeid et al's classification is important because of the definition of coronal imbalance and its guidance in surgical treatment.[12]

Accordingly, modifiers have been defined.

- Mobility of the main coronal curvature (Flexible/Rigid).
- Mobility of the lumbosacral junction (Flexible/Rigid).
- Degeneration of the lumbosacral junction (Little or no/Advanced).

Basically, correction of the main curvature in concave curves corrects coronal imbalance, while correction of the main curvature in convex curves increases coronal imbalance[12] (**Fig. 13.4** and **Fig. 13.5**).

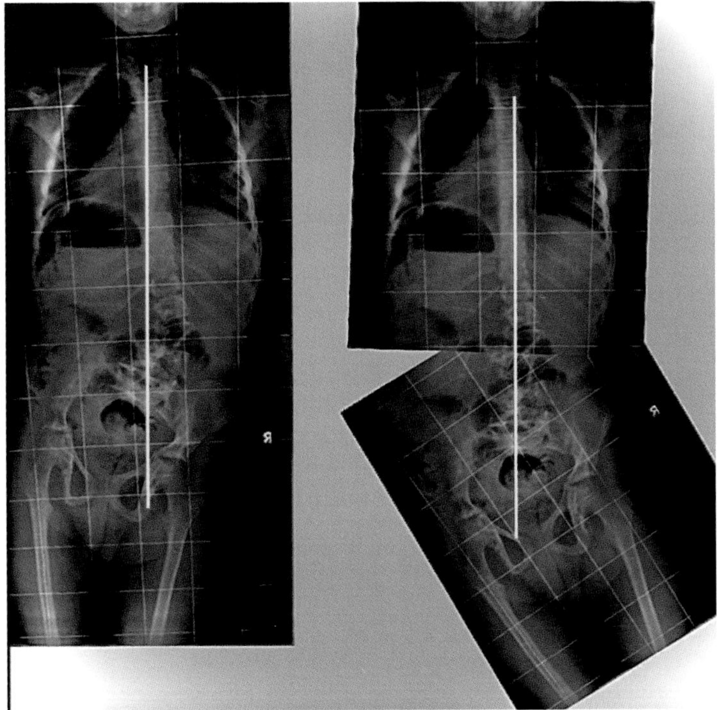

Fig. 13.4 Type 1 concave coronal imbalance. When the main curvature is corrected, the coronal curvature is corrected.

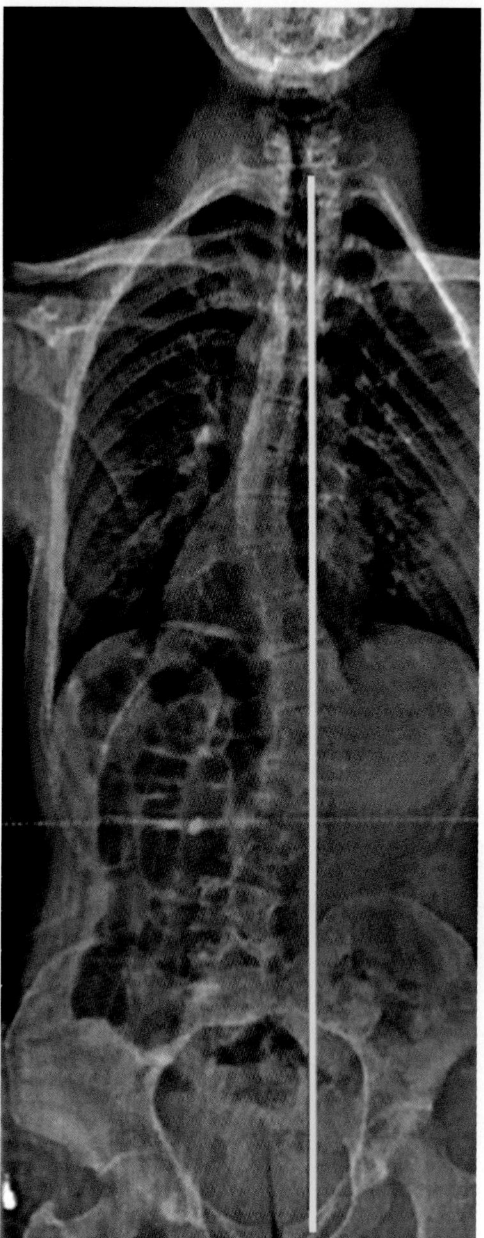

Fig. 13.5 Type 2 convex coronal imbalance. The coronal curvature is further increased when the main curvature is corrected.

Type 1 Concave Coronal Imbalance[12]

It is divided into two subgroups according to the location of the main coronal curvature.

Type 1A: The main curvature is located in the lumbar or thoracolumbar region. (Apex is between T12 and L4.)

Type 1B: The main curvature is located in the thoracic or cervicothoracic region. (Apex is above T12.)

According to the above-mentioned mobility, according to the movement of the main curvature located in the lumbar or thoracolumbar region, it is defined as Type 1A1 if it is mobile, and Type 1A2 if it is nonmobile. In Type 1A1, which is mobile, stabilization with posterior relaxation is sufficient, while in Type 1A2, which is rigid, correction is required with three-column osteotomies[12] (**Fig. 13.6** and **Fig. 13.7**).

In Type 1B, where the main curvature is located in the thoracic or cervicothoracic region, osteotomy of three columns is usually recommended for correction.[12]

Type 2 Convex Coronal Imbalance[12]

It is divided into two subgroups according to the location of the main coronal curvature.

Type 2A: The main curvature is located in the lumbar or thoracolumbar region. (Apex is between T12 and L4.)

Type 2B: The main curvature is at L4 and below.

The lumbosacral junction mentioned above was defined according to mobility: Type 2A1 if mobile and Type 2A2 if rigid. Type 2A1, which is flexible, requires correction of the main curvature by posterior relaxation, whereas Type 2A2, which is rigid, requires correction by three-column osteotomies. In Type 2B, it is recommended to correct the lumbosacral junction as a short segment with three-colon osteotomy[12] (**Fig. 13.8**).

Pearls

- Direct correction of type II (convex coronal imbalance) will progress coronal imbalance following the surgery.
- Fractional curve should be considered.

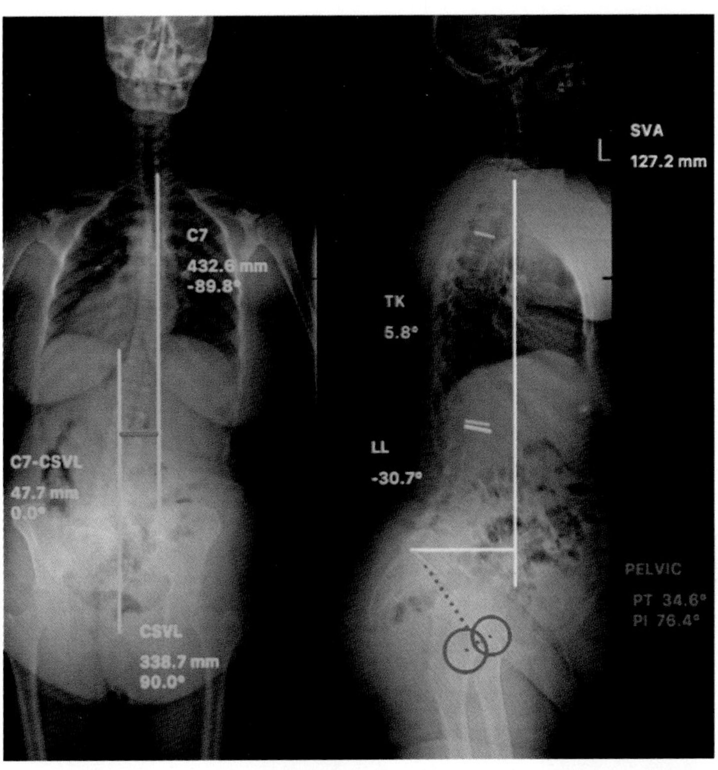

Fig. 13.6 A 49-year-old female patient has increasing complaints of lower back and leg pain. Type 1A1 concave coronal imbalance along with sagittal imbalance was detected on the scoliosis radiographs of the patient. The main curvature of the patient was in the lumbar region (Type 1A) and the main curvature was seen to be flexible on the lateral bending radiographs (Type 1A1). In this patient, it is suggested that the main curvature can be corrected by posterior relaxation. CSVL, central sacral vertical line; LL, lumbar lordosis; PT, pelvic tilt; PI, pelvic incidence.

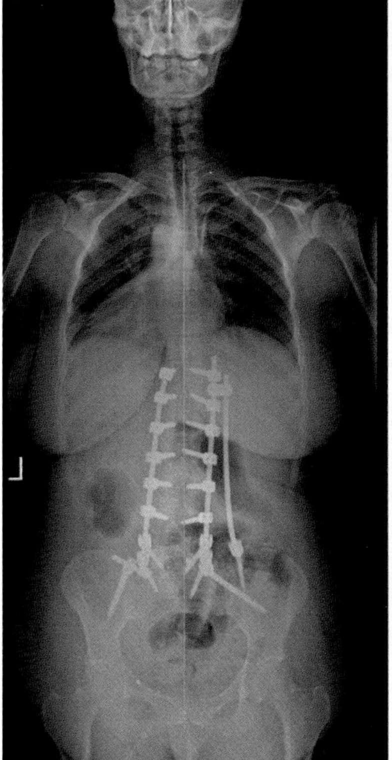

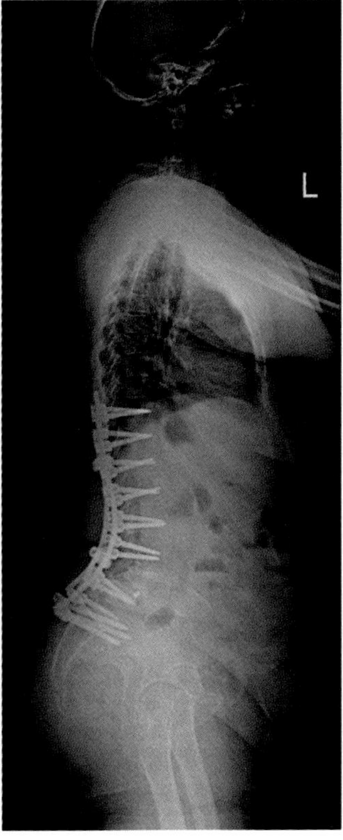

Fig. 13.7 Because the patient needed more lumbar lordosis due to the high pelvic incidence (PI) and sagittal vertical axis (SVA) was 12.7 cm, the patient underwent L4 corner osteotomy and posterior relaxation to other levels. Coronal and sagittal balance of the patient is provided after surgery.

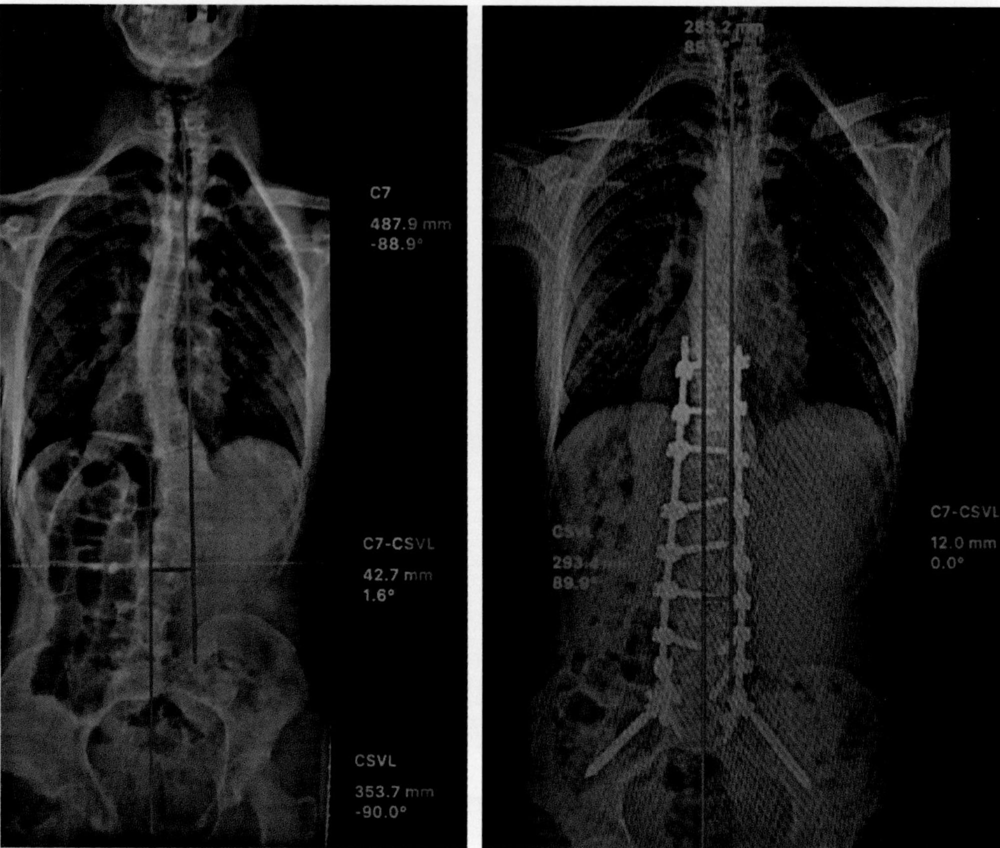

Fig. 13.8 A 37-year-old male patient with late period adolescent idiopathic scoliosis (AIS). The patient has a convex coronal imbalance on the Anterior Posterior (AP) scoliosis radiograph. On the side-bending scoliosis graph, the lumbosacral (LS) junction was mobile (Type 2A1). Coronal curvature and coronal imbalance of the patient were corrected by posterior relaxation. Coronal imbalance, which was 4 cm before surgery, was detected as 1.2 cm after surgery. CSVL, central sacral vertical line.

Coronal Balance Correction Techniques

Asymmetric pedicle subtraction osteotomy (PSO) and interbody cage application are effective methods that can be used to correct coronal imbalance.[12,13] These are also recommended for combined imbalance or rare pure coronal imbalance. However, there are some disadvantages such as high complication rates and high pseudoarthrosis rates.[25]

Kickstand Rod Technique (KRT) and Tie Rod Technique (TRT)

In order to correct coronal imbalance, Makhni et al described these techniques.[26] In the coronal plane, forces applied during the distraction maneuver cause the loss of lordosis in the sagittal plane. If lumbar lordosis is provided, kickstand rod is sufficient.[27] However, in patients where lumbar lordosis cannot be achieved, the application of

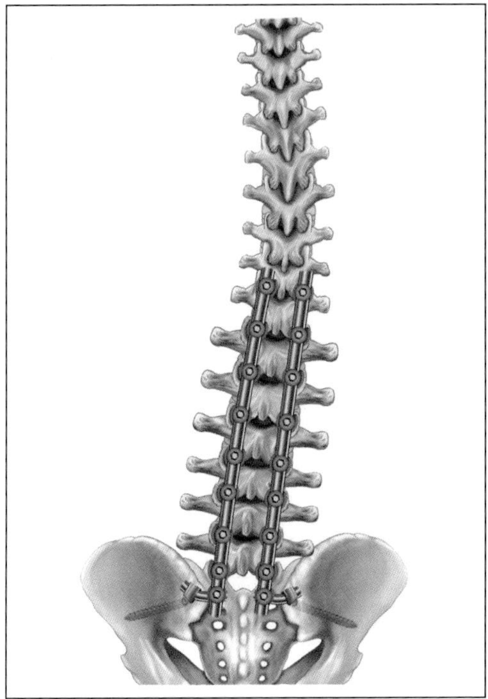

Fig. 13.9 Iliac wing screw placed on the patient's right iliac wing with coronal balance toward the right side.

compression forces on the rod placed on the other side (tie rod) will correct the coronal plane, as well as correct the lumbar lordosis in the sagittal plane.[27] The iliac wing screw is placed perpendicular to the right iliac wing of the patient, where the coronal imbalance is shifted to the right side, for example (**Fig. 13.9**).

A new rod is placed on the screw placed in the iliac wing, and this rod is combined with the previously placed rod using an open domino at the thoracolumbar junction (**Fig. 13.10**).

The screw heads on the rod that were placed earlier are loosened (for the rod placed on the right side, and not for the extra rod placed on the iliac wing) (**Fig. 13.11**).

The screw head on the domino side of the extra rod placed in the iliac wing is loosened and the distal end is tightened. Distraction is done with the help of a strong rod holder (**Fig. 13.12**). The screw head located inside the Domino and the rod that had been placed before is tightened. With intraoperative fluoroscopy, coronal balance and the level

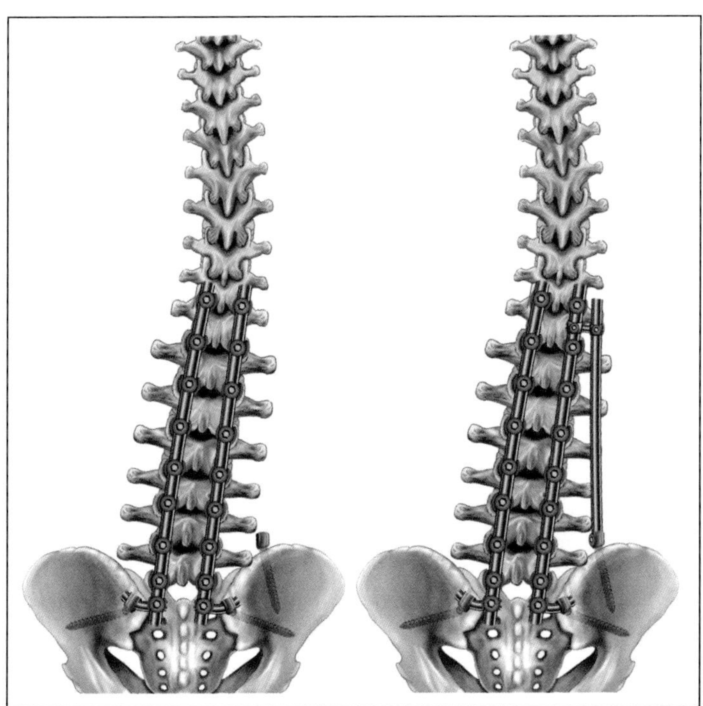

Fig. 13.10 Additional rod placement. The open-top domino is placed in the thoracolumbar junction to increase the force arm.

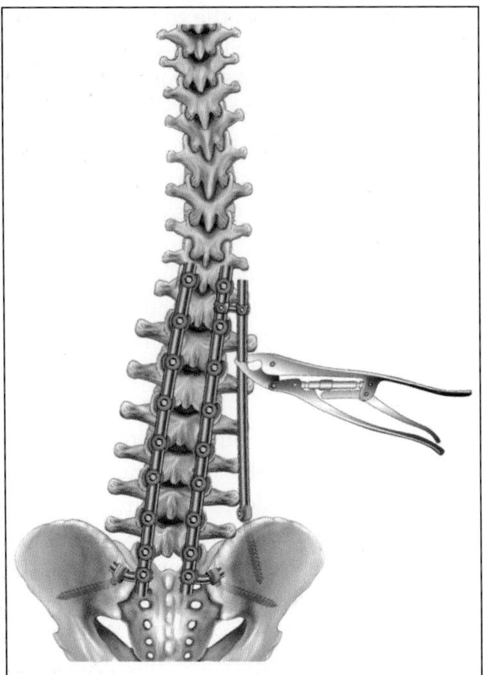

Fig. 13.11 Strong rod holder is placed on the extra placed rod.

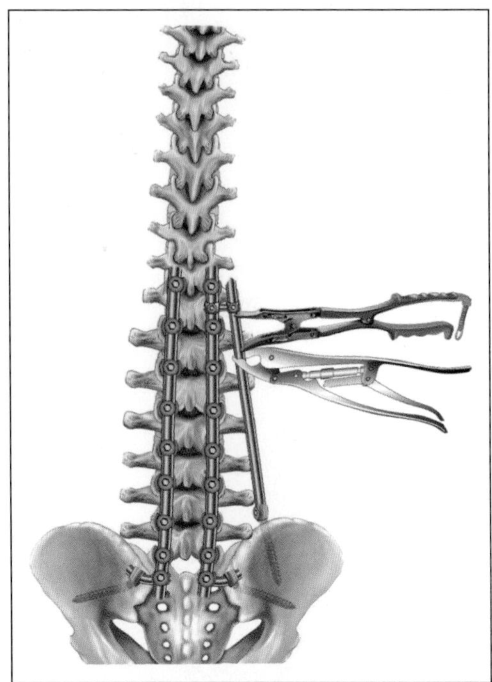

Fig. 13.12 The coronal imbalance is corrected by distracting the rod placed in the iliac wing.

of iliac wings are checked. Pre- and postoperative images of the patient whose coronal imbalance was corrected with kickstand rod technique are provided in **Fig. 13.6** and **Fig. 13.7**.

Pearl

Kickstand and tie rod techniques are useful techniques to correct coronal imbalance.

References

1. Schwab FJ, Hawkinson N, Lafage V, et al; International Spine Study Group. Risk factors for major peri-operative complications in adult spinal deformity surgery: a multi-center review of 953 consecutive patients. Eur Spine J 2012;21(12):2603–2610
2. Lafage V, Schwab F, Patel A, Hawkinson N, Farcy JP. Pelvic tilt and truncal inclination: two key radiographic parameters in the setting of adults with spinal deformity. Spine 2009;34(17):E599–E606
3. Ploumis A, Simpson AK, Cha TD, Herzog JP, Wood KB. Coronal spinal balance in adult spine deformity patients with long spinal fusions: a minimum 2- to 5-year follow-up study. J Spinal Disord Tech 2015;28(9): 341–347
4. Moal B, Schwab F, Ames CP, et al; International Spine Study Group. Radiographic outcomes of adult spinal deformity correction: a critical analysis of variability and failures across deformity patterns. Spine Deform 2014;2(3):219–225
5. Bao H, Yan P, Qiu Y, Liu Z, Zhu F. Coronal imbalance in degenerative lumbar scoliosis: prevalence and influence on surgical decision-making for spinal osteotomy. Bone Joint J 2016;98-B(9):1227–1233
6. Scheer JK, Tang JA, Smith JS, et al; International Spine Study Group. Reoperation rates and impact on outcome in a large, prospective, multicenter, adult spinal deformity database: clinical article. J Neurosurg Spine 2013; 19(4):464–470

7. Acaroğlu E, Guler UO, Olgun ZD, et al; European Spine Study Group. Multiple regression analysis of factors affecting health-related quality of life in adult spinal deformity. Spine Deform 2015;3(4):360–366
8. Koller H, Pfanz C, Meier O, et al. Factors influencing radiographic and clinical outcomes in adult scoliosis surgery: a study of 448 European patients. Eur Spine J 2016; 25(2):532–548
9. Daubs MD, Lenke LG, Bridwell KH, et al. Does correction of preoperative coronal imbalance make a difference in outcomes of adult patients with deformity? Spine 2013; 38(6):476–483
10. Acaroğlu E, Guler UO, Yavu Y, et al; European Spine Study Group. Multiple regression analysis of factors affecting HRQL in adult spinal deformity. In: 20th IMAST, 2013; Vancouver, Canada
11. Ploumis A, Liu H, Mehbod AA, Transfeldt EE, Winter RB. A correlation of radiographic and functional measurements in adult degenerative scoliosis. Spine 2009;34(15): 1581–1584
12. Obeid I, Berjano P, Lamartina C, Chopin D, Boissière L, Bourghli A. Classification of coronal imbalance in adult scoliosis and spine deformity: a treatment-oriented guideline. Eur Spine J 2019;28(1):94–113
13. Cecchinato R, Berjano P, Aguirre MF, Lamartina C. Asymmetrical pedicle subtraction osteotomy in the lumbar spine in combined coronal and sagittal imbalance. Eur Spine J 2015;24(Suppl 1):S66–S71
14. Lewis SJ, Keshen SG, Kato S, Dear TE, Gazendam AM. Risk factors for postoperative coronal balance in adult spinal deformity surgery. Global Spine J 2018;8(7):690–697
15. Sitte I, Kathrein A, Pfaller K, et al. Morphological differences in adolescent idiopathic scoliosis: a histological and ultrastructural investigation. Spine 2013;38(19):1672–1680
16. Kim YJ, Bridwell KH, Lenke LG, Rhim S, Kim Y-W. Is the T9, T11, or L1 the more reliable proximal level after adult lumbar or lumbosacral instrumented fusion to L5 or S1? Spine 2007;32(24):2653–2661
17. Cho K-J, Suk SI, Park SR, et al. Risk factors of sagittal decompensation after long posterior instrumentation and fusion for degenerative lumbar scoliosis. Spine 2010;35(17): 1595–1601
18. Le Huec JC, Aunoble S, Philippe L, Nicolas P. Pelvic parameters: origin and significance. Eur Spine J 2011;20(Suppl 5):564–571
19. Kelly MP, Lenke LG, Bridwell KH, Agarwal R, Godzik J, Koester L. Fate of the adult revision spinal deformity patient: a single institution experience. Spine 2013;38(19):E1196–E1200
20. Charosky S, Guigui P, Blamoutier A, Roussouly P, Chopin D; Study Group on Scoliosis. Complications and risk factors of primary adult scoliosis surgery: a multicenter study of 306 patients. Spine 2012;37(8):693–700
21. Maruo K, Ha Y, Inoue S, et al. Predictive factors for proximal junctional kyphosis in long fusions to the sacrum in adult spinal deformity. Spine 2013;38(23):E1469–E1476
22. Yagi M, Hosogane N, Okada E, et al; Keio Spine Research Group. Factors affecting the postoperative progression of thoracic kyphosis in surgically treated adult patients with lumbar degenerative scoliosis. Spine 2014;39(8):E521–E528
23. Yagi M, Akilah KB, Boachie-Adjei O. Incidence, risk factors and classification of proximal junctional kyphosis: surgical outcomes review of adult idiopathic scoliosis. Spine 2011;36(1):E60–E68
24. Berjano P, Lamartina C. Classification of degenerative segment disease in adults with deformity of the lumbar or thoracolumbar spine. Eur Spine J 2014;23(9):1815–1824
25. Obeid I, Boissière L, Vital J-M, Bourghli A. Osteotomy of the spine for multifocal deformities. Eur Spine J 2015;24(Suppl 1): S83–S92
26. Makhni MC, Cerpa M, Lin JD, Park PJ, Lenke LG. The "Kickstand Rod" technique for correction of coronal imbalance in patients with adult spinal deformity: theory and technical considerations. J Spine Surg 2018;4(4): 798–802
27. Redaelli A, Langella F, Dziubak M, et al. Useful and innovative methods for the treatment of postoperative coronal malalignment in adult scoliosis: the "kickstand rod" and "tie rod" procedures. Eur Spine J 2020;29(4): 849–859

14 Osteotomies in Adult Spinal Deformity

Paul Page, Eric Momin, and Nathaniel P. Brooks

Introduction

The ultimate objective when considering the correction of spinal deformities is to obtain normal upright spinal balance. In cases of severe spinal imbalance or rigid spine deformities, osteotomies are frequently necessary to achieve an adequate correction. Rigid deformities may by present in a variety of spondyloarthropathies, such as ankylosing spondylitis, and iatrogenically from prior spinal fusions. While osteotomies are rarely necessary in the pediatric population, these are commonly necessary in the adult population as these curves are typically inflexible as compared to their pediatric counterparts. Adult spinal deformity is highly prevalent, with some studies citing up to 68% of asymptomatic patients aged 60 years or older meeting radiographic criteria for an underlying spinal deformity.[1] With the relatively recent characterization of spinopelvic parameters, numerous studies have demonstrated the high correlation with pain and disability when these parameters are abnormal. Correction of these parameters have additionally been shown to result in improved pain and disability scores in health-related quality of life scales, especially in regard to sagittal imbalance.[2,3] As a result of these studies, when considering surgical correction most adults should be corrected to have a sagittal vertical axis of less than or equal to 5 cm, pelvic tilt less than 25 degrees, and lumbar lordosis within 10 degrees of the pelvic incidence.[4,5] When considering the evaluation and treatment of the aging population, it is crucial for spine surgeons to have a complete and modern understanding of osteotomies and their use in the correction of spinal deformities.

History of Spinal Osteotomies

Spinal deformity is one of the oldest pathologies recorded in history. Prior to safe surgical intervention for these pathologies, the vast majority of these treatments were done nonoperatively with a variety of spinal traction or bracing devices. Given the significant challenges to surgical intervention for spinal deformity, it wasn't until the advancement of surgical techniques in the late nineteenth and early twentieth centuries that surgical intervention became a viable option. The first described osteotomy was described in 1922 by Mac-Lennan as a vertebral column resection (VCR) for severe scoliosis.[6] Shortly following this, in 1945 Smith-Petersen described a novel extension, or chevron, osteotomy to allow for lordosis correction without the invasiveness of a full VCR. The Smith-Petersen osteotomy was initially described as an open-wedge osteotomy involving multiple levels through previously fused articular processes of L1, L2, and L3 as well as adjacent spinous processes.[7] Due to the mobility requirement of the anterior column with the Smith-Petersen technique, in 1985 Thomasen and colleagues introduced the now widely popular pedicle subtraction osteotomy (PSO).[8] The mid to late 1900s were marked by dramatic advancements in spinal instrumentation. Subsequently, a variety of combination osteotomies have been described as well as predictive data to assist the surgeon in decision-making regarding the number and location of osteotomies to be performed.

Schwab Anatomic Osteotomy Classification

The Schwab Anatomic Classification System was developed in 2013 as an anatomic classification for osteotomies in order to provide a consistent classification based upon the amount of bony resection and degrees of correction received from each. Prior to this classification system, a large number of spinal osteotomies had been previously described; however, no consensus regarding their classification had been developed. This grading system ranges from Grade 1 (partial facet joint resection) to Grade 6 (multiple VCRs) (**Table 14.1** and **Fig. 14.1**). In addition, modifiers have been added to denote the surgical approaches but not the column of the spine that has been destabilized.[9] In its original study, it demonstrated high rates of intraobserver and interobserver reliability.

Table 14.1 The Schwab anatomic classification system

Schwab classification	Description
Grade 1	Partial facet joint resection
Grade 2	Complete facet joint resection
Grade 3	Pedicle and partial body resection
Grade 4	Pedicle, partial body, and disc resection
Grade 5	Complete vertebra and disc resection
Grade 6	Multiple adjacent vertebrae and disc resection

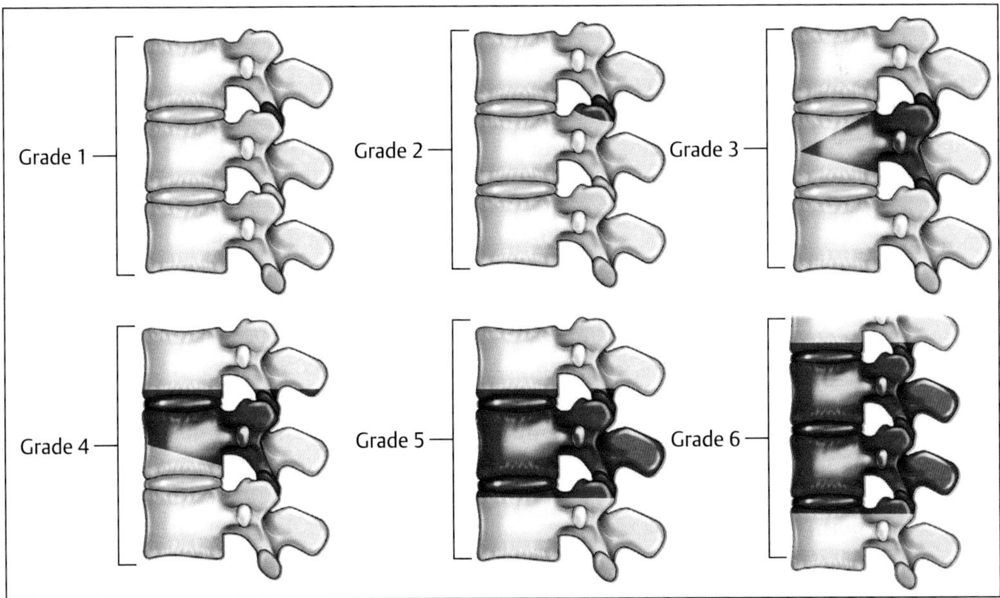

Fig. 14.1 Schwab classification system of spinal osteotomies. Adapted from Schwab et al 2015.[9]

Facet Osteotomy

Posterior facet osteotomies, also sometimes called Smith-Petersen osteotomies (SPO) or wedge osteotomies, create an osteotomy through the facet without disruption of the underlying pedicle. These facet osteotomies can be classified as type I or type II in the Schwab classification system. The type I posterior column osteotomy (PCO) is commonly employed to increase fusion surface area, assist in mobilization of flexible curves, and uncover the pedicle entry sites. The type I PCO involves resection of the inferior facet and joint capsule alone. Ultimately these provide little change in correction, with some studies citing anywhere from 5 degrees to 10 degrees per level. Other terms to describe this type of osteotomy include the Chevron osteotomy and extension osteotomy.

Comparatively, the type II osteotomy is also a facet osteotomy; however, this osteotomy involves resection of both inferior and superior facets as well as the ligamentum flavum, and other posterior elements including the lamina. As in grade 1 osteotomies, the mobility of the disc space is key. Some degree of anterior column mobility is mandatory in order to obtain any degree of correction. While this is primarily conducted through a posterior approach, this may be combined with an anterior approach to allow for sectioning of the anterior longitudinal ligament (ALL) and/or disc space. Similar to a type II osteotomy, the Ponte osteotomy or Ponte procedure is the resection of multiple facet joints along with resection of the spinous processes as well as posterior column ligaments and, critically, extension of the anterior column via a fracture through the disc space to afford deformity correction. Originally, this osteotomy was described in use for Scheuermann kyphosis and adolescent idiopathic scoliosis. A recent review of 240 patients who underwent true Ponte osteotomies at every level of their kyphosis demonstrated that a large degree of correction can be achieved ranging from 80 degrees to 31 degrees when conducted correctly at a large number of levels.[10]

Pedicle Subtraction Osteotomy (PSO)

The PSO is a wedge closing osteotomy affecting all three columns. This osteotomy involves resection of the posterior elements and creation of a V-shaped bony wedge through the pedicle extending into the posterior aspect of the vertebral body. In this osteotomy, the disc spaces above and below remain intact. This osteotomy results in shortening of the posterior and middle columns without significantly altering the length of the anterior column. Once the osteotomy is completed, the remaining bony elements collapse down on themselves, producing the desired lordosis. The PSO has classically been described to create approximately 30 to 40 degrees of lordosis per level. While the traditional PSO is a grade 3 osteotomy according to the Schwab classification, extension into the disc space can be achieved to increase the resultant lordosis and would resultantly be classified as a grade 4 osteotomy. Inclusion of the disc space in the osteotomy is believed to result in less stretching of the great vessels anteriorly. Variants include the circumferential wedge bone resection described by Shimode et al.[11]

Given the versatility of this osteotomy, it has become a very popular choice for the correction of adult spinal deformities. In general, short angular deformity, positive global sagittal balance greater than 6 cm, and coexistent coronal deformity are considerations for PSO. The PSO also is indicated in patients with no anterior mobility at the level of the planned osteotomy and those with a prior circumferential fusion. Although the level of the PSO does not directly affect the total global sagittal balance, it can have beneficial effects on pelvic tilt when conducted at more caudal levels. An asymmetric PSO also can be useful in the correction of combined sagittal and coronal imbalances.

In addition to the versatility of the PSO, it provides the advantage of three-column bone-on-bone contact, resulting in very high rates of fusion. This high degree of bony contact is advantageous in cases of smokers and diabetics. Despite the high versatility associated with it, complication rates are widely variable between studies. In a recent retrospective review of 423 patients, the overall complication rate was cited as high as 42%, with the most common postoperative complication being an unplanned return to the operating room (OR) in 19% of cases.[12] In addition to relatively high complication rates, a study comparing PSO versus posterior spinal fusion without PSO demonstrated similar operative times, higher estimated blood loss, similar number of new neurologic deficits, and similar rates of medical complications.[13]

Vertebral Column Resection (VCR)

The greatest degree of bony resection and the osteotomy with the most capability for correction is the VCR. The VCR is defined as resection of the entire vertebral segment including the spinous process, lamina, pedicles, vertebral body, and disc above and below the vertebral body. The VCR is primarily utilized when the deformity is severe and fixed with trunk translation. It has also been described for the treatment of spinal column tumors, spondyloptosis, congenital kyphosis, and hemivertebral excision. In the thoracic region, it is vital to include resection of the rib head in order to achieve adequate motility. This procedure is usually performed through posterior approach only, but can also be done via a combined anterior and posterior approach. A cage or other type of anterior column support is always required in this procedure.

Despite the extreme amount of reduction possible with VCR, these techniques are rarely utilized because of high complication rates. Complication rates for VCR have been cited as high as 34% with neurologic compromise occurring in 17%; however, rates vary dramatically between authors.[14] During the posterior reconstruction, a high degree of spinal instability is present. Given this high degree of instability, subluxation, buckling, or compression of the spinal cord, it is not uncommon that severe neurologic compromise occurs. In addition to neurologic compromise, additional complications such as pneumothorax, hardware failure, and postoperative pulmonary complications are also relatively common. Given the risk of neurologic compromise, most authors recommend use of intraoperative neuromonitoring, and some evidence suggests this information may reduce rates of neurologic injury.[14]

Anterior Column Release

Posterior osteotomies combined with an anterior column release (ACR) are a relatively new approach. The ACR is an extension of the previously described anterolateral lumbar interbody fusion techniques by incorporating division of the ALL. Sectioning the ALL allows for a greater manipulation of the anterior and middle columns across the disc space. When combined with posterior osteotomies, the use of ACR allows for mobilization of all three columns through a minimally invasive approach. Early studies have demonstrated increases of up to 30 degrees of segmental lordosis as well as 16 to 31 degrees increase in mean global lordosis. In a recent review of 41 patients by Xu et al, it was found that the global lumbar lordosis increased on an average by 16.7 degrees and the pelvic incidence and lumbar lordosis mismatch reduced by an average of 15.1 degrees.[15] In this series, 37% of patients who developed proximal junctional kyphosis occurred with a threshold of 5 degrees and 9.8% with a threshold of 20 degrees. In their series, there were no reported vascular or neurologic complications. In 2018, Uribe et al produced a classification system of ACR with varying degrees of associated osteotomies.[16] This classification ranges from ACR with placement of a hyperlordotic cage to VCR with sectioning of the ALL (**Table 14.2**).

Table 14.2 Anterior column release classification of osteotomies

ACR classification	Description
Grade A	ALL release with hyperlordotic cage and intact posterior elements
Grade 1	ALL release with hyperlordotic cage and inferior facetectomy
Grade 2	ALL release with hyperlordotic cage and PCO (Schwab grade 2)
Grade 3	ALL release with hyperlordotic cage and three-column osteotomy through the adjacent vertebral body
Grade 4	ALL release with hyperlordotic cage and three-column osteotomy placed two vertebrae distal to the ACR implant
Grade 5	Vertebrectomy with ALL release

Abbreviations: ACR, anterior column release; ALL, anterior longitudinal ligament; PCO, posterior column osteotomy.

Pearls

- Facet osteotomies provide approximately 5 to 10 degrees of correction per level.
- Facet osteotomies are typically done at multiple levels if utilized to achieve correction.
- The PSO creates approximately 30 to 40 degrees of lordosis per level.
- VCR is associated with high rates of morbidity and mortality.

Surgical Technique in Osteotomies

In addition to the usual preparation for a deformity procedure, we recommend several additional steps to prepare for osteotomies. First, the use of a Jackson table is sufficient, but achieving the desired lordosis with a Jackson table can sometimes require either intraoperative repositioning maneuvers or significant persuasion on the rods. Primarily, repositioning can be done by extending the hips by placing additional padding under the thighs. A hinged table that allows adjustment of lordosis may be helpful but is not necessary. Second, for grade 3 osteotomies and above, we recommend careful measurement of the depth of the cuts to be made on a preoperative computed tomography (CT) and marking these measurements on the osteotome. These deep cuts are often made blindly, with the aorta and great veins on the opposite side, so a solid understanding of the depth of these cuts will provide peace of mind. Third, for grade 3 osteotomies and above, we recommend saving the osteotomy for later in the procedure. There is significant blood loss from any osteotomy involving the vertebral body, and if done first, this would slow down subsequent portions of the procedure. Finally, for grade 3 osteotomies and above, pedicle screws must already be placed as a temporary rod should be used contralateral to the working side to stabilize the spine and prevent translation or unplanned reduction. Surgical techniques used in our practice are described below.

Grade 1: Partial Facet Joint Resection

A ¾-inch osteotome (or drill) is placed with one tip at the pars and another tip at the lateral and inferior border of the lamina. Cutting here will release the facet of the inferior articulating process. Twist the osteotome to separate any remaining connections, and remove the inferior facet with a grabbing instrument. Alternately, the inferior facet can be drilled away (**Fig. 14.2**).

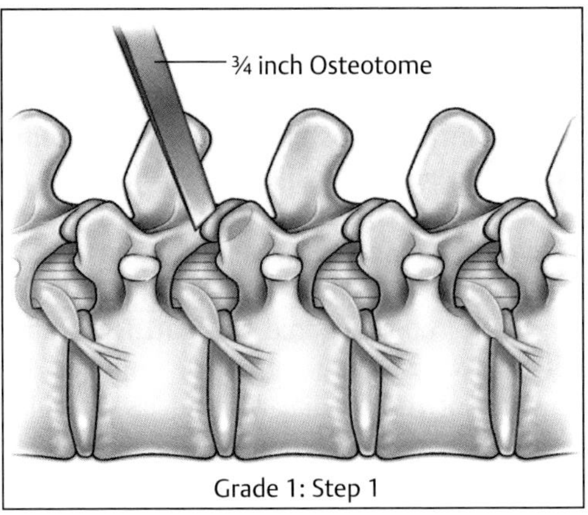

Fig. 14.2 Step one of grade 1 spinal osteotomy. An osteotome is placed with one tip in the pars and the other tip in the inferior border of the lamina. Cutting here removes the inferior facet.

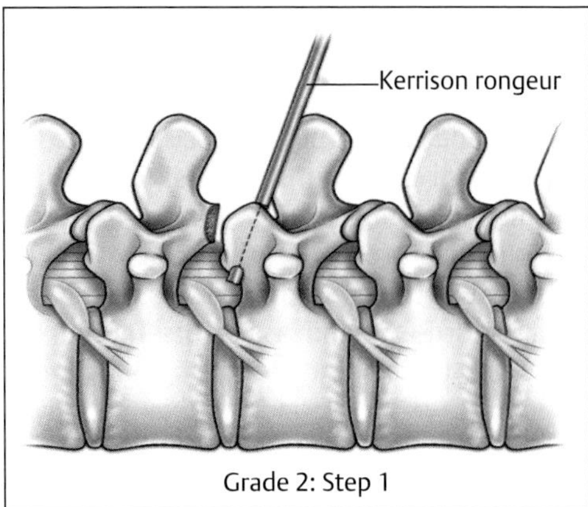

Fig. 14.3 Following removal of the inferior articular facet as described in **Fig. 14.2**, thinning of the crest of the superior facet with a drill can occur. After thinning of the superior facet, the remaining facet can be removed using a ronguer or biting instrument.

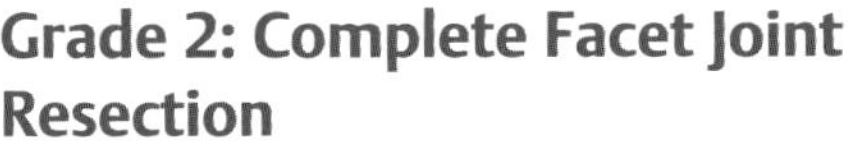

Grade 2: Complete Facet Joint Resection

Start with grade 1 osteotomy as described above and expose until the superior tip of the superior facet is visible. Dissect and expose the medial border of the superior facet. Thin the crest of the superior facet with drill and rongeur. Then place a punch underneath the overhang of the superior facet and remove pieces of bone. The punch follows a superior trajectory, hugging the medial wall of the pedicle, and then curving out laterally to hug the superior wall of the pedicle, unroofing the foramen (**Fig. 14.3**).

Grade 3: Pedicle and Partial Body Resection

Perform all instrumentation before starting this procedure. Perform a laminectomy and complete facet removal at the level above and below the planned osteotomy. Remove all bone until both pedicles are visible, like towers protruding from the vertebral body. Create a plane under each transverse process, and remove the transverse processes with a punch. Affix a temporary rod to the contralateral side. Establish a clear plane between the neural elements, and the bone and disc, with special attention to defining the area where the nerve root curves inferior to the pedicle. Use a small Cobb to establish a plane ventral to the vertebral body, and push a gauze sponge into this cavity in order to protect the ventral structures. Retract the thecal sac to the opposite side. Use an osteotome or bone scalpel in order to make a wedge-cut above the pedicle and then another wedge-cut below the pedicle. If using an ultrasonic bone drill (e.g., bone scalpel), we suggest connecting it to the navigation. If using an osteotome, we suggest making the cuts with use of frequent C-Arm X-rays to ensure the osteotome does not travel too ventrally. Remove pieces of bone from the wedge with a grabbing instrument. Switch temporary rods and then work on the contralateral side. It is not uncommon to be left with a bridge of bone centrally; this can be addressed with an osteotome from each side, and then with a down-pushing instrument. Once the wedge is created, the deformity needs to be corrected by closing the wedge. Ask neuromonitoring staff to monitor closely for any change in motor-evoked potentials (MEPs) or somatosensory-evoked potentials (SSEPs). The surgeon holds the hips and the temporary rod is loosened to allow compression but still resist translation. If using a Jackson table, the authors perform the following procedure: the surgeon slowly extends the thighs in order to establish the desired lordosis, and assistants in the OR will stack towels under the thighs in order to hold the new position. As this maneuver is being performed, the surgical assistant watches the thecal sac and nerve roots to look for any compression. In addition, it is important to watch for subluxation and rotation. This maneuver often fractures the last remaining fragment of bone just anterior to the wedge, causing a loud crack (**Fig. 14.4**). Alternatively, the new desired lordosis can be set by adjusting a mechanical table.

Grade 4

All posterior elements are removed from the inferior facet of the level above to the superior facet of the level below. A Discectomy is performed at the level above. Then, using techniques as described for the grade 3 osteotomy, a cut through the vertebral body is made, creating a wedge. The wedge is then closed using the same technique described for the grade 3 osteotomy (**Fig. 14.5**).

Grade 5

For the thoracic spine, practice of the authors is to perform this osteotomy via a posterior-only transpedicular approach. All posterior elements are removed from the inferior facet of the level above to the superior facet of the level below. The thecal sac is exposed and the nerve root is ligated and cut. The transverse processes are removed, followed by removal of the medial rib and its articulation at the costovertebral joint. The pedicles are eggshelled by drilling within, then the walls are carefully peeled away in a lateral direction. Discectomies are performed above and below. The vertebral body is drilled away. In the lumbar spine, we perform a 360-degree approach. This involves instrumentation first, then removal of the posterior elements, transverse processes, and pedicles via a posterior approach, then locking the instrumentation. Then the vertebral body is removed via a retroperitoneal exposure and a cage is placed. Finally, the back is opened again, and the instrumentation adjusted to achieve sagittal balance and coronal alignment (**Fig. 14.6**).

Grade 6

The technique is similar to that described for grade 5, except applied to multiple levels.

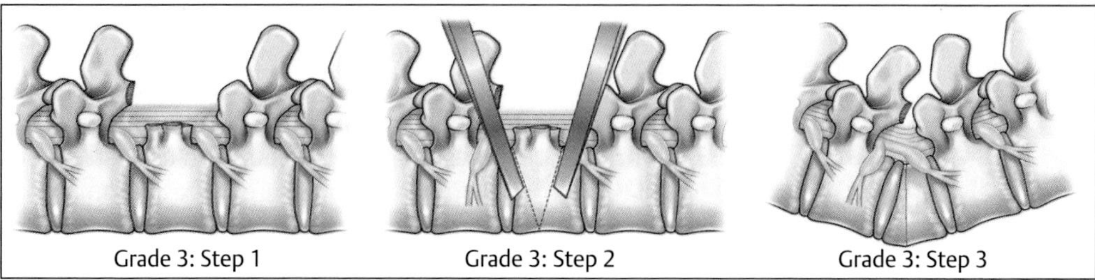

Fig. 14.4 Step 1 involves resection of the superior and inferior facets as described in the figures. Following removal of the facets, a portion of the pedicle is additionally resected bilaterally. Step 2 involves using an osteotome or bone scalpel to make a wedge-cut above and below the remaining pedicle into the vertebral body. Neuronavigation or frequent C-Arm X-rays may be utilized to ensure the body is not breached ventrally. Step 3 involves allowing deformity to close on itself, restoring lordosis by loosening the temporary rod that was placed earlier in the procedure.

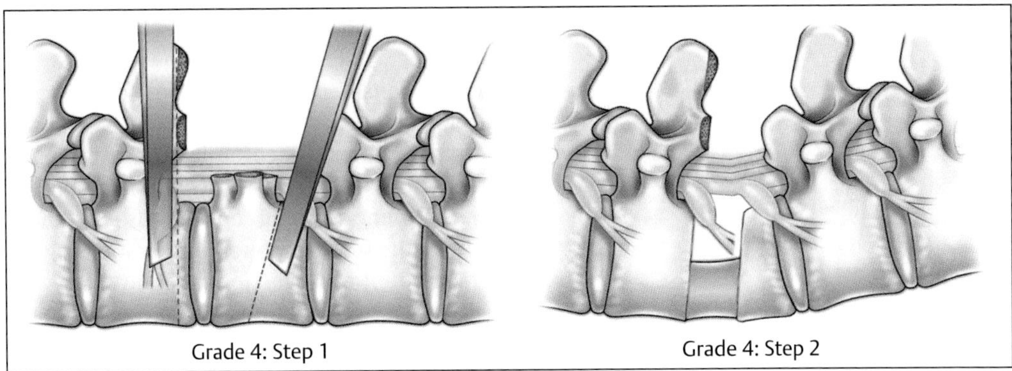

Fig. 14.5 Step 1 involves resection of the superior and inferior facets as well as part of the pedicle bilaterally. This is typically, as described in prior figures, utilizing an osteotome to remove the inferior articular facet, and the superior facet may be removed with a drill followed by a Rongeur. The majority of the pedicle is then resected as well. Step 2 involves completion of a discectomy at the level above the proposed osteotomy and a cut through the vertebral body to produce a wedge. The cut through the body can be conducted using a high-speed drill with a combination of neuronavigation or serial X-rays.

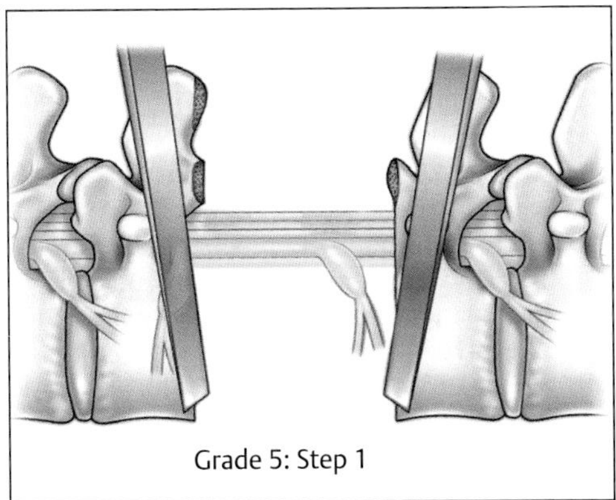

Fig. 14.6 Resection of the superior and inferior articular facets as well as the pedicle as described in other figures. Once the pedicles are resected, superior and inferior discectomies can be completed, followed by complete resection of the vertebral body. Prior to vertebral body resection, temporary rods are placed above and below the area of corpectomy to ensure a control reduction. Again, neuronavigation or serial X-rays may be utilized to limit the risk to the great vessels anteriorly.

When performed near the thoracolumbar junction, we prefer to obtain a spinal angiogram at this level in order to ensure that the recurrent anastomotic anterior spinal artery ("Artery of Adamkiewicz") is not sacrificed during the anterior corpectomy (**Fig. 14.7**).

Complication Avoidance in Osteotomies

Complication in spinal osteotomies is an unfortunate but common issue. In a recent 2014 study comparing posterior spinal fusion to patients undergoing three column osteotomies, rates of medical complications were reported as high as 73.7%.[13] Given the high percentage of medical complications in this group, a prolonged course of conservative therapy should be completed and a full preoperative risk evaluation should be performed prior to any elective three-column osteotomy including an evaluation of cardiovascular risk, obesity, smoking status, nutrition, diabetes, osteoporosis, and frailty.

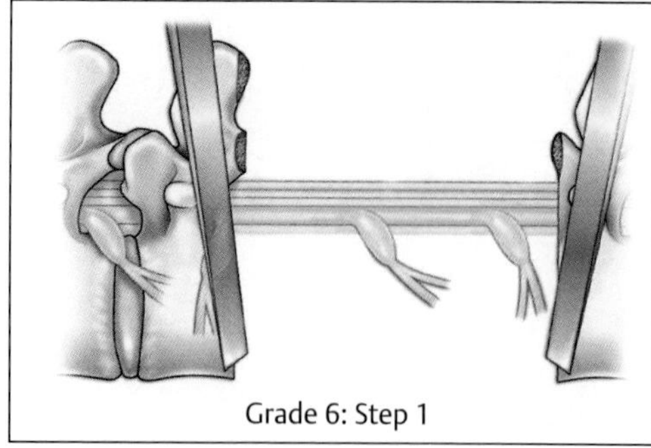

Fig. 14.7 Complete resection of multiple vertebrae as described in **Fig. 14.6**. Temporary rod placement is vital to ensure a controlled reduction. Neuromonitoring should be watched closely during reduction.

In addition to medical complications, neurologic complication avoidance is critical. As previously described, a variety of preventative strategies have been developed to reduce the incidence of neurologic complications. In one retrospective review of 43 patients undergoing posterior VCR, the use of monitoring identified seven patients (18%) who lost intraoperative neurogenic monitoring-evoked potentials during their correction. With this information, prompt intraoperative techniques were able to return them to their baseline without neurologic deficit as the conclusion of the case.[14] This is in direct comparison to studies which have not routinely utilized monitoring. Comparatively, one study by Suk et al, who did not use monitoring demonstrated neurologic complications in up to 25% of patients.[17] In authors' experience, neuromonitoring should be routinely used for any deformity correction.

Pearls

- Neurologic monitoring is recommended for cases of deformity correction.
- A full preoperative risk evaluation should be obtained prior to any deformity correction.

Conclusion

When considering osteotomies for complex rigid deformity correction, decisions are often complex. Osteotomies range dramatically from mild to great destabilizing potential. When deciding on the use of these procedures, a thorough understanding of the amount of correction is required, as well as risk and benefits to the various osteotomies is critical for surgical planning. Given the complexity of these procedures as well as high risk for severe complications, these procedures should be reserved for those with experience in complex deformity correction.

References

1. Schwab F, Dubey A, Gamez L, et al. Adult scoliosis: prevalence, SF-36, and nutritional parameters in an elderly volunteer population. Spine 2005;30(9):1082–1085
2. Blondel B, Schwab F, Ungar B, et al. Impact of magnitude and percentage of global sagittal plane correction on health-related quality of life at 2-years follow-up. Neurosurgery 2012;71(2):341–348, discussion 348
3. Daubs MD, Lenke LG, Bridwell KH, et al. Does correction of preoperative coronal imbalance make a difference in outcomes of adult patients with deformity? Spine 2013; 38(6):476–483
4. Glassman SD, Bridwell K, Dimar JR, Horton W, Berven S, Schwab F. The impact of positive sagittal balance in adult spinal deformity. Spine 2005;30(18):2024–2029
5. Schwab F, Lafage V, Patel A, Farcy JP. Sagittal plane considerations and the pelvis in the adult patient. Spine 2009;34(17):1828–1833
6. Meredith DS, Vaccaro AR. History of spinal osteotomy. Eur J Orthop Surg Traumatol 2014; 24(1, Suppl 1):S69–S72
7. Smith-Petersen MN, Larson CB, Aufranc OE. Osteotomy of the spine for correction of flexion deformity in rheumatoid arthritis. Clin Orthop Relat Res 1969;66(66):6–9
8. Thomasen E. Vertebral osteotomy for correction of kyphosis in ankylosing spondylitis. Clin Orthop Relat Res 1985; (194):142–152
9. Schwab F, Blondel B, Chay E, et al. The comprehensive anatomical spinal osteotomy classification. Neurosurgery 2015;76(Suppl 1): S33–S41, discussion S41

10. Ponte A, Orlando G, Siccardi GL. The true Ponte osteotomy: by the one who developed it. Spine Deform 2018;6(1):2–11
11. Shimode M, Kojima T, Sowa K. Spinal wedge osteotomy by a single posterior approach for correction of severe and rigid kyphosis or kyphoscoliosis. Spine 2002;27(20): 2260–2267
12. Bianco K, Norton R, Schwab F, et al; International Spine Study Group. Complications and intercenter variability of three-column osteotomies for spinal deformity surgery: a retrospective review of 423 patients. Neurosurg Focus 2014;36(5):E18
13. Kelly MP, Lenke LG, Shaffrey CI, et al. Evaluation of complications and neurological deficits with three-column spine reconstructions for complex spinal deformity: a retrospective Scoli-RISK-1 study. Neurosurg Focus 2014;36(5):E17
14. Lenke LG, Sides BA, Koester LA, Hensley M, Blanke KM. Vertebral column resection for the treatment of severe spinal deformity. Clin Orthop Relat Res 2010;468(3):687–699
15. Xu DS, Paluzzi J, Kanter AS, Uribe JS. Anterior column release/realignment. Neurosurg Clin N Am 2018;29(3):427–437
16. Uribe JS, Schwab F, Mundis GM, et al. The comprehensive anatomical spinal osteotomy and anterior column realignment classification. J Neurosurg Spine 2018;29(5): 565–575
17. Suk SI, Chung ER, Kim JH, Kim SS, Lee JS, Choi WK. Posterior vertebral column resection for severe rigid scoliosis. Spine 2005; 30(14):1682–1687

15 Osteotomies and Other Strategies for Cervical Deformity Correction

Mehmet Zileli and Salman Sharif

Introduction

Deformity of the cervical spine is a more difficult task than other regions of the spine. Reasons for these are most of the nerve roots in this region are eloquent, they cannot be sacrificed, and the vertebral artery should be preserved. Thrombosis or kinking of the dominant vertebral artery or both vertebral arteries can result in a catastrophic brainstem ischemia. Rigid fixation of the cervical spine would produce significant disability due to restriction of the head movements. Extensive anterior surgery of the cervical spine may create significant site-related complications (i.e., swallowing difficulty, dysphonia, respiratory problems).

Preoperative Planning

Before surgery, sagittal balance measurements should be done.[1] The main measures are cervical lordosis, the sagittal vertical axis (SVA), T1 slope, and chin-brow vertical angle (CBVA). Cervical lordosis (C2–C7) should be maintained less than 15 degrees, SVA should be less than 40 mm, CBVA must be between −10 and +20 degrees (**Table 15.1**).[2–4]

Table 15.1 Cervical deformity classification system proposed by Ames et al.[3]

Deformity descriptors	
C: Primary sagittal deformity apex in the cervical spine	
CT: Primary sagittal deformity apex at the cervicothoracic junction	
T: Primary sagittal deformity apex in the thoracic spine	
S: Primary coronal deformity (C2–C7 Cobb angle ≥15 degrees)	
CVJ: Primary craniovertebral junction deformity	
Five modifiers	
C2–C7 sagittal vertical axis (SVA)	**Horizontal gaze: chin-brow vertical angle (CBVA)**
0: <4 cm	0: CBVA 1 to 10 degrees
1: 4–8 cm	1: CBVA −10 to 0 degree or 11 to 25 degrees
2: >8 cm	2: CBVA <−10 or >25 degrees
Cervical lordosis minus T1 slope (TS-CL)	**Myelopathy (mJOA)**
0: TS-CL <15 degrees	0: mJOA = 18 (none)
1: TS-CL 15 to 20 degrees	1: mJOA = 15–17 (mild)
2: TS-CL >20 degrees	2: mJOA = 12–14 (moderate)
	3: mJOA = <12 (severe)
SRS–Schwab classification	
T, L, D, or N: Curve type	
0, +, or ++: PI minus LL	
0, +, or ++: Pelvic tilt	
0, +, or ++: C7–S1 SVA	

There are many modifiers of cervical kyphosis affecting our decision making, including (**Flowchart 15.1**):

- Flexibility of the deformity. This can be defined by having hyperflexion and hyperextension lateral radiographs.
- Neurological symptoms. Presence of one or multiple level canal compression.
- Level (location) of the kyphosis. C7 or lower versus C6 and upper.
- Kyphosis angle and presence of sharp/smooth angled kyphosis.[5]
- Patient's age and comorbidities.

We should evaluate dynamic X-rays, magnetic resonance imaging, and computed tomography to understand these details. The most crucial factor is the rigidity of the kyphosis. In rigid kyphosis, a posterior release or an osteotomy (anterior or posterior) will be necessary.

In flexible cases, a posterior-only surgery will be sufficient. Lateral mass screws can do it with some rigid orthosis or pedicle screw fixation, which is a more rigid fixation.

However, in rigid cases, the decision should be based on neurologic deficits and spinal cord compression. In case of neurologic deficits and rigid kyphosis, the surgery must contain anterior decompression of the spinal canal. If there are no neurological deficits but rigid kyphosis, an anterior or posterior osteotomy is possible. Anterior osteotomy should be chosen if the apex of the kyphosis is at C6 or more cranial, or if the kyphosis angle is very sharp and more than 90 degrees. A posterior osteotomy should be chosen if the apex of the kyphosis is at C7 or lower levels if it is a soft-angled kyphosis, or the reason for the kyphosis is ankylosing spondylitis.

Pearl

The most important determinant of cervical deformity surgery is its flexibility.

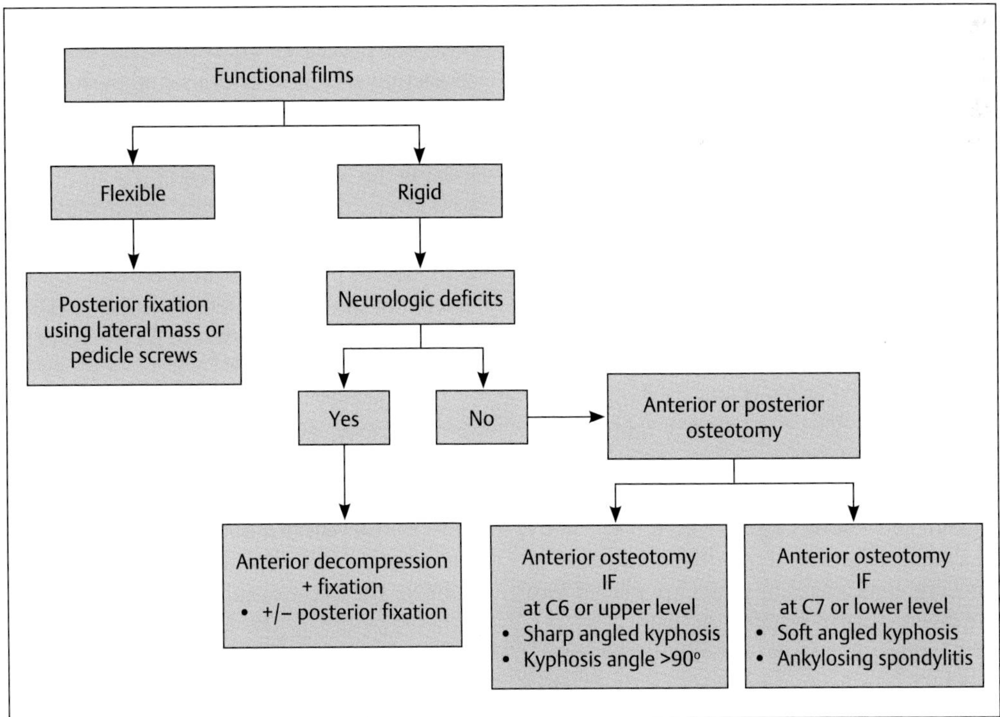

Flowchart 15.1 Algorithm to be used to manage cervical kyphosis.

Type of Surgery

Although very severe cervical deformities need both anterior and posterior combined approaches, you can choose anterior or posterior surgery in some instances. There are always gray zones that only anterior or posterior surgery may provide good deformity correction.[6]

Here we will summarize anterior and posterior techniques for cervical deformity correction and comment on when a combined surgery should be chosen.

Anterior Approaches

Most cervical deformities are with kyphosis. A ventral approach to any kyphosis will be safer than a dorsal approach. So, the surgeon should decide the goals of deformity surgery: deformity correction, restoration of horizontal gaze, decompression of the spinal cord and roots, etc.[7]

Anterior Cervical Discectomy and Fusion (ACDF) with Plate

Anterior cervical Discectomy and fusion or corpectomy and fusion with a plate are good techniques for cervical kyphotic deformity. Both methods can provide preservation or restoration of cervical lordosis, especially in flexible cases. However, if anterior cervical Discectomy and fusion are planned, anterior osteotomies will be necessary in rigid kyphotic cases. If applied at multiple levels, ACDF with a lordotic plate can still result in pseudoarthrosis, which may additionally require posterior fixation.

Preparation of disc spaces with curettes should be done using vertebral body spreaders. After the sequential distraction of the spreaders, cages or grafts are placed into the disc spaces to provide lordosis.

A lordotic plate can further help the reduction by first placing the screws on the cranial and caudal ends of the construct, then pulling the cervical spine ventrally with more central screws. However, this maneuver should not exert too many forces; otherwise, a correction loss with screw loosening will follow.

Pearl

Multilevel anterior cervical Discectomy, distraction using vertebral body spreaders, then disc cages, and placing a lordotic plate is effective in flexible cervical kyphosis.

Anterior Cervical Corpectomy (ACCF) with Plate

Corpectomy should be preferred in cases with cord compression at the vertebral body level or significant cord compression, patients with neurologic deficits, and subjects with a very sharp-angled kyphosis.

Anterior Osteotomy

Anterior cervical osteotomy is an effective technique for cervical deformity correction.[8,9] Anterior osteotomy can be done by drilling uncinate processes on both sides, carefully dissecting vertebral arteries, and performing anterior foraminotomies to decompress cervical roots. Although some authors prefer to have the head suspended in the air during supine position, the author use a Mayfield head holder to fix the patient's head as extended as possible. After osteotomy, more extension can be provided, and anterior strut grafts plus a plate are used to fix the spine in extension.

In some very kyphotic patients, intubation can be tricky, even with using a fiberoptic intubation device.

If the kyphosis angle is more than 70 degrees, the curve's apex is very deep into the wound, and dissection is very hard to achieve. The anterior tubercle of the foramen transversarium is the lateral border of the uncinate process, a landmark for the vertebral artery. The drilling must not go beyond lateral to the uncinate. After drilling, an osteotomy may further correct kyphosis by releasing the head-holder and compressing again.

In an anterior osteotomy, distractive forces should be applied to correct the deformity, and a graft or cage must be placed into the disc space to maintain correction (**Fig. 15.1**). It can be done in multiple levels to provide a significant reduction in kyphosis (**Fig. 15.2** and **Fig. 15.3a–e**).

Pearls

- Anterior cervical corpectomy is necessary if the kyphosis tip is at the body level, and in case of severe sharp-angled kyphosis.
- Anterior cervical osteotomy should involve uncinate processes and can be done at all subaxial levels.

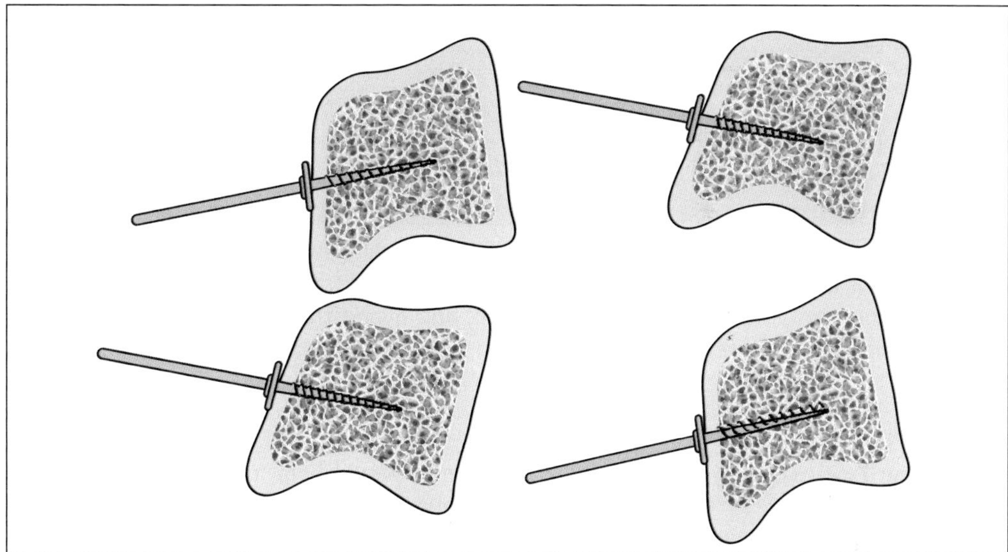

Fig. 15.1 Vertebral body distractor pins can help in reduction in kyphosis. The distraction of the pins opens the disc space, which should be supported by strut grafts or cages.

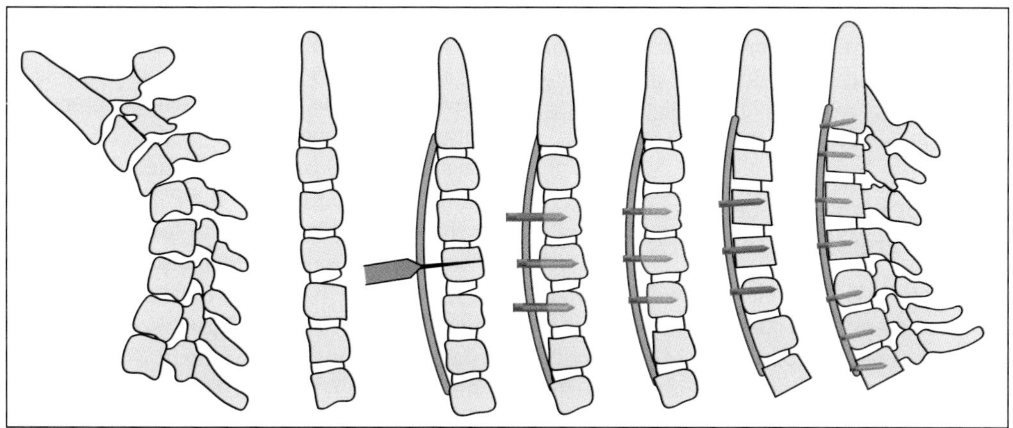

Fig. 15.2 Sequential reduction of cervical kyphosis using the anterior cervical screws and plate system.

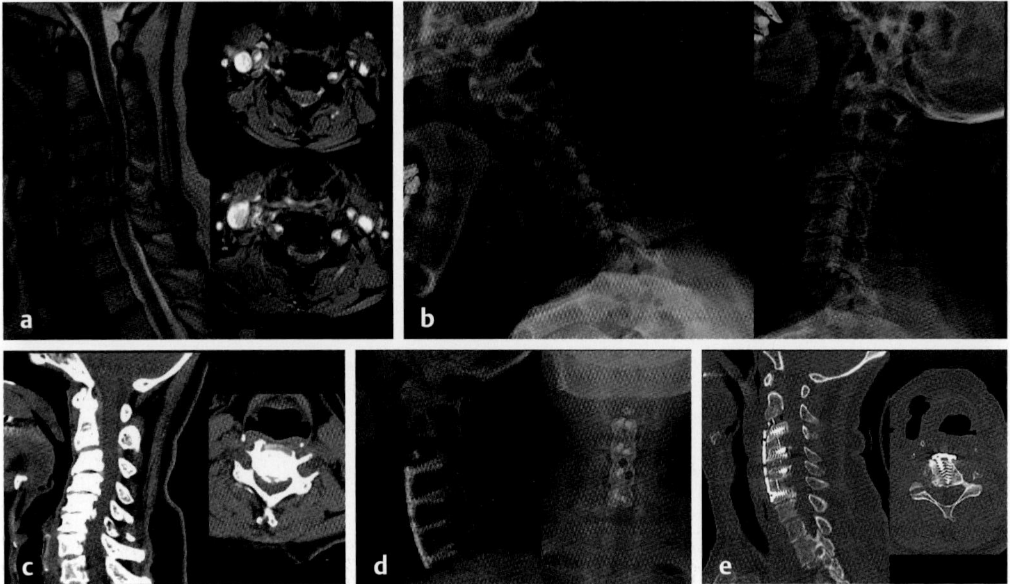

Fig. 15.3 (a–e) Multilevel anterior cervical Discectomy and fusion (ACDF) and plating for cervical sagittal imbalance (CSM) and kyphosis. A 59-year-old female had neck pain and right arm pain, motor weakness of flexors of right arm, and hypoesthesia. A four-level ACDF with cages and a lordotic plate corrected deformity and provided adequate decompression.

Posterior Techniques

Posterior Instrumentation and Fusion

This is a routine procedure for many spine surgeons. In flexible curves, lateral mass screws may be correct. However, if there is a more rigid curve, cervical pedicle screws will apply greater forces for reduction. Another option is to add some osteotomies (facet-lamina resection or pedicle subtraction osteotomy) for correction.[10]

Posterior Lamina-Facet Osteotomies (Smith-Petersen Osteotomy)

In the midcervical levels, removing laminae, spinous process, and part of facet joints is an option. In this case, pedicles, vertebral body, and transverse process are left intact, causing no compression or kinking to the vertebral artery. In the end, posterior compressive forces are applied to reduce the deformity. To provide more forces on compression, pedicle screws would help much than lateral mass screws. The surgeon must be aware that the nerve root is not compressed under the superior articular facet or pedicle.

Pedicle Subtraction Osteotomy (PSO)

PSO is safe at the caudal levels where the vertebral artery is not at the transverse foramen. This is primarily C7 or T1 level.[11,12] However, if the vertebral artery enters the foramen transversarium at C7 (5% of the cases), the PSO can be performed at T1.[10]

In the earlier cases,[13] the PSO was done in a sitting position and under local anesthesia. The advantage of this technique was neurologic monitoring of the awake patient and avoiding difficulties of intubation. However, many surgeons use prone position either with traction using Gardner-Wells tongs or fixation with a Mayfield head clamp[14] (**Fig. 15.4**). The authors' personal preference is to use the Mayfield head clamp; after finishing the osteotomy, release the clamp

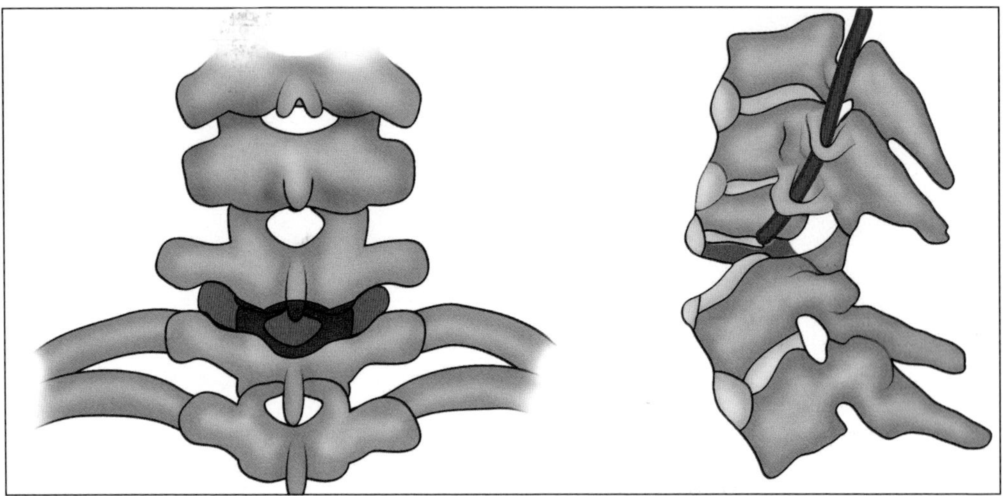

Fig. 15.4 C7 pedicle subtraction osteotomy. At the C7–T1 level, the vertebral artery does not create a problem.

and manually extend the head by closing the posterior gap (**Fig. 15.5a–e**).

Pearls

- Posterior cervical pedicle subtraction osteotomy should be done at the levels in which vertebral artery is not present in foramen transversarium (C7 and below).
- Posterior lamina-facet osteotomies (Smith-Petersen type) can be done at any subaxial level.

Combined Approaches

In the case of severe deformity and multilevel disease, combined approaches are more effective to achieve sufficient decompression and a rigid fixation (**Fig. 15.6a–f**).

Pearl

Combined anterior-posterior approaches may be necessary for severe rigid deformities.

Conclusion

Cervical spine deformity is challenging to treat the condition. The aim of the surgery must be to correct the deformity and decompress the spinal cord and nerve roots without causing complications. Preoperative planning must involve sagittal balance measurements and functional lateral radiographs. There are multiple anterior and posterior surgical techniques to achieve a good correction. Anterior and posterior osteotomies can be used in rigid deformities.

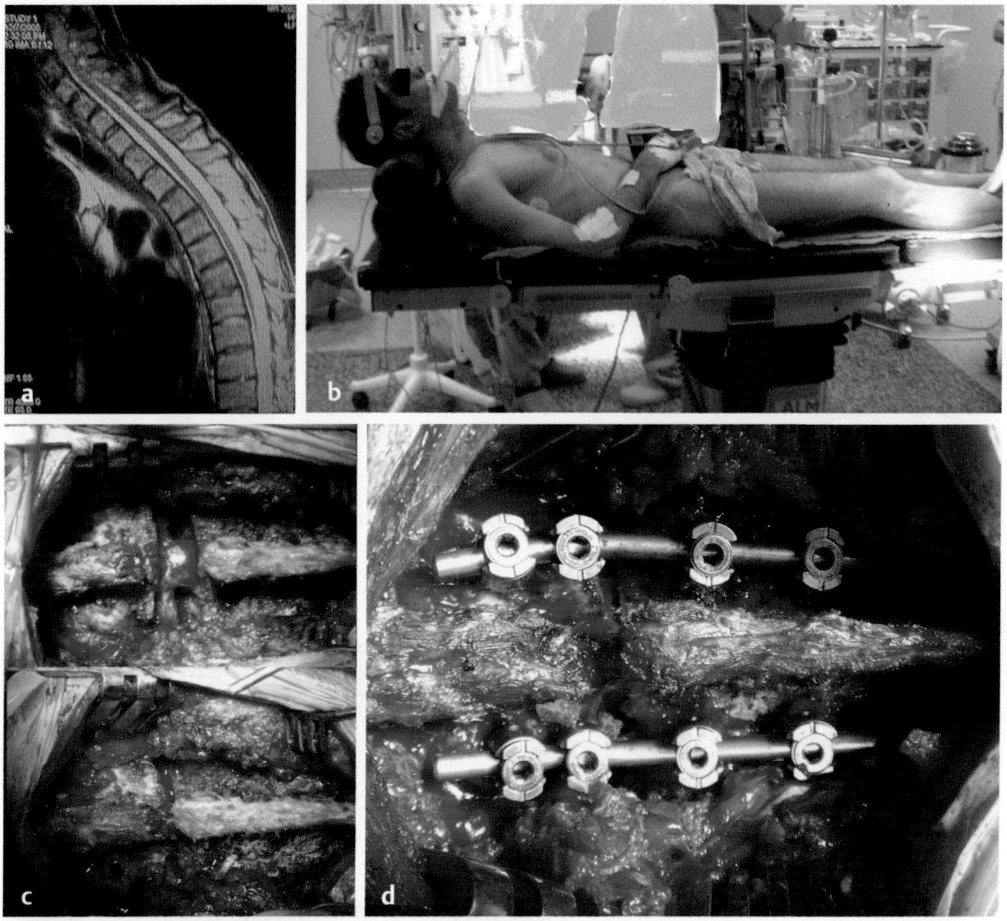

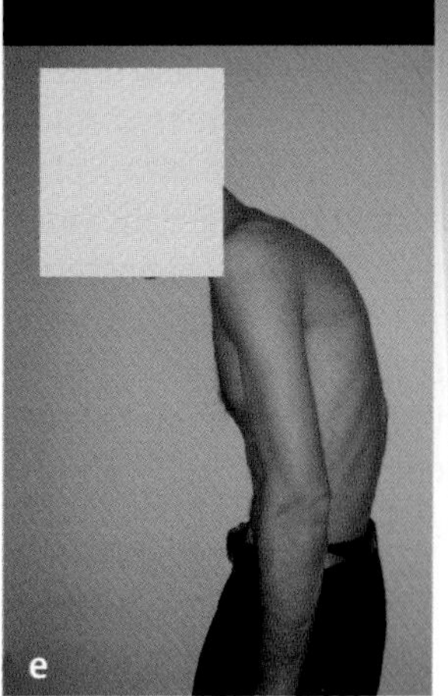

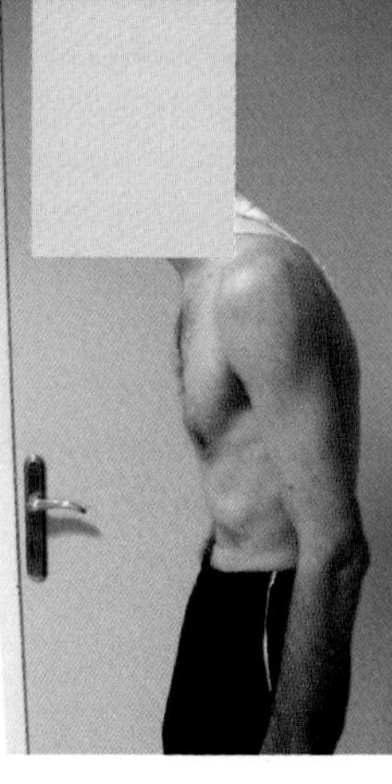

Fig. 15.5 (a-e) C7 Osteotomy for ankylosing spondylitis. This is a 34-year-old male diagnosed with ankylosing spondylitis for 10 years **(a)**. He had both cervicothoracic and upper lumbar kyphosis. **(b)** The kyphosis is more prominent in the supine position on the operating table **(c)**. A C7 posterior osteotomy was done. The osteotomy gap was closed by releasing the Mayfield head holder and extension of the head **(d)**. A short fixation using C5–C6 lateral mass and T1–T2 pedicle screws was performed **(e)**. Restoration of the gaze orientation is seen after surgery.

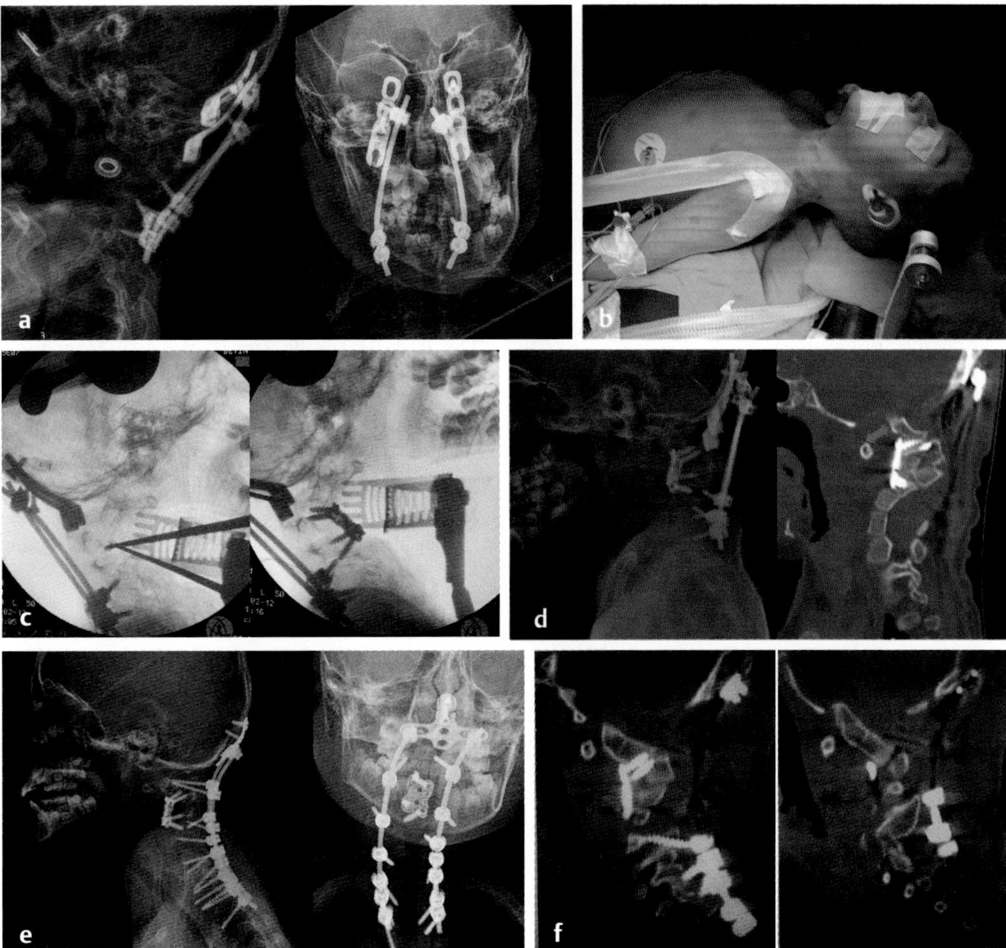

Fig. 15.6 (a) An 11-year-old male patient. He had surgery at 2 years of age due to neurofibromatosis and neurofibroma at C2, C3, C4 levels. After developing cervical kyphosis and scoliosis, he had an occipitocervical fixation surgery when he was 6-years old. Due to implant failure, he was placed in a Halo when he was 7. Halo was removed one year later. When admitted, he was tetraparetic, unable to walk, and wheelchair dependent. Magnetic resonance imaging (MRI) showed basilar invagination, atlantoaxial dislocation, and severe kyphosis at the C3–C4 level. Lateral radiographs showed failed and dislocated posterior fixation implants **(b)**. A two-stage surgery was performed: Firstly using an anterior approach with traction and neck extension **(c)**, C3–C4 disc space was entered. Partial decompression was performed, followed by graft and plate application **(d)**. Radiographs after first surgery showing an increase in atlantoaxial dislocation **(e)**. The second stage was a posterior approach, with removal of previous implants, a C4–C5 Smith-Petersen osteotomy and occiput to T4 fixation **(f)**. Postoperative computed tomography (CT) scans show a reduction in atlantoaxial dislocation and partial reduction in cervical kyphosis.

References

1. Diebo BG, Shah NV, Solow M, et al. Adult cervical deformity: radiographic and osteotomy classifications. Orthopade 2018;47(6):496–504
2. Tan LA, Riew KD, Traynelis VC. Cervical spine deformity-Part 1: biomechanics, radiographic parameters, and classification. Neurosurgery 2017;81(2):197–203
3. Ames CP, Smith JS, Eastlack R, et al; International Spine Study Group. Reliability assessment of a novel cervical spine deformity classification system. J Neurosurg Spine 2015;23(6):673–683
4. Gillis CC, Kaszuba MC, Traynelis VC. Cervical radiographic parameters in 1- and 2-level anterior cervical discectomy and fusion. J Neurosurg Spine 2016;25(4):421–429
5. Zileli M. Surgery for kyphosis. Adv Tech Stand Neurosurg 2014;41:71–103
6. Dru AB, Lockney DT, Vaziri S, et al. Cervical spine deformity correction techniques. Neurospine 2019;16(3):470–482
7. Tan LA, Riew KD, Traynelis VC. Cervical spine deformity-Part 2: management algorithm and anterior techniques. Neurosurgery 2017;81(4):561–567
8. Kim HJ, Piyaskulkaew C, Riew KD. Anterior cervical osteotomy for fixed cervical deformities. Spine 2014;39(21):1751–1757
9. Safaee MM, Tan LA, Riew KD. Anterior osteotomy for rigid cervical deformity correction. J Spine Surg 2020;6(1):210–216
10. Tan LA, Riew KD, Traynelis VC. Cervical spine deformity-Part 3: posterior techniques, clinical outcome, and complications. Neurosurgery 2017;81(6):893–898
11. Park JH, Lee JB, Kim IS, Hong JT. Transdiscal C7 pedicle subtraction osteotomy with a strut graft and the correction of sagittal and coronal imbalance of the cervical spine. Oper Neurosurg (Hagerstown) 2020;18(3):271–277
12. Wollowick AL, Kelly MP, Riew KD. Pedicle subtraction osteotomy in the cervical spine. Spine 2012;37(5):E342–E348
13. Urist MR. Osteotomy of the cervical spine; report of a case of ankylosing rheumatoid spondylitis. J Bone Joint Surg Am 1958;40-A(4):833–843
14. Traynelis VC. Total subaxial reconstruction. J Neurosurg Spine 2010;13(4):424–434

16 Deformity Correction Surgery Using Long Fixation: Where to Stop?

Abdelfattah Saoud

Introduction

Deformity correction is not a new technique. However, one of the major aspects of deformity correction is to identify the length of the construct—to be more specific, whether to stop at L5 or extend the construct up to the pelvis. It has been observed that many surgeons tend to refrain from ending fixation at L5 because of the distinct anatomical properties of the sacrum and ilium. These anatomical barriers include the thin cortical shell of the sacrum where it is significantly difficult to insert the screw (except the anterosuperior part of S1 and the thick lateral part of the sacral ala), wide pedicles, and the Anterior Posterior (AP) depth below S1, which tapers rapidly causing the screw span to fall short (**Fig. 16.1**). Although multiple fixation points can be used to strengthen the construct, doing so can lead to overcrowding of the hardware. In addition to these properties, other structures are at risk of injury during sacropelvic instrumentation.

Among the vascular structures, the arteries that could be injured during lumbopelvic fixation include the middle sacral vessels and the common iliac vessels. The sacral vessels are likely to get injured where the S1 screws converge. Common iliac vessels begin at L4, then pass along the lateral surface of the L5 vertebral body to bifurcate at the lumbosacral junction into internal and external iliac arteries. These arteries are ventral and lateral to the iliac veins, providing relatively safe heaven away from the spine. The internal iliac artery is in close proximity to the bony surface of ala, but psoas muscles separate the external iliac artery. The other vessel that is at a high risk of severing is the superior gluteal artery if the iliac screws are improperly placed, thereby increasing the chances of breaching the sciatic notch.

Other structures that could be injured include the lumbosacral trunk formed by the ventral branches of L4 and L5 roots that are joined by sacral nerves on the ventral surface of ala. The sympathetic chain might be endangered with anterior lumbar interbody fusion, long converging S1 screws, and finally, the colon, especially with S2 screws (**Fig. 16.2**).

Indications of Going Further than L5

In certain occasions, it would deem necessary to go further than L5. That is if L5 and S1

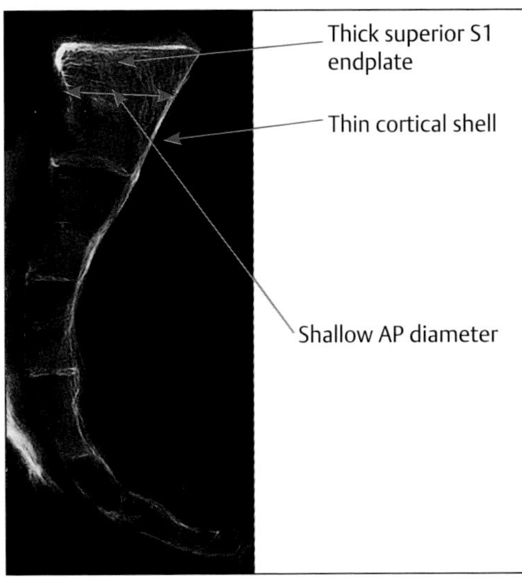

Fig. 16.1 The anatomical properties of sacrum that must be kept in mind during instrumentation.

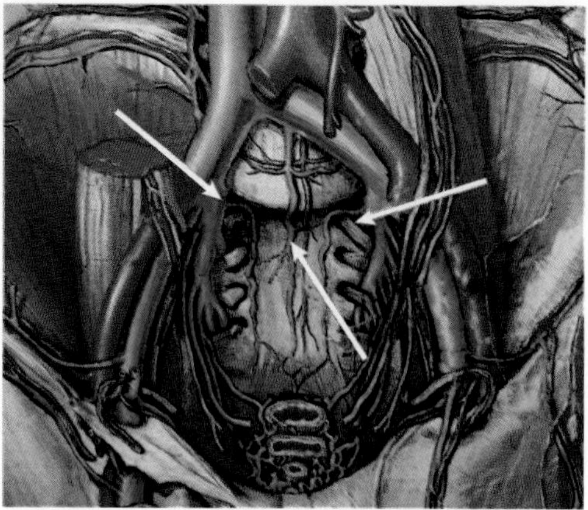

Fig. 16.2 Various vascular structures are at risk of injury with improper placement of sacral screws. The three *white arrows* correlate with common iliac veins and median sacral vein.

are part of the deformity that needs correction (pelvic obliquity correction), especially if it contributes significantly to the loss of lordosis (e.g., Flatback syndrome), when multisegmental fixation is required to add to the strength of construct or in a setting of significant osteoporosis in lumbosacral spine. In addition, the following are considered: radiological instability at L5–S1 level (pathologic or iatrogenic instability), L5–S1 dysfunctional motion segment that has failed conservative management, trauma with an unstable L5 fracture, sacral fractures especially, and tumors of L5 or sacrum.

Outcomes of Stopping at L5

Brown and colleagues in 2004[1] and Polly et al[2] in 2006 gave similar conditions for the success of stopping fusion at the L5 level. They stated that patients with adult scoliosis with good preoperative sagittal balance could preserve the L5–S1 disc height or lumbar lordosis with good postoperative fractional curve correction. Edwards and colleagues reported twice on long fusions to L5. One showed 61% degeneration at L5–S1 on 2 years follow-up, whereas the other showed 67% degeneration. The analysis by Brown and colleagues also exhibited that at least three revisions were required in 16 patients who went through long L5 fusions as they showed 38% degeneration at L5–S1. Kuhns et al in 2007[3] evaluated 31 consecutive patients with an average age of 45 years, who went through fusion from the thoracic spine till L5, over a mean follow-up of 9.4 years. They concluded that advanced L5–S1 degeneration developed in 69% of deformity patients after long fusions to L5 over 5 to 15 years of follow-up.

What is really overlooked in these studies is the sagittal alignment. However, other studies have considered this. Harding et al in 2008[4] concluded that disc degeneration occurred below an arthrodesis for adult scoliosis at L4–L5 or L5–S1 and that revision surgery for adjacent segment disease (ASD) was relatively uncommon in this population. In their conclusion, they stated that "whether degeneration occurs de novo with time or is related to the altered biomechanical environment is not clear, although this and previous studies would suggest that imbalance and/or malalignment of the spine following fusion are factors that contribute to adjacent segment degeneration." Similarly, a prospective study of 53 patients conducted by Saoud et al in 2010 showed that patients with preoperative disc degeneration at an adjacent segment were more at risk for the development of ASD. Their prospective series proved that keeping lordotic alignment decreased the incidence of both symptomatic and nonsymptomatic ASD. The disturbance of this alignment increased the incidence of symptomatic and nonsymptomatic ASD in the segments directly above and below fusion hypolordotic alignment.

Pearls

- Harding et al in 2008[4] concluded that disc degeneration does occur below an arthrodesis for adult scoliosis at L4–L5 or L5–S1 levels and that revision surgery for ASD is relatively uncommon.
- Whether degeneration occurs de novo with time or is related to the altered biomechanical environment is not clear, although this and previous studies would suggest that imbalance and/or malalignment of the spine following fusion are factors that contribute to adjacent segment degeneration.
- Stopping at L5 is not the best decision for long fusions, and it worsens when sagittal alignment is not achieved.

Alternatives to Stopping at L5

If fixation is extended until the pelvis, three important biomechanical facts should be considered; the lumbosacral pivot point (**Fig. 16.3**) as described by McCord et al in 1993.[5] It is described as the axis of rotation at the lumbosacral junction at the intersection of the middle osteoligamentous column and L5–S1 disc. The clinical importance of this is that only those constructs that cross the lumbosacral junction ventrally provide a significant advantage over the rigidity of fixation. This is shown in **Fig. 16.3**.

O'Brien in 2003[6] classified fixation zones into three categories (**Fig. 16.4**).

Accordingly, Zone 1 consists of the S1 vertebral body with cephalad margins of sacral ala where fixation is carried out using converging S1 screws, bilateral L5/S1 transfacet screws, and augmentation with anterior augmentation support.

Zone 2 includes the inferior margins of sacral alae, S2, and the area till the tip of the coccyx. This zone fixation is achieved by the use of alar screws, hooks, and sublaminar wires. This is the least effective zone of fixation because of poor bone stock and other anatomic constraints.

Zone 3, which is the most efficient biomechanical anchor, includes both the ilia. Although this is the best option for fixation, it is difficult to get optimum fusion at this level. This difficulty is largely attributed to the presence of a deep slope between the L5 and S1 iliac screw, which leads to high-stress levels at this point. This also explains the high chances of pseudarthrosis due to the range of motion (about 17 to 18 degrees of flexion and extension). There are also high chances of implant failure with these constructs as the implants tend to move posteriorly to the

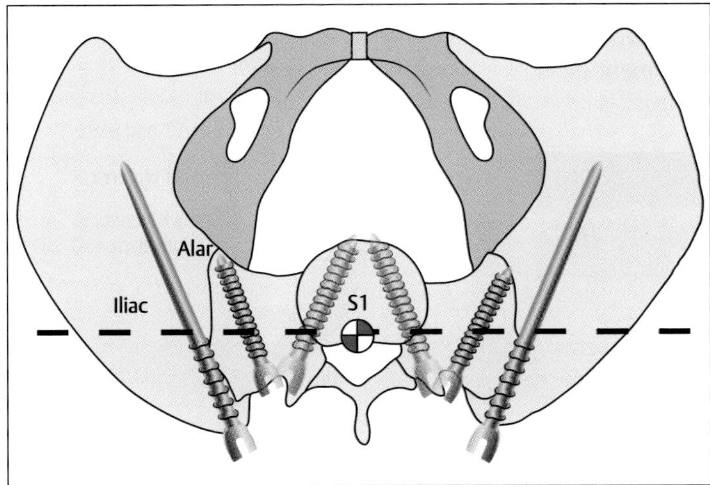

Fig. 16.3 It shows the McCord Pivot point (13) and how various forms of instrumentation are carried anterior to it to achieve good stable construct.

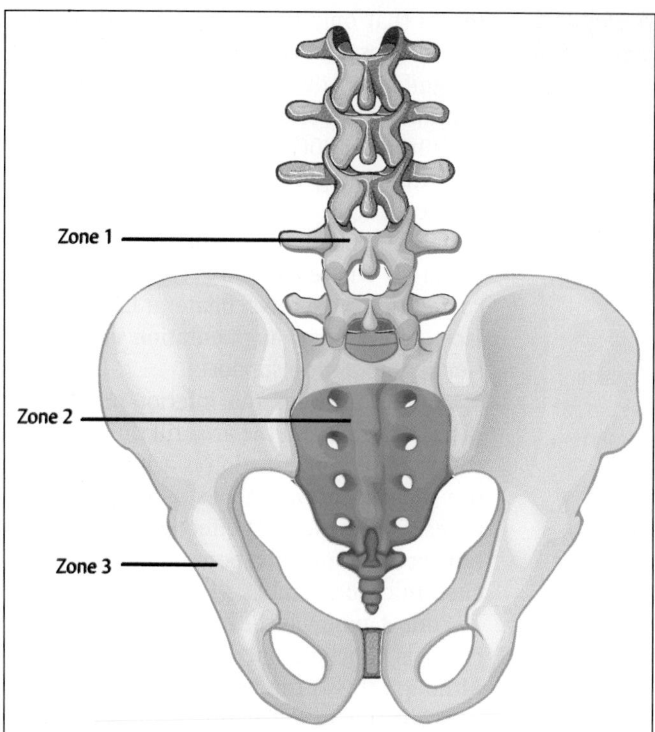

Fig. 16.4 Fixation zones as pointed out by O'Brian.

center of gravity during flexion and extension. Poor bone quality is another factor that leads to implant failure; hence, bone mineral density (BMD) represents the most important factor in determining the strength of construct,[7] with the superior sacral end plate having the highest BMD.[8]

The best solution to enhance fusion at the LS junction is biological enhancement using carpentry, grafting, and mechanical enhancement using the aforementioned fixation points for a strong construct.

Pearl

Bone mineral density is the most important factor in fixation.

Sacral Fixation

This type of fixation can be achieved in three possible manners (**Fig. 16.5**). One is to tighten the S1 screws medially to achieve bicortical purchase through the anterior cortex

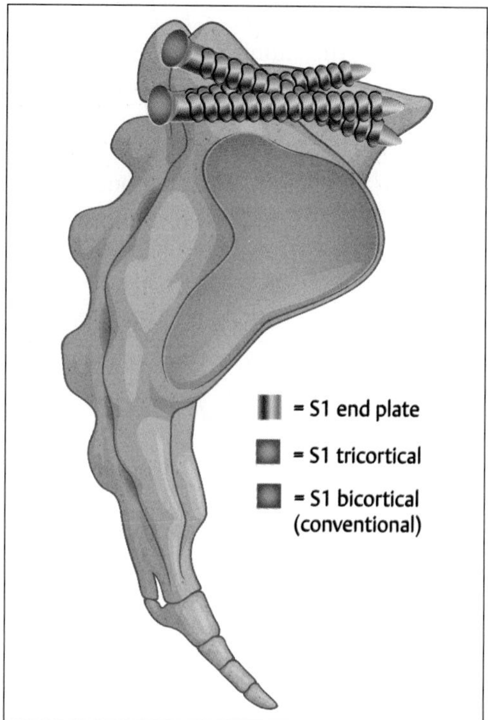

Fig. 16.5 Various forms of screws that could be placed in sacrum.

of S1. This is a relatively safe zone with only a median sacral vessel to spare (**Fig. 16.6**). The second option is to place the screws in the direction of the end plate where BMD is the highest. In a setting of tricortical purchase, the direction should be through the tip of the promontory using both the cortex and the end plate.

Laterally Directed S1 or S2 Screws

Another way of fixation is to tighten the S1/S2 screws 20 to 45 degrees laterally while keeping them unicortical in the process. The old assumption of a lateral safe zone for laterally directed screws was proven wrong by Doh et al in 1998.[9] This study shows that bicortical placement of S1 screws into the sacral ala presents unnecessary risks to the neurovascular structures; therefore, bicortical, laterally directed sacral screws in any direction between 20 and 50 degrees puts the sacroiliac joint, lumbosacral trunk, internal iliac vein, and iliolumbar artery at risk (**Fig. 16.7**).

Anterior Constructs: For Anterior Interbody Fusion

This construct is performed by using grafts or bone substitutes placed in disc space or utilizing a fibular graft, passed from the body of L5 to the sacrum (Rene P. Louis)[10] (**Fig. 16.8**). Another method is to use a mesh that is filled with bone graft supplemented

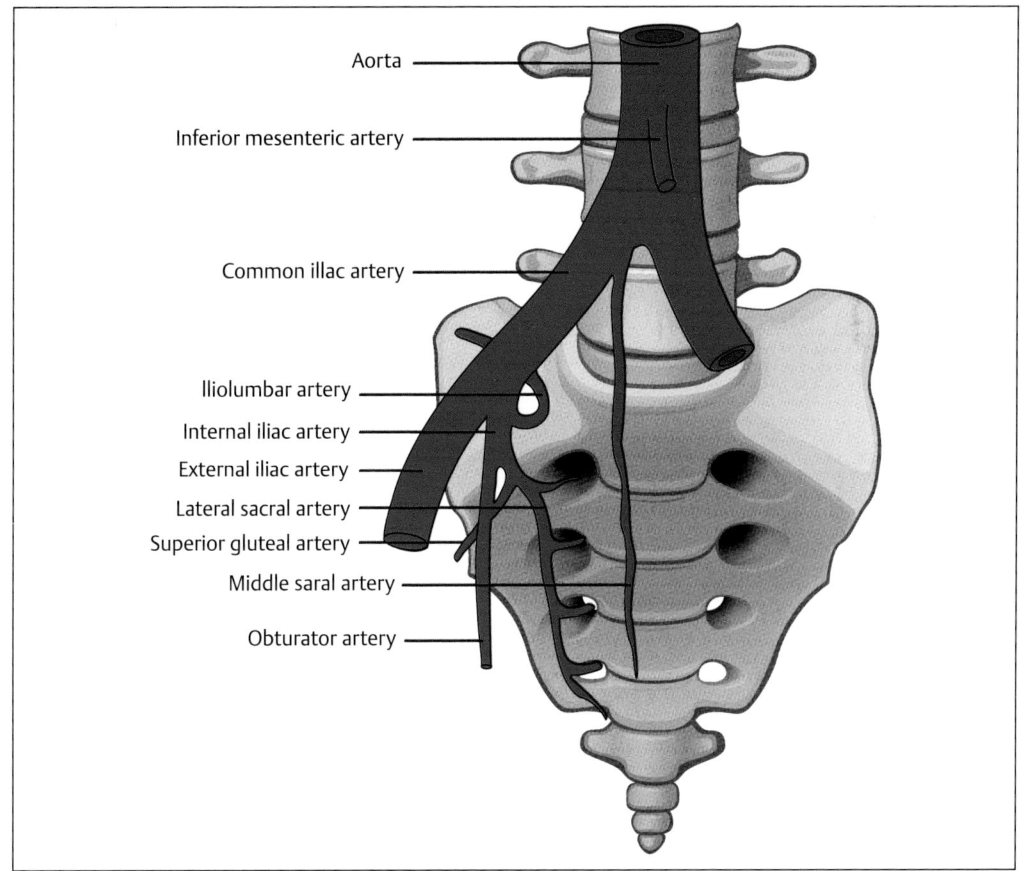

Fig. 16.6 Medial safe zone as there is only one small vessel in midline relative to multiple vessels placed laterally.

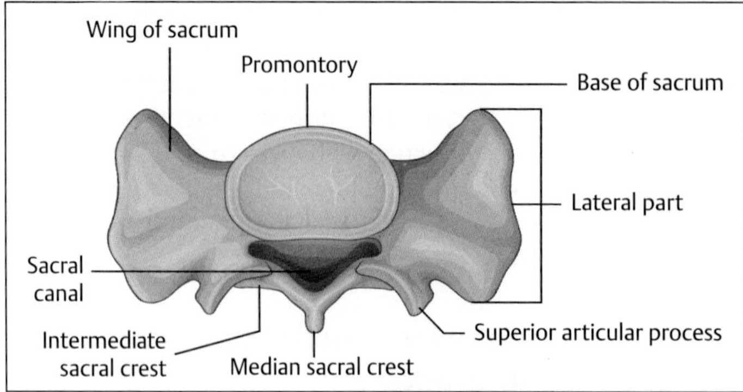

Fig. 16.7 Laterally directed S1 or S2 screws carry risk of injuring lateral vessels and sacroiliac joint.

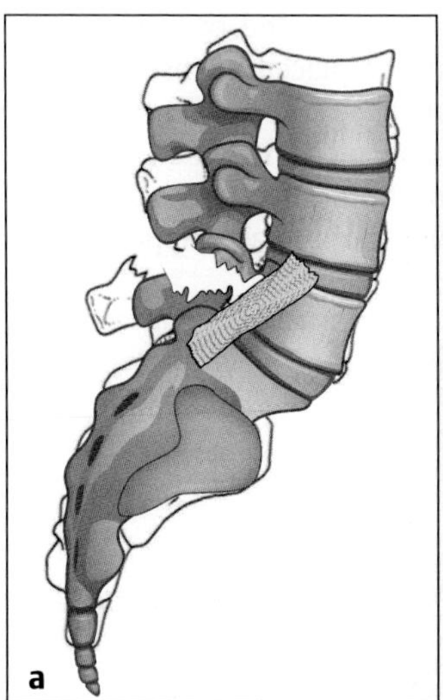

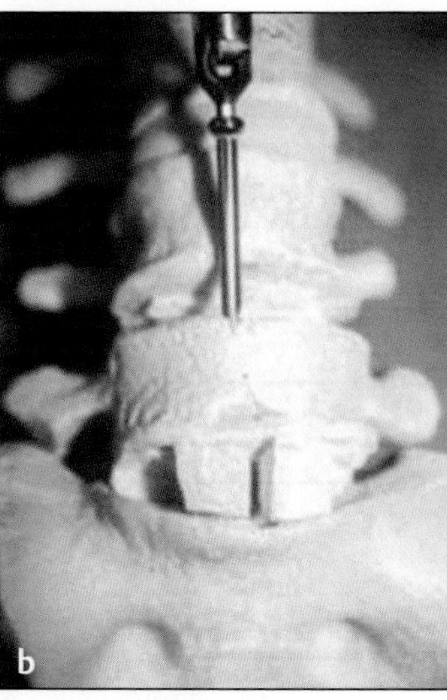

Fig. 16.8 (a, b) A fibular graft is used to get 360-degree fusion in conjunction with posterior fixation.

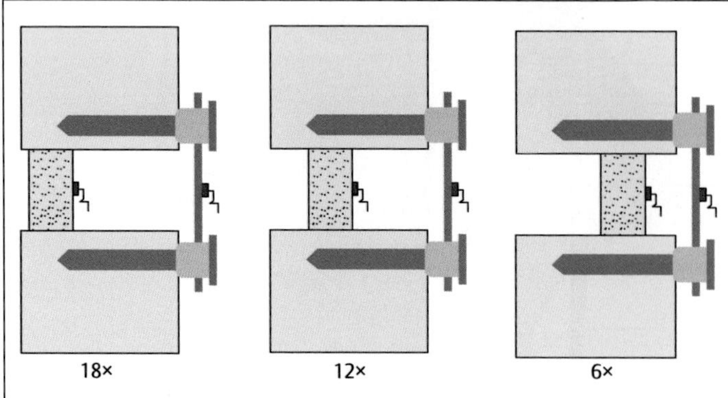

Fig. 16.9 Location of the interbody support is important and the more anterior it is, the more rigidity we get for the whole construct. Rigidity of simultaneous anterior and posterior fixation and carpentry increases by 18% with anterior placement of the interbody support and decreases by going back to about 6%.

by posterior-pedicular fixation. Similarly, cages filled with graft (stand-alone or with posterior fixation) can also be used. This helps in attaining 360-degree fusion in conjunction with posterior fixation. The location of placement of the interbody support is important—the more anterior it is, stronger the construct is. The durability of both the anterior and posterior fixations and carpentry increase by 18% with the anterior placement of the interbody and decreases by going back to about 6% (**Fig. 16.9**).

Transdiscal Fixation of L5–S1

This type of fixation has become quite popular and is done by entering at 1 cm distal and 1 cm medial to the standard S1 screw. It is then passed through S1, followed by the disc space and finally the L5 body with the help of fluoroscopy. Posterolateral fusion is usually added to achieve in situ fusion (**Fig. 16.10** and **Fig. 16.11**).

Facetal/Translaminar Screws

Magerl developed facetal translaminar screws in 1983.[11] In order to get the left-sided screw, it is necessary to begin from the right side of the spinous process. The anterior column should be intact or supported by a cage or graft, and the lamina should be unscathed (**Fig. 16.12**).

> **Pearl**
>
> Magerl, in 1983,[11] developed the modern translaminar facet screws.

Sacral Hooks

These are used only as an adjunct to other forms of instrumentation. Laminar, alar, or sacral foraminal hooks and sublaminar wires and cables lack significant biomechanical

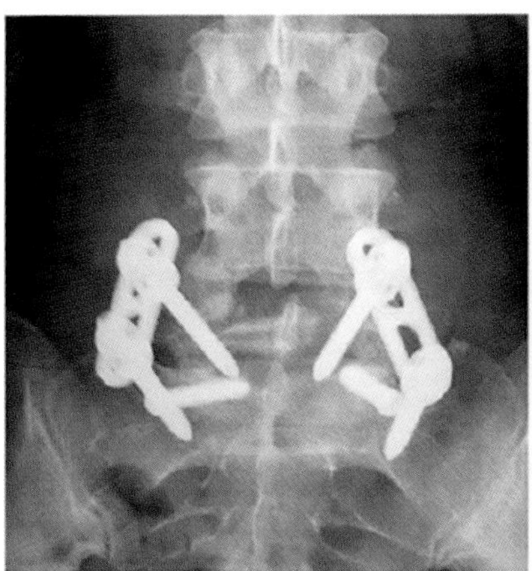

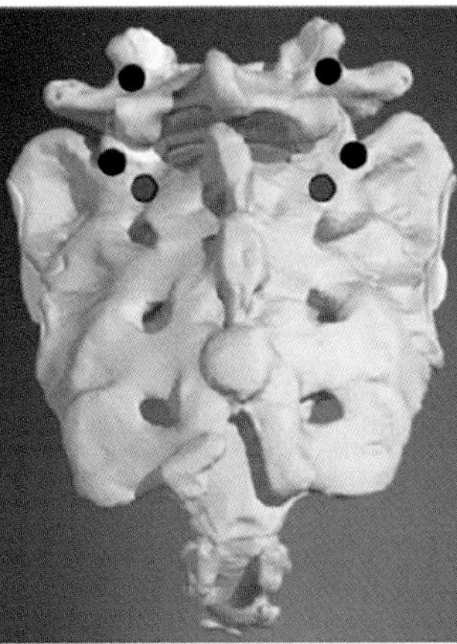

Fig. 16.10 Transdiscal fixation of L5–S1.

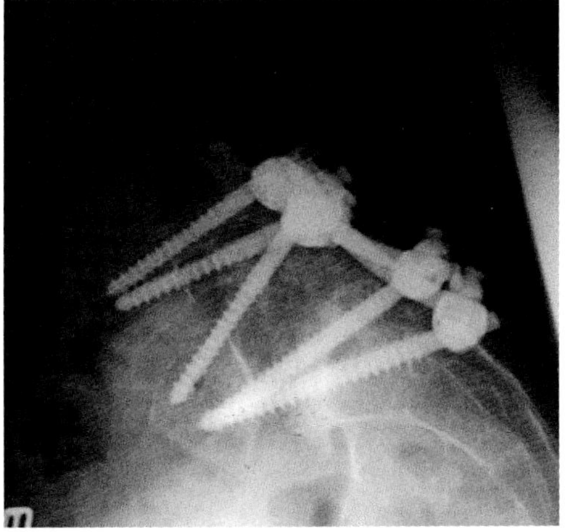

Fig. 16.11 Entry point for transdiscal fixation.

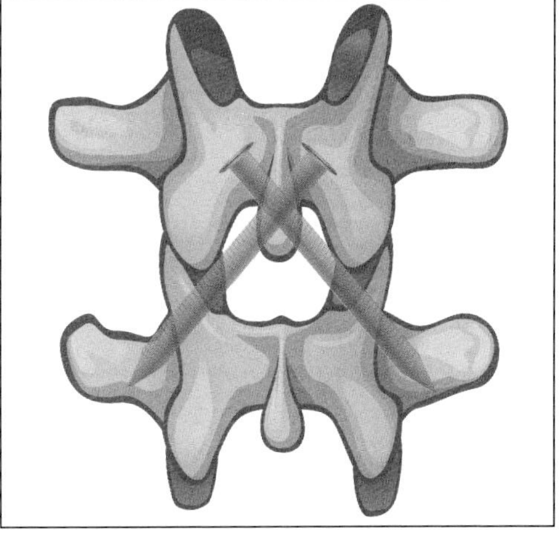

Fig. 16.12 Translaminar screws.

strength as these implants are dorsal to the McCord point. The only exception is at S1 in Zone 1 due to the presence of strong bone (**Fig. 16.13**).

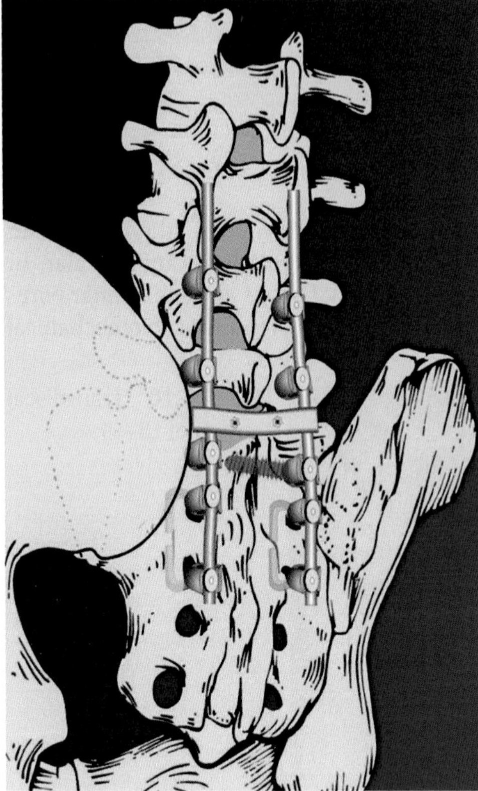

Fig. 16.13 Sacral hooks.

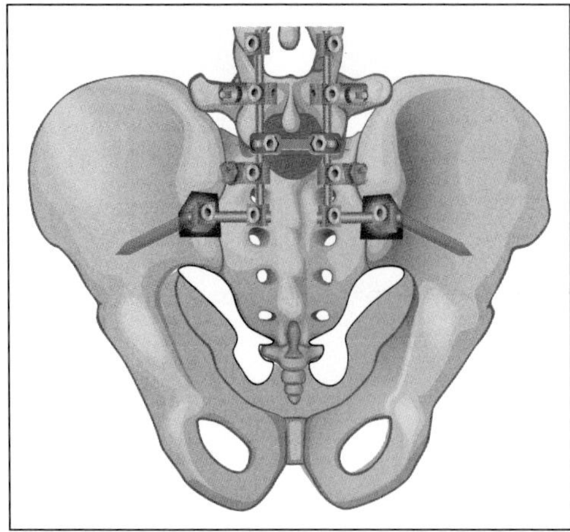

Fig. 16.14 Iliac screws connected with lumbosacral fixation.

Iliac Screws

Iliac screws are biomechanically effective according to both parameters. They are partially anterior to the McCord point and best in Zone 3 for fixation (**Fig. 16.14**). They can be connected to the rest of the fixation by various connectors. For this fixation to work, the iliac screws need to be placed exactly medial to the posterior superior iliac spine (PSIS) and other positioning methods so that they can be kept connected to the rest of the construct (**Fig. 16.15**).

S2 Alar Iliac Screws

These were made to avoid the above-mentioned issues. Iliac fixation through the S2 ala provides a starting point in line with the S1 pedicle screw. The starting point is 1 to 2 mm lateral and 1 to 2 mm distal to the S1 dorsal sacral foramen (**Fig. 16.16**).

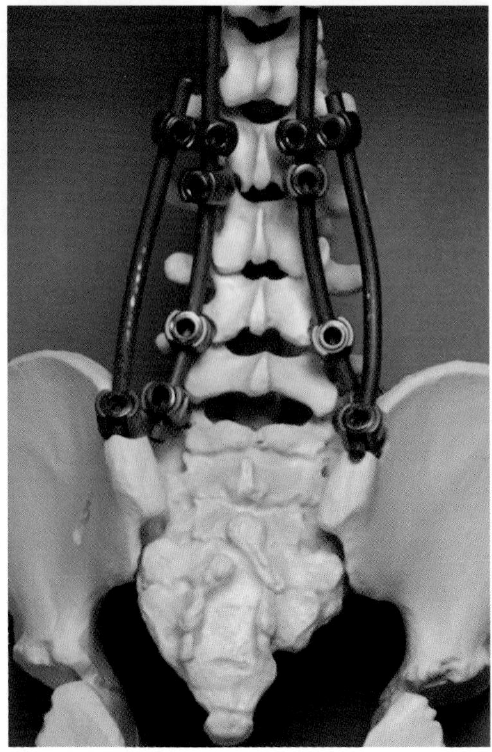

Fig. 16.15 Flying buttress connection of iliac screws to deformity constructs.

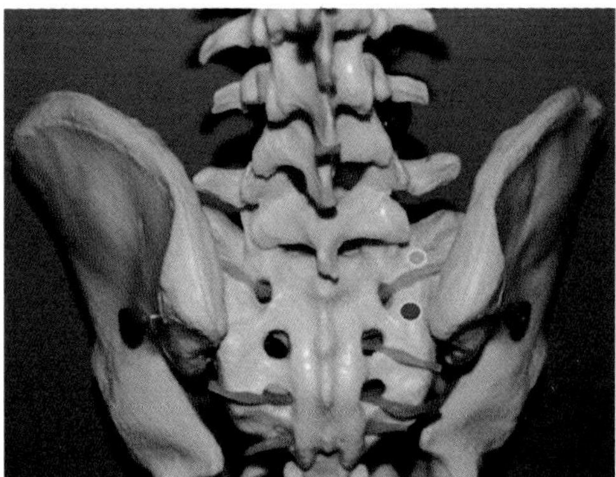

Fig. 16.16 The starting point is 1 to 2 mm lateral and 1 to 2 mm distal to the S1 dorsal sacral foramen.

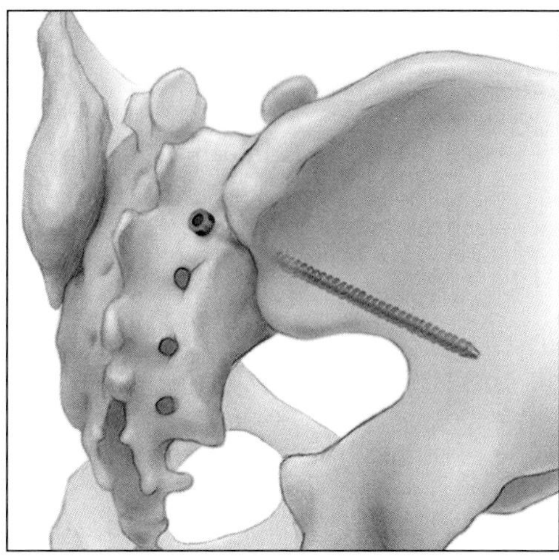

Fig. 16.17 Direction of S2 alar iliac screws.

The real trajectory is 40 degrees anterior to the horizontal plane and 20 to 30 degrees caudal from being directly lateral (**Fig. 16.17**).

Iliosacral Screw Fixation

This is actually a sacral screw but passes through the ilium to increase the purchase. Traversing three cortices that helps in gaining better purchase, the screw is connected to the construct at the part exposed between the sacrum and the iliac bone using connectors (**Fig. 16.18**). Both iliac and sacroiliac screws can be used simultaneously (MW Construct).

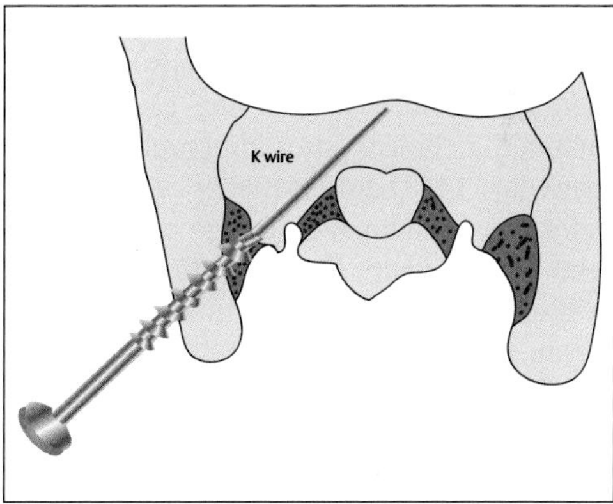

Fig. 16.18 Direction of iliosacral screw and the used part to connect to lumbar fixation.

Outcomes of Stopping at the Sacrum for Long Constructs for Deformity

Correction

Many factors suggest that stopping at the sacrum for those long deformity constructs might not be the best decision for patients. In an interesting article in 2007, Swamy et al[12] compared the use of L5 and S1 as an ending point of long fusions for idiopathic scoliosis. Advantages and disadvantages to long fusion to L5 and S1 are listed in **Box 16.1** and **Box 16.2**, respectively.

Box 16.1 Advantages and disadvantages to long fusions to L5

Advantages

- Save motion at L5–S1
- Avoid risk of pseudarthrosis at L5–S1
- Avoid possible anterior surgery at L5–S1
- Lower medical complication rate

Disadvantages

- Potential for subsequent degeneration at L5–S1
  - ➢ Loss of sagittal plane correction
  - ➢ Pain
- Poor purchase in L5 pedicle, leading to implant loosening

Box 16.2 Advantages and disadvantages to long fusions to S1

Advantages

- Avoid potential subsequent degeneration at L5–S1
- Maintain sagittal plane correction, particularly in case of major preoperative sagittal plane imbalance

Disadvantages

- Loss of L5–S1 motion
  - Possible gait abnormality
  - Possible difficulty with perineal care
- High complication rate
  - Medical complications
  - Pseudarthrosis
- Potential sacroiliac (SI) joint arthrosis

Kim et al[13] conducted a study on pseudarthrosis in long adult spinal deformity instrumentation and fusion to the sacrum that included a clinical and radiographic assessment of 144 adult patients with spinal deformity with an average age of 52.0 years who underwent long (5–17 vertebrae, average 11.9) spinal instrumentation and fusion to the sacrum at a single institution with a minimum of 2-years follow-up. They concluded that the overall prevalence of pseudarthrosis following long adult spinal deformity instrumentation and fusion to S1 was 24%.

Chen et al[14] in 2018 analyzed the data on stopping at sacrum versus nonsacral vertebra in long fusion surgery for adult spinal deformity by doing a meta-analysis of revision with a minimum 2-year follow-up. They concluded that the total revision rate in ASD patients is 11.38%, with implant failure, ASD, and proximal junctional kyphosis being the common factors. They also stated that stopping at sacrum in long fusion surgery of ASD patients increases the incidence rate of revisions and pseudarthrosis.

Pearls

- Kim et al[13] studied pseudarthrosis in long adult spinal deformity instrumentation and fusion to the sacrum and suggested that the overall prevalence of pseudarthrosis following long adult spinal deformity instrumentation and fusion to S1 was 24%.
- Chen et al[14], in 2019, analyzed the literature data on stopping at sacrum versus nonsacral vertebra in long fusion surgery for adult spinal injury and stated that stopping at sacrum in long fusion surgery of ASD patients appears to increase the incidence rate of revisions and pseudarthrosis.

The transdiscal fusion procedures are tested biomechanically by some authors.

Minamide et al[15] introduced and performed a biomechanical study with this screw using a cadaveric model of L5–S1 spondylolisthesis. They inferred that transdiscal L5–S1 fixation was 1.6 to 1.8 times more rigid than the traditional pedicle screw fixation and that it was similar to a combination of interbody and screw fixation. However, only a few case series studies were done on this technique. Logroscino et al in 2012[16] published on transdiscal fixation for dysplastic L5–S1 listhesis against standard posterior lumbar intertransverse fusion (PLITF) and found that it gave faster fusion and symptom resolution. Palejwala et al[17] also presented a single case with 14 months fusion of an adolescent with grade IV spondylolisthesis treated by transdiscal fixation. He had significant pain improvement with overall good outcome. Similarly, Collados-Maestre et al[18] published a retrospective case-control study where he compared 25 consecutive patients who underwent transdiscal fixation with 31 patients undergoing standard pedicle screw fixation. They were both clinically and radiographically compared. They concluded that the L5–S1 transdiscal screw fixation provided better functional and radiographic outcomes at medium-term than conventional pedicle fixation for high-grade spondylolisthesis even though transdiscal sacral screws are difficult to place in the correct position. Adding anterior fusion to L5–S1 fixation definitely adds to the biomechanical advantage.

The Outcomes of Going Anterior

Kostuik et al back in 1998[19] proved in a biomechanical study how anterior fixation statistically increased rigidity of the constructs, but on the clinical perspective, Khan et al[20] studied outcomes of combined anterior and posterior surgery in lumbar degenerative scoliosis which showed that it is an effective method. However, clinical outcomes were characterized by a 35% increase in the rate of complications and the need for revision surgery.

Pearl

L5–S1 transdiscal screw fixation provides better functional and radiographic outcomes at medium-term than conventional pedicle fixation for high-grade spondylolisthesis, along with anterior fusion to L5–S1 fixation.

Outcomes of Going to the Ilium

Theoretically, a higher rate of loosening of the ilial fixation implants (due to stresses of movements at sacroiliac joint) was caused by the posterior lever arm forces along with the higher rate of sacroiliac joint arthritis (as this does limit the movement of the joint with increased wear and tear of its cartilage), but this is doubtful. Lebwohl et al in 2002[21] and Nguyen et al in 2019[22] concluded that iliac screws were an effective method of spinopelvic fixation that had high rates of lumbosacral fusion and far lower complication rates than previously reported. Collectively, these findings argue that iliac screw fixation should remain a favored technique for spinopelvic fixation.

Pearl

Ohtori et al[23] studied about the "clinical incidence of sacroiliac joint arthritis and pain after sacropelvic fixation for spinal deformity" and showed that the pain scores significantly improved after surgery. Patients showed bone union at final follow-up while degeneration of sacroiliac joints was reduced considerably.

Tsuchiya et al in 2006[24] published a minimum 5-year analysis of L5–S1 fusion using sacropelvic fixation (bilateral S1 and iliac screws) for spinal deformity. A total of 67 patients were analyzed for radiographic and clinical outcomes. This study showed no cases of sacral screw failure (i.e., screw loosening, partial screw pullout, or fracture of the sacral screw). Therefore, iliac screws were effective in protecting the sacral screws from failure. There were five cases of nonunion at L5–S1. Of these five cases, three did not have anterior column support at L5–S1. There were seven cases of iliac screw breakage whereas iliac screw halos were observed in 29 patients. No sacroiliac osteoarthritis was observed on the true anteroposterior pelvis films in 5 to 10 years of follow-up. The conclusion for iliac screws is that they cause breakage and failure.

Ohtori et al[23] studied the clinical incidence of sacroiliac joint arthritis and pain after sacropelvic fixation for spinal deformity. This study analyzed the results of 20 patients who were preoperatively diagnosed with degenerative scoliosis. In this study, seven patients showed failed back syndrome, six patients exhibited destructive spondyloarthropathy, whereas three patients developed Charcot spine. All patients underwent posterolateral fusion surgery incorporating lumbar, S1, and iliac screws. Their pain scores, bone union, and degeneration of sacroiliac joints were evaluated by X-ray imaging and computed tomography before and 3 years after surgery. The evaluation of lower back and buttock pain (which were thought to arise from sacroiliac joints 3 years after surgery) was done by administering lidocaine in order to examine pain relief. This resulted in significant improvement in pain scores after surgery. All patients showed bone union at final follow-up, and degeneration of sacroiliac joints was not visible in 20 patients 3 years postoperatively. Patients that showed slight lower back and buttock pain 3 years after surgery and were not relieved with the lidocaine injection into the sacroiliac joint indicated that their pain did not originate from sacroiliac joints.

Studies on the use of S2 alar iliac screws have been reported, but they have a short-term follow-up. Sponseller[25] used S2 alar iliac screws in the pediatric population and had improved results at 2-years follow-up. Ramos et al[26] in a meta-analysis study on iliac screws versus S2 alar iliac screw fixation in adults concluded that S2 alar iliac screw fixation in adults has a significantly lower mechanical failure and complication rate than iliac screws.

There is little data on the MW technique (**Fig. 16.19**). Carroll et al[27] study shows better correction of coronal deformity and pelvic obliquity using the MW construct in a limited number of patients with neuromuscular scoliosis. Literature suggests that there is no specific order in which all the screws mentioned above can be used for a better outcome. There is not enough evidence to show that iliac screws increase the chances of sacroiliac joint arthritis. It has been reported that there has been loosening and breakage in some cases.

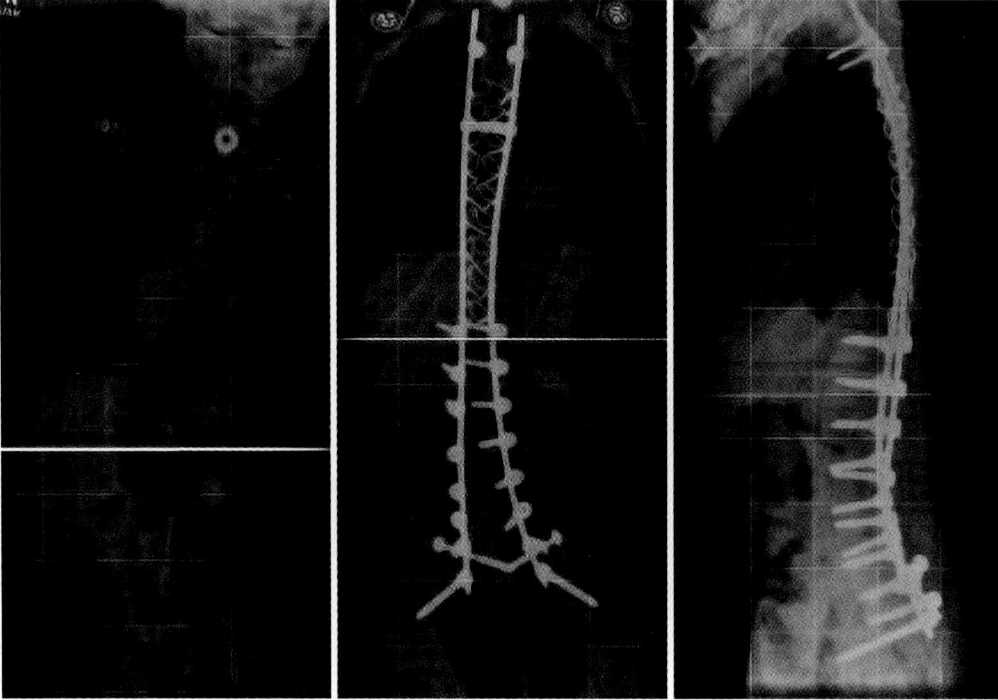

Fig. 16.19 MW technique.

Conclusion

The pelvic approach for fixation can be done safely. To do so, it is important to avoid the temptation of stopping at L5, which causes various postoperative complications, especially revision. Both sagittal and coronal alignment should be restored to achieve better outcomes. Fusion at the L5–S1 level is difficult. It is pertinent to mention that to achieve good fusion, it is necessary to perform biological enhancement and good fixation (decortication and grafting of the surfaces intended for fusion like transverse processes, facets, or interbody). Adding anterior support to the area of fixation is helpful, but one has to be precise as to where to put it (the more it is anterior, the better). When the pelvis is reached, it seems that stopping at S1 would give a superior result for the patient and that the addition of iliac screws is a better option (though they have more chance of pullout and breakage, and need of removal). The addition of iliac screws would lower the rate of L5–S1 nonunion and reduce S1 screw failure without arthritis of the sacroiliac joint.

References

1. Brown KM, Ludwig SC, Gelb DE. Radiographic predictors of outcome after long fusion to L5 in adult scoliosis. J Spinal Disord Tech 2004;17(5):358–366
2. Polly DW Jr, Hamill CL, Bridwell KH. Debate: to fuse or not to fuse to the sacrum, the fate of the L5-S1 disc. Spine 2006; 31(19, Suppl): S179–S184
3. Kuhns CA, Bridwell KH, Lenke LG, et al. Thoracolumbar deformity arthrodesis stopping at L5: fate of the L5–S1 disc, minimum 5-year follow-up. Spine 2007;32(24):2771–2776
4. Harding IJ, Charosky S, Vialle R, Chopin DH. Lumbar disc degeneration below a long arthrodesis (performed for scoliosis in adults) to L4 or L5. Eur Spine J 2008;17(2):250–254
5. McCord DH, Cunningham BW, Shono Y, Myers JJ, McAfee PC. Biomechanical analysis of lumbosacral fixation. Lumbar Fusion and Stabilization. Springer; 1993:259–277
6. O'Brien MF. Sacropelvic fixation in spinal deformity. Spinal deformities: the comprehensive text. New York: Thieme; 2003; 2003:601–614
7. Zindrick MR, Wiltse LL, Widell EH, et al. A biomechanical study of interpeduncular screw fixation in the lumbosacral spine. Clin Orthop Relat Res 1986;203(203):99–112
8. Zheng Y, Lu WW, Zhu Q, Qin L, Zhong S, Leong JC. Variation in bone mineral density of the sacrum in young adults and its significance for sacral fixation. Spine 2000;25(3):353–357
9. Doh JW, Benzel EC, Lee KS, et al. Anatomical safe zone of sacral ala for ventrolateral sacral (S1) screw placement: re-evaluation of its effectiveness. J Korean Neurosurg Soc 1998; 27(3):291–298
10. Saoud AMF. Lumbo sacral pelvic fixation techniques. Spine Review comprehensive spine course. Cleveland, Ohio, USA. 2020
11. Magerl FP. Stabilization of the lower thoracic and lumbar spine with external skeletal fixation. Clin Orthop Relat Res 1984; (189):125–141
12. Swamy G, Berven SH, Bradford DS. The selection of L5 versus S1 in long fusions for adult idiopathic scoliosis. Neurosurg Clin N Am 2007;18(2):281–288
13. Kim YJ, Bridwell KH, Lenke LG, Rhim S, Cheh G. Pseudarthrosis in long adult spinal deformity instrumentation and fusion to the sacrum: prevalence and risk factor analysis of 144 cases. Spine 2006;31(20):2329–2336
14. Chen S, Luo M, Wang Y, Liu H. Stopping at sacrum versus nonsacral vertebra in long fusion surgery for adult spinal deformity: meta-analysis of revision with minimum 2-year follow-up. World Neurosurg 2018; 124:e380–e6
15. Minamide A, Akamaru T, Yoon ST, Tamaki T, Rhee JM, Hutton WC. Transdiscal L5–S1 screws for the fixation of isthmic spondylolisthesis: a biomechanical evaluation. J Spinal Disord Tech 2003;16(2):144–149
16. Logroscino CA, Tamburrelli FC, Scaramuzzo L, Schirò GR, Sessa S, Proietti L. Transdiscal L5–S1 screws for the treatment of adult spondylolisthesis. Eur Spine J 2012; 21(1, Suppl 1) S128–S133
17. Palejwala A, Fridley J, Jea A. Transsacral transdiscal L5–S1 screws for the management of high-grade spondylolisthesis in an adolescent. J Neurosurg Pediatr 2016;17(6): 645–650

18. Collados-Maestre I, Lizaur-Utrilla A, Bas-Hermida T, Pastor-Fernandez E, Gil-Guillen V. Transdiscal screw versus pedicle screw fixation for high-grade L5–S1 isthmic spondylolisthesis in patients younger than 60 years: a case-control study. Eur Spine J 2016;25(6): 1806–1812
19. Kostuik JP, Valdevit A, Chang H-G, Kanzaki K. Biomechanical testing of the lumbosacral spine. Spine 1998;23(16):1721–1728
20. Khan SN, Hofer MA, Gupta MC. Lumbar degenerative scoliosis: outcomes of combined anterior and posterior pelvis surgery with minimum 2-year follow-up. Orthopedics 2009;32(4):249–259
21. Lebwohl NH, Cunningham BW, Dmitriev A, et al. Biomechanical comparison of lumbosacral fixation techniques in a calf spine model. Spine 2002;27(21):2312–2320
22. Nguyen JH, Buell TJ, Wang TR, et al. Low rates of complications after spinopelvic fixation with iliac screws in 260 adult patients with a minimum 2-year follow-up. J Neurosurg Spine 2019;30(5):1–9
23. Ohtori S, Sainoh T, Takaso M, et al. Clinical incidence of sacroiliac joint arthritis and pain after sacropelvic fixation for spinal deformity. Yonsei Med J 2012;53(2):416–421
24. Tsuchiya K, Bridwell KH, Kuklo TR, Lenke LG, Baldus C. Minimum 5-year analysis of L5–S1 fusion using sacropelvic fixation (bilateral S1 and iliac screws) for spinal deformity. Spine 2006;31(3):303–308
25. Sponseller P. The S2 portal to the ilium. Semin Spine Surg 2007;2:83–87
26. De la Garza Ramos R, Nakhla J, Sciubba DM, Yassari R. Iliac screw versus S2 alar-iliac screw fixation in adults: a meta-analysis. J Neurosurg Spine 2018;30(2):253–258
27. Carroll EA, Shilt JS, Jacks L. MW construct in fusion for neuromuscular scoliosis. Eur Spine J 2007;16(3):373–377

17 Correction of Deformity Using Minimally Invasive Surgical Techniques

Ziev B. Moses, Matthew H. Trawczynski, Brian T. David, and Richard G. Fessler

Introduction

Adult spinal deformities constitute a wide range of pathologies including progressive adolescent idiopathic scoliosis extending into adulthood, de novo scoliosis either from iatrogenic sagittal deformity or degenerative disc disease, and secondary degenerative scoliosis.[1] The average age of presentation of de novo scoliosis in adults is 70.5 years with an approximate prevalence of 6% in adults older than 50 years.[2] Given the acceleration of the global aging population, it is expected that the prevalence of adult spinal deformity patients will only continue to rise.[3] Pain and disability have been linearly correlated with the degree of spinal deformity,[4] and in at least one cost-effectiveness study comparing operative versus nonoperative treatment of adult lumbar scoliosis reported that operative treatment was cost-effective in the first 3 years and improved over time to be highly cost-effective at 5 years.[5] This impetus to operate has resulted in a rising number of patients undergoing corrective surgery for adult spinal deformity.

One of the challenges in treating adult spinal deformity is that traditional open deformity surgery is a major insult to the human body and complication rates have been reported to reach 39% in at least one multicenter study, with almost half of patients requiring a reoperation at 49 months if their construct was extended to the sacrum.[6] Another study found a rate of neurologic complications to be 17.6%, the majority of which included radiculopathy and motor deficits.[7] Minimally invasive techniques have been developed over the past 10 years to reduce the morbidity of open surgery,[8] and one recent retrospective multicenter review of open compared with minimally invasive surgery (MIS) revealed that MIS surgery was associated with significantly less blood loss and need for transfusion as compared to open surgery.[9] In addition, patients required shorter stays in the ICU postoperatively. The focus of this chapter is to highlight the possibilities of minimally invasive techniques to correct adult spinal deformity.

Preoperative Assessment and Management

After a history and physical examination, 36-inch-long standing X-rays are required to understand the deformity, including the spinopelvic parameters. Bending X-rays can help assess for flexibility and instability. Often, coronal imbalances that correct >30% on lateral bending films are considered flexible and do not necessitate osteotomies.[10] A magnetic resonance imaging (MRI) is obtained and can help determine the degree of spinal stenosis; in addition, it can identify sequestered disc fragments which may be a contraindication for indirect decompression of the lumbar spine. If there is concern for a fused segment, a computed tomography (CT) can be obtained to search for any areas that may impede correction of the deformity through the interbody spacer.

A bone density scan is also obtained and in patients with a T-score of >3, a deformity correction is typically contraindicated. If the T-score is between −2 and −3, an endocrinology referral is made. Patients can often be started on preoperative teriparatide, if no contraindications exist.

Pearl

Coronal imbalances that correct >30% on lateral bending films often do not necessitate osteotomies. Assessment of bone density is critical prior to undergoing MIS deformity surgery.

Radiographic Considerations for Diagnosis and Surgical Planning

The minimally invasive spinal deformity surgery (MISDEF) algorithm was created to assist spine surgeons in choosing an appropriate surgical approach for patients undergoing MIS deformity surgery.[11] The MISDEF divides general surgical approaches into three classes. It bases the surgical approach on known spinopelvic parameters and whether the deformity is flexible or rigid. Eleven fellowship-trained spine surgeons validated this algorithm using a series of 20 example cases previously published in the literature that were resurveyed by the same surgeons at least 2 months later. Interobserver kappa values were found to be 0.58 initially and 0.69 following the repeat survey, indicating substantial agreement among surgeons. See **Fig. 17.1** for a breakdown of the algorithm.

Class I

This approach is reserved for patients with a sagittal vertical axis (SVA) <6 cm, pelvic tilt (PT) <25 degrees, pelvic incidence-lumbar lordosis (PI-LL) mismatch <10 degrees, lateral listhesis <6 mm, and a coronal Cobb <20 degrees. These patients are generally mildly affected by their deformity and often present with symptoms of either neurogenic claudication or radiculopathy. The primary goal of surgery is to decompress the neural elements via an MIS approach rather than correct their mild spinal deformity. Preoperative dynamic radiographs should be obtained to rule out a Meyerding grade II spondylolisthesis; at most, a grade I spondylolisthesis should be treated with this approach using a single-level MIS fusion, either via a transforaminal lumbar interbody fusion (TLIF), lumbar interbody fusion (LIF), or anterior lumbar interbody fusion (ALIF). The LIF or ALIF may be enhanced with MIS posterior fixation.

Class II

These patients have an SVA >6 cm, PT <25 degrees, lateral listhesis >6 mm (Meyerding class I or 2 spondylolisthesis or lateral listhesis), LL-PI mismatch >10 degrees and <30 degrees, and a thoracic kyphosis <60 degrees. Their curves are also flexible, displaying some correction on lateral bending films. They are more symptomatic from their axial back pain in addition to symptoms arising from neural element compression. With this approach, a main goal of surgery is to correct the deformity by extending the fusion at more than one level and either over the apex or all involved levels of the major curve. This approach utilizes a combination of MIS TLIF, lateral lumbar interbody fusion (LLIF), and/or ALIF supplemented by posterior fixation.

Class III

This surgical approach includes patients with rigid curves, SVA >6 cm, PT >25 degrees, PI-LL greater than 30 degrees, and thoracic kyphosis >60 degrees. These patients are debilitated by their substantial sagittal and/or coronal curves. Given their major deformities, open surgery with the potential for multilevel osteotomies and/or three-column osteotomies is recommended, given

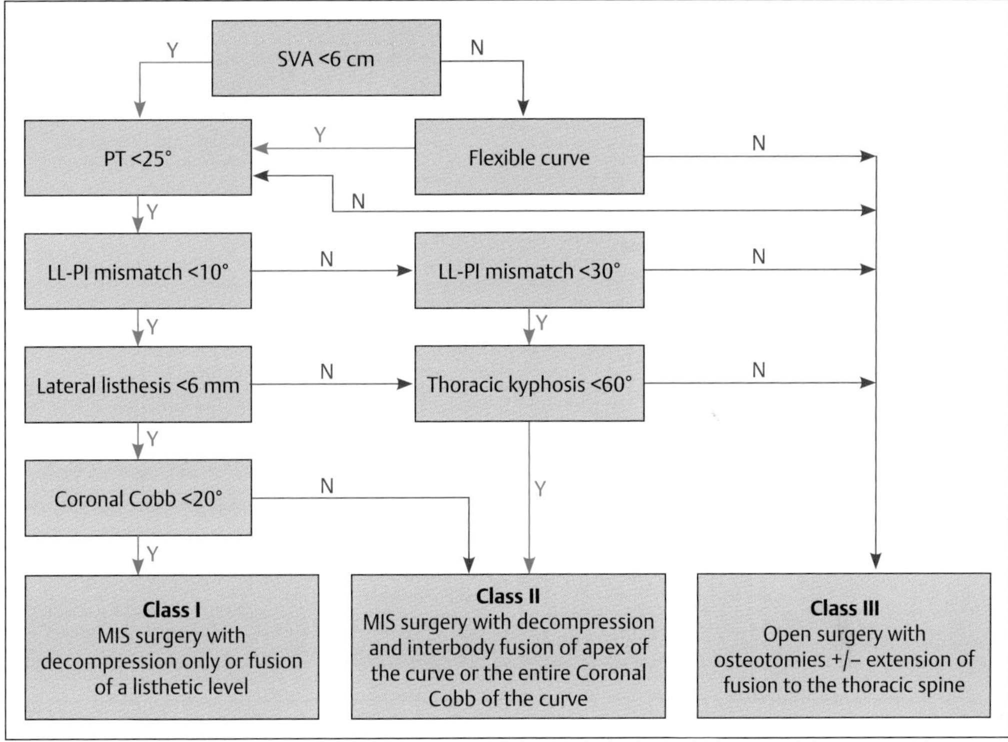

Fig. 17.1 Minimally invasive spinal deformity algorithm for decision making when considering less invasive correction techniques. N = no; Y = yes; SVA, sagittal vertical axis; PT, pelvic tilt; LL-PI, pelvic incidence-lumbar lordosis.

that current MIS techniques cannot reliably achieve the correction goals.

Importantly, since the introduction of the revised MISDEF algorithm in 2014, MIS techniques have continued to advance with the incorporation of new devices and techniques to augment the degree of sagittal correction achievable through an MIS approach. These include lordotic interbody cages as well as expandable cage technology that lengthen the anterior column and approaches such as the Lateral transpsoas release of the anterior longitudinal ligament.[12] Combined with circumferential MIS approaches, a proposed update to the MISDEF algorithm was recently introduced.[13] This revised algorithm (**Fig. 17.2**) introduces a fourth class reserved for cases where more than five levels need to be fused, including L5–S1, or >10 segments need treatment, and/or multilevel instrumentation needs to be revised. The revised MISDEF algorithm is currently undergoing reliability evaluation at this time.

Pearl

MISDEF is a helpful reference for categorizing surgical strategies into three options for deformity patients. The revised algorithm is still undergoing evaluation at this time.

Keys to Surgical Planning

The circumferential MIS protocol (cMIS protocol) is a staged protocol for surgical correction of adult sagittal deformity[14] (**Fig. 17.3**). Stage I begins with MIS interbody fusions at all levels to be included in the deformity correction, in a distal-to-proximal fashion. This is typically either done in one position with LLIFs at all levels, including an

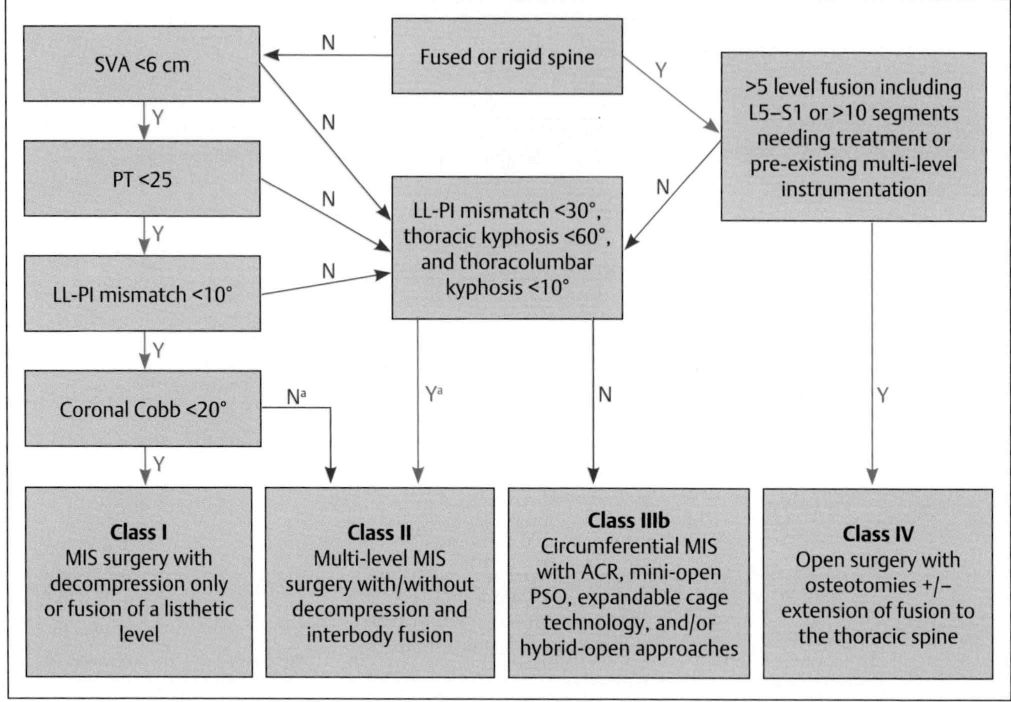

Fig. 17.2 Revised minimally invasive spinal deformity surgery (MISDEF) algorithm for the correction of adult spinal deformity. [a]For curved greater than 60, double major curves, consider class III. [b]For experienced MIS surgeons. SVA, sagittal vertical axis; PT, pelvic tilt; LL-PI, pelvic incidence-lumbar lordosis; ACR, anterior column realignment; N, no; PSO, pedicle subtraction osteotomy; Y, yes. (From Choy et al[13])

oblique ante-PSOAS approach to access the L5–S1 disc space if incorporating this segment in the construct. Otherwise, depending on surgeon preference, ALIFs can be performed at L4–L5 and L5–S1, the patient repositioned in a lateral decubitus position, and then LLIFs performed in the remaining cephalad levels. At L5–S1, removal of the posterior longitudinal ligament allows for improved disc height restoration and lordotic correction. With the use of multilevel interbody cages, routine anterior longitudinal ligament release is not needed. From L5–S1 to L2–L3, 12-degree or greater cages are typically used, whereas at more cephalad levels either 6- or 12-degree cages can be used depending on the patient's radiographic measurements.

Stage 2 of the cMIS protocol calls for the assessment of radicular symptoms and radiographic parameters following stage I. Thirty-six-inch standing radiographs are obtained to determine the new alignment parameters. This is typically done on the second or third postoperative day. Patients with new or persistent radicular symptoms can undergo an MRI and if a region of stenosis is seen, decompression of that segment can be performed during the next stage. If an appropriate degree of correction has been achieved via Stage 1, which is considered to be an SVA of less than 5 to 8 cm (depending upon patient age) and a PI-LL mismatch of less than 10 degrees, then Stage 2 consists of MIS posterior instrumentation with techniques such as aggressive rod contouring and reduction. If a persistent deformity exists, MIS tubular partial facetectomies can be performed at all levels

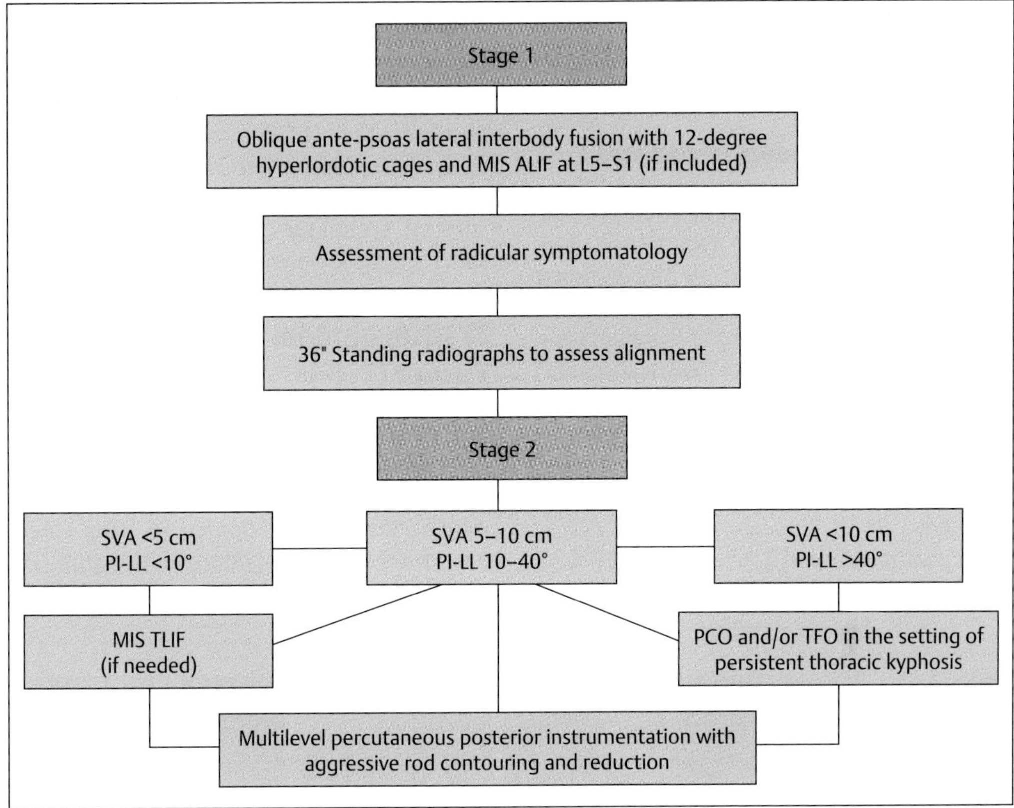

Fig. 17.3 Staged surgical protocol for CMIS correction of ASD. MIS, minimally invasive surgery; ALIF, anterior lumbar interbody fusion; SVA, sagittal vertical axis; PI-LL, pelvic incidence lumbar lordosis mismatch; TLIF, transforaminal lumbar interbody fusion; PCO, posterior column osteotomy; TFO, transforaminal osteotomy. (From Anand et al[14])

posteriorly prior to placement of the pedicle screws. A chevron-type osteotomy is made, and lordosis can be further enhanced with compression maneuvers.

Pearl

The cMIS protocol is a surgical strategy recommended in patients undergoing MIS deformity correction.

Typical Case to Start With

It is critical to become familiar with each individual surgical approach prior to combining multiple approaches into a two-stage approach. Therefore, a straightforward case would involve a MISDEF Class I approach with minimal deformity correction. Mastering the workhorse techniques including single-level ALIF, TLIF, and LLIF is first recommended prior to commencing multilevel interbody fusions with percutaneous posterior fixation.

Typical Case to Avoid When Starting the Procedure and not Very Experienced

Most revised MISDEF Class III and all MISDEF Class IV surgical approaches should be avoided for those starting MIS deformity procedures. These include cases with significant spinopelvic parameter misalignment and/or rigid deformities.

Cases for Advanced in the Area

Class III approaches in the revised MISDEF algorithm are reserved for experienced MIS surgeons. Familiarity with all the building block surgical techniques (e.g., ALIF, TLIF, LLIF, partial facetectomies, and negotiating long-rod constructs in the subfascial plane) is required prior to proceeding with these cases. In addition, in select cases, anterior column release strategies and miniopen pedicle subtraction osteotomies may be required.

An example case of a revised MISDEF class III approach is shown in **Fig. 17.4**.

Surgical Positioning: Important Points

Positioning for MIS deformity cases is critical to achieve appropriate spinopelvic parameter optimization. Given each individual surgical technique has its own particular specifications, we will discuss these in turn.

Transforaminal Lumbar Interbody Fusion (TLIF)

The patient is positioned prone on a radiolucent Wilson frame on a flat Jackson table, or alternatively on an open Jackson table which allows the abdomen to hang freely and decrease intraabdominal pressure. An open Jackson table also allows for additional

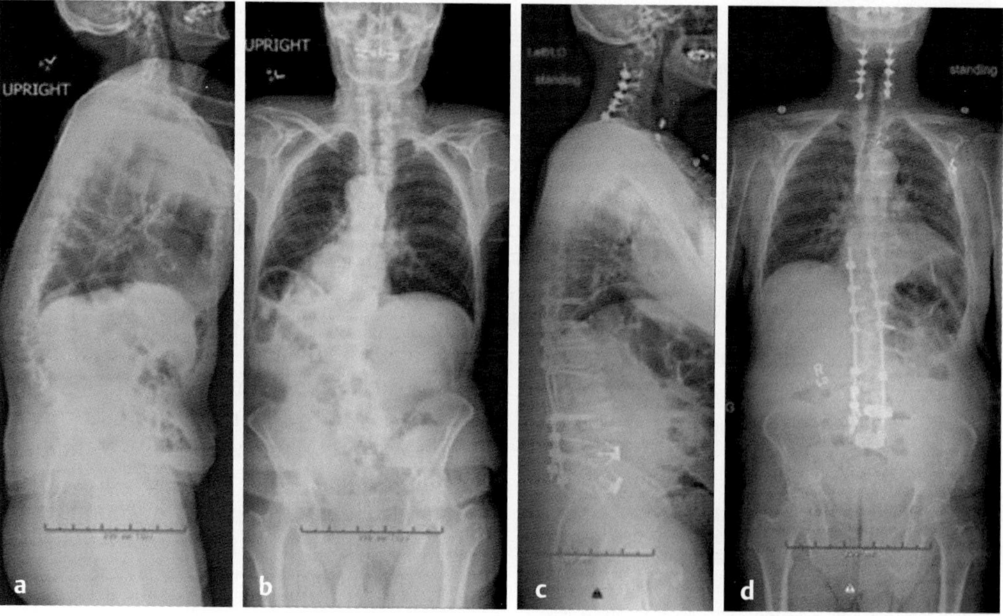

Fig. 17.4 Standing 36-inch scoliosis X-rays in a 68-year-old man with several years of incapacitating back pain. Preoperative **(a)** sagittal and **(b)** anterior–posterior views revealing a sagittal vertical axis (SVA) of 10.1 cm and coronal Cobb angle of 28.9 degrees. Other spinopelvic parameters including a pelvic incidence of 44.0 degrees, lumbar lordosis of 15.2 degrees. Postoperative **(c)** sagittal and **(d)** anterior–posterior views revealing an improved SVA of 4.8 cm and coronal Cobb angle of 9.8 degrees. Lumbar lordosis was increased to 39.9 degrees with near resolution of the PI-LL mismatch. The patient required no blood transfusions.

restoration of lumbar lordosis. Both Jackson tables allow easy maneuverability of the imaging equipment compared with a standard operating table. Gentle taping of the hips and shoulders can assist in reducing coronal plane deformity. If there are unilateral radicular symptoms, the ipsilateral side should be approached with the bed-mounted tubular retractor arm and fluoroscopy machine based on the opposite side of the table. We employ neuromonitoring for all TLIF procedures.

Lateral Lumbar Interbody Fusion (LLIF)

The patient is positioned on a breakable radiolucent table in a true lateral decubitus position. The thoracolumbar curve can either be approached from the convex or concave side. At least two retrospective studies have found no statistical difference in postoperative complication rates regardless of approach side.[15,16] Our preference is to approach the concavity in order to reach all the intended treatment levels through a minimal opening. A bean bag is used to support the patient and pad all pressure points. The top leg is bent to relax the PSOAS muscle and aid in the dissection. The bean bag can also be used to pad the axilla or alternatively an axillary roll can be used. Tape is also used around the legs, hips, and upper torso to secure the patient to the bed. The optimal position of the break in the bed is above the iliac crest. It is important to maximize the interval between the iliac crest and lower thoracic rib cage using the bed controller. Fluoroscopy is then used to confirm a true lateral position which involves having the spinous process in the midline, observing sharp end plates, and seeing the pedicle shadows equidistant laterally from the midline. The bed is adjusted so as to ensure a true lateral projection while the fluoroscopy unit stays perpendicular to the floor. We employ neuromonitoring including triggered and continuous electromyography (EMG) for all LLIF procedures.

Anterior Lumbar Interbody Fusion (ALIF)

The patient is positioned supine on a flat Jackson table. In order to augment lumbar lordosis, a roll or bump can be placed under the lumbar spine. In addition, the patient is placed in slight reverse Trendelenburg to help shift the abdominal contents superiorly and away from the working space. The arms are placed on arm boards in a cruciform position to allow for maximal working space. Neuromonitoring is not routinely used for ALIF procedures.

Pearl

Positioning is critical for optimizing correction of deformity in MIS cases. Each surgical approach has its own unique details as described above.

Surgical Procedure—Tips and Tricks

Transforaminal Lumbar Interbody Fusion (TLIF)

After prepping and draping the patient, the appropriate level is localized. It is important to have good fluoroscopic images including true lateral and anteroposterior (AP) views. A skin incision is made 2 to 3 cm lateral to midline (depending upon the specific interbody cage selected) and its length varies on the number of levels. For a single level, 2.5 cm should be sufficient to allow for placement of a 24-mm tube. After dissection down to the lumbosacral fascia, a linear incision is sharply made along the length of the fascia. The first dilator is then advanced to the depth of the bony margin of the facet and lamina. This is confirmed with fluoroscopy and additional dilators are placed up until the final tubular retractor is placed and secured to the table mounted arm.

Depending on surgeon preference, either loupe magnification, an endoscope, or the operating microscope can be used to perform the facetectomy. First, the edge of the inferior lamina of the rostral level is identified with straight and angled curettes. A hemilaminotomy is then made with Kerrison rongeurs, followed by a facetectomy with either an osteotome or a high-speed drill. An osteotome is preferred as it facilitates saving of the bony facet to be used later as an autograft. Following removal of the facet, the ligamentum flavum is removed. It is recommended to leave the ligamentum flavum intact until after the bony removal is complete as it helps prevent dural tears. The ligamentum flavum is then released using straight and angled curettes, followed by removal using a Kerrison rongeur.

After removal of the ligamentum flavum, the thecal sac and traversing nerve root are exposed medially, whereas the exiting nerve root is traveling superiorly. A radical discectomy is performed. It is helpful to use a nerve root retracting suction tip to protect the thecal sac during the interbody work. The discectomy is performed with paddle shavers, curettes, and end plate scrapers. It is critical to prepare the end plates well to optimize arthrodesis, while minimizing end plate violation which can lead to subsidence. Sequential trials are placed, and an appropriate vertical and horizontal length as well as lordotic angle are obtained. An interbody graft is chosen based on the maximum allowable size that does not tear the anterior longitudinal ligament or jut out posteriorly behind the annulus. The graft is typically filled with a small amount of bone morphogenic protein (BMP, off-label use), morselized autograft, and/or demineralized bone matrix (DBM). After confirming the graft is in the proper position using AP and lateral fluoroscopy, hemostasis is obtained, and the tubular retractor is removed. The placement of posterior fixation is discussed below. The wound is irrigated with antibiotic solution and closed in layers.

Pearl

It is advisable to leave the ligamentum flavum intact until after the bony removal is complete as it helps prevent dural tears.

Lateral Lumbar Interbody Fusion (LLIF)

A radiopaque instrument is used to mark the surgical mid-disc zone. If several levels are being treated, a longer mark is made that will allow access to all the surgical levels. Typically, at least two levels can be reached with each incision. A small incision is made over the mark and blunt retractors are used to reach the fibers of the internal and external oblique muscles which are bluntly split. Blunt retractors are used to open the transversalis fascia and reach the retroperitoneal space, followed by blunt dissection past the retroperitoneal fat onto the PSOAS muscle. The EMG probe is passed through the PSOAS into the anterior half to third of the disc, with adjustments made if activity is detected with the free-run EMG. A guidewire is passed through the EMG probe. Then, the first dilator is guided onto the PSOAS muscle directly over the intended surgical disc level. Triggered EMG is then used to safely dock the first dilator on the intervertebral space. This is confirmed with AP fluoroscopy. Sequential dilation ensues and the retractor is brought into final position. After confirming no activation of the lumbar plexus with triggered EMG, the retractor is secured using pins or shims into the superior and inferior vertebral bodies.

A discectomy is performed under direct visualization using straight and angled curettes, pituitary rongeurs, rasps, and trials. A wide Cobb instrument is used to break through the contralateral annulus with regular fluoroscopy during this maneuver. Sequential trial upsizing is used until a final implant size is chosen. The end plates are then prepared, and the implant is placed and checked for final position with fluoroscopy. Hemostasis is obtained and the tubular retractor is removed. The wound is irrigated with antibiotic solution and closed in layers, ensuring closure of the transversalis fascia and external oblique fascia to prevent hernia.

Pearl

The preference of the authors is to approach the concavity in order to reach all the intended treatment levels through a minimal opening.

Anterior Lumbar Interbody Fusion (ALIF)

Lateral fluoroscopy is used to mark the surgical levels. There are several possible opening incisions. We prefer to use a horizontal incision if one level is being targeted. The approach to the L5–S1 disc space can be quite steep, requiring the incision to be close to the pubic symphysis. If two or more levels are being operated on, a vertical incision is made on the left near the linea semilunaris. We prefer a left-sided retroperitoneal approach and use an access surgeon in these cases. The anterior rectus sheath is incised, and the rectus muscles are bluntly split until the posterior rectus sheath which is then divided. The PSOAS muscle is then encountered laterally, and the peritoneal contents are bluntly swept medially. The left ureter and iliac vessels are identified. A fixed Omni retractor system is used to circumferentially position and protect the peritoneal contents and vessels. At L4–L5, occasionally the iliolumbar vein requires ligation, whereas at L5–S1, the middle sacral vessels require ligation. In addition, at L4–L5, the aorta and vena cava can be retracted medially, whereas at L5–S1, the disc space can be accessed between the great vessels. A spinal needle is used to localize the appropriate level using lateral fluoroscopy.

After confirming the correct disc level, an annulotomy is made with a #11 blade. A discectomy is performed in standard fashion using curettes, pituitary rongeurs, and Kerrison rongeurs. A large Cobb elevator is used to remove the cartilaginous end plate from the vertebral bodies. Care must be taken to remove sufficient disc to allow for maximal lordosis, while preventing subchondral bone removal and increasing the risk of subsidence. Trials are sequentially used to appropriately size a final implant. Once the implant is positioned, screws/pins are used to secure the implant to the superior and inferior vertebral bodies. A final lateral and AP X-ray is used to confirm the proper position. The retractors are sequentially released, and hemostasis is obtained with careful bipolar cautery. The anterior rectus sheath and abdominal fascia are closed in layers.

Pearl

The authors prefer a left-sided retroperitoneal approach and use an access surgeon in these cases.

Posterior Instrumentation

The patient is positioned prone on either a flat Jackson table with radiolucent Wilson frame or an open Jackson table to optimize lordosis. If a prior midline incision is present, or if more than three levels are to be posteriorly instrumented, a midline incision is used. Otherwise, multiple small skin incisions are used to access the pedicles. If pelvic fixation is required, iliac screws can be placed minimally invasively with an incision over the posterior superior iliac spine. With a midline incision, a transfascial muscle-sparing approach is used.

In cases that require aggressive correction, partial facetectomies can be performed via the tubular retractor. Pedicle screws are placed using either an AP view technique, biplanar fluoroscopy, or using image-guidance. Facet fusion is performed at all levels that have not undergone interbody fusion. A nasal speculum or tubular retractor system can be used to access the facet in the intermuscular plane used for placement of the pedicle screws. Rods are contoured in the sagittal plane to provide for additional sagittal correction and are kept straight in the coronal plane. This allows for derotation of the spine as the spine is reduced and translates onto the rod. Titanium alloy rods are preferred over cobalt-chrome to lessen the risk of screw backout during the reduction.

It is important to use a percutaneous rod reduction system that allows for aggressive rod reduction. It is important to pass the contoured rod in the subfascial space from cranial to caudal. The tulips of the screws are used as anchor points to reduce the rod, beginning with reduction at the apex of the lordosis to prevent flattening of the rod. Careful sequential reduction is undertaken at each tulip to maximize sagittal restoration. Following placement of the rod, final X-rays are taken to ensure there is rod above and below the superior and inferiormost screws. The set screws are then fastened and finally tightened. After decortication of the facet and pars, local bone graft, BMP, and demineralized bone matrix are packed into the drilled regions. The wound is copiously irrigated with antibiotic solution, hemostasis is obtained, and the wound is closed in layers.

Pearl

The authors recommend performing facet fusion at all levels that have not undergone interbody fusion.

Surgical Procedure: Complications and Their Avoidance

Transforaminal Lumbar Interbody Fusion (TLIF)

The most common complication of TLIF is durotomy. While exposure is limited when using a tubular retractor, a primary repair can be achieved with 4–0 or smaller suture, using a right-angled probe to push the knot down and hold it in place with a micropituitary. A dural sealant can be used for smaller tears that cannot be repaired primarily. Nerve root injury is another possible complication of TLIF. This typically occurs if there is excessive retraction on the nerve root during placement of the interbody graft. Therefore, it is important to minimize retraction of the nerve root by carefully visualizing and conserving the appropriate trajectory. Pseudoarthrosis and subsidence are both potential complications of TLIF. These are minimized by carefully preparing the end plates without violating them and using as large a graft as possible. Graft displacement and retropulsion are other potential complications that can be minimized by using as large a graft as possible and ensuring the pedicle screws are locked down in compression. Vascular injury is a potential complication during discectomy and it is critical to maintain awareness of the integrity of the anterior longitudinal ligament at all times. Another complication inherent to all procedures is wound infection and dehiscence.

Lateral Lumbar Interbody Fusion (LLIF)

Neurologic complications following LLIF are the main concern, given the proximity to the lumbosacral plexus during the approach. One systematic review found the incidence of transient neurologic deficits to be 36.07% and the incidence of persistent neurologic deficit to be 3.98%.[17] These included PSOAS weakness, thigh hypoesthesia, and anterior thigh pain. Having the tubular retractor docked more superficially on the PSOAS muscle is intended to reduce the risk of these deficits. Minimizing retraction time also decreases the incidence of hypoesthesia. Injury to the segmental artery is rare but can result in significant blood loss. Use of bipolar cautery and hemostatic agents can stop the blood loss, should this arise during surgery. Other complications common to retroperitoneal approaches include injury to the peritoneum, bowel, and kidney.

Anterior Lumbar Interbody Fusion (ALIF)

Neurological complications following ALIF are rare, given there is usually no attempt made at a direct decompression of the neural elements and the epidural space is not entered. Given the retroperitoneal approach to the lumbar spine, several complications including injury to the bowel, ureter, and presacral neural plexus are possible. Careful dissection and sufficient exposure are encouraged to minimize these risks. Hernias are also possible if the peritoneum or transversalis fascia are violated—it is best to repair these during the initial surgery. Retrograde ejaculation can occur if the presacral neural plexus is injured. Therefore, minimizing the use of monopolar cautery, particularly during L5–S1 ALIF, is encouraged. The left common iliac vein is at risk of tear, resulting in large blood loss. Tears can usually be repaired using fine suture material with the assistance of vascular surgery. Iliac vein thrombosis is another potential complication with prolonged retraction. Pulse oximetry of the bilateral lower extremities can detect differences in oxygen saturation. Should a thrombosis be detected, intravenous heparin and an open thrombectomy is performed. Subsidence is a potential complication that can be minimized by carefully preparing the end plates without being overly aggressive.

Pearl

Each surgical approach has its own particular risk profile: durotomy is most common in TLIF, neurological complications following LLIF, and vascular complications during ALIF.

Postoperative Care

In patients undergoing LLIF or ALIF, a complete blood count is obtained in the recovery area and on the morning following surgery to survey for retroperitoneal hematoma. All patients are mobilized on their first postoperative day and no bracing is needed. Standing 36-inch scoliosis X-rays are obtained prior to discharge. In patients with posterior instrumentation, a CT scan is obtained to ensure satisfactory placement of screws. Most patients are discharged for home or to inpatient rehabilitation by postoperative days 3–5.

Follow-up

Patients are seen in clinic at 2 weeks, 2 months, 6 months, 1 year, and 2 years after surgery. Standing X-rays and flexion-extension views are obtained at each visit to ensure adequate radiographic fusion progression.

Future Perspectives: Vision for Further Development

As MISS techniques continue to evolve, future advances—namely, novel neuronavigation, robotic, and expandable cage technologies—will further drive preoperative, intraoperative, and postoperative care, resulting in both improved operative efficiency and morbidity outcomes. Thus so far, the use of neuronavigation,[18–21] robotics,[22–24] and various expandable intervertebral cage innovations[25] in combination with MISS techniques for deformity correction has been proved safe, but few studies have conclusively shown superior patient outcomes with MISS surgery over conventional methods. Future advances and trials are needed before a clear gold standard is established and the high cost of these technologies is warranted.[26]

The combination of MISS and neuronavigation has resulted in several improved surgical and complication outcome parameters, but future advances are needed to realize full potential. Current neuronavigation technology comprises cone-beam CT, which generates three-dimensional images intraoperatively.[20] In the context of MISS deformity correction, the use of neuronavigation has two advantages over traditional fluoroscopic techniques; potentially increased accuracy in pedicle screw placement and decreased radiation exposure to the surgeon/patient relative to fluoroscopy.[27,28] For example, Bourgeois et al calculated a 99% decrease in MISS pedicle screw breach when using three-dimensional neuronavigation.[27] Some groups have also reported decreased estimated blood loss and decreased reports of postprocedural pain after neuronavigation-assisted MISS correction of Lenke Type 5C adolescent idiopathic scoliosis.[18] This being said, this same study found that total operative time was found to be increased by an average of 62 minutes for neuronavigation-assisted MISS group. In contrast, other groups have reported blood loss equivalent to standard techniques, especially in pre-PSOAS oblique lumbar interbody fusion (OLIF).[28] Thus, only some groups report morbidity improvements, and future advances are needed to decrease complication rates.

In addition to improving pedicle screw placement and patient morbidity, recent advances in neuronavigation-assisted MISS have allowed for new surgical approaches and trajectories. For example, intraoperative neuronavigation can be vital for novel or challenging surgical approaches like pre-PSOAS OLIF, where the surgical trajectory may be unfamiliar.[29] Other groups have reported successful neuronavigation-assisted MISS using novel, portable CT technologies like the Brainlab Airo, which help streamline all stages of TLIF including planning, accurate screw placement, and cage placement.[30] Airo has also recently been used to predict positioning of interbody cages and to eliminate the need for K-wires, further reducing potential postsurgical complications.[31] Overall, neuronavigation for MISS deformity correction has rapidly progressed, but overall patient outcomes remain largely unchanged when comparing neuronavigation MISS and traditional techniques.[28] Before they fully are implemented and utilized, these technologies, possibly in combination with others like robotics, must first provide a clear patient outcome benefit.

Recent advances in robotics and expandable cage technologies also hold significant potential for neuronavigation-assisted MISS in the context of deformity correction. Like with neuronavigation alone, robot-assisted pedicle screw placement has also been reported to result in increased accuracy and safety in the correction of idiopathic adolescent scoliosis, especially when combined with image-guided techniques.[24] Other studies have shown safe and feasible deformity correction using robot-guided S2-alar-iliac screw insertion.[22] Robot-assisted TLIF for adult degenerative scoliosis, in combination with analgesic sponges, resulted in shorter hospital stays and successful long-term clinical outcomes.[23] Other studies have demonstrated feasible MIS-ALIF using da Vinci surgical systems.[32,33] New expandable cage technologies used for MIS-TLIF have also yielded encouraging results. In one study, expandable cage MIS-TILF showed increased disc height longevity, foraminal height, and segmental lordosis than static cages.[25] This being said, other studies have found opposite results.[34] Thus, further trials are needed before conclusive results can be obtained.

The progression of new technologies for MISS deformity correction has resulted in decreased complication rates and an increase in more accurate surgical techniques. As others have mentioned, cost-benefit analysis will continue to be performed when evaluating the utility of these technologies.[26] Other technologies not mentioned in this section include neurosurgical augmented reality, such as Google Glass or HoloLens, which are currently being tested.[35] Such technologies hold tremendous potential and may someday be used in combination with the above-mentioned neuronavigation, robotics, and expandable cage technology.

References

1. Aebi M. The adult scoliosis. Eur Spine J 2005; 14(10):925–948
2. Diebo BG, Shah NV, Boachie-Adjei O, et al. Adult spinal deformity. Lancet 2019; 394(10193):160–172
3. Lutz W, Sanderson W, Scherbov S. The coming acceleration of global population ageing. Nature 2008;451(7179):716–719
4. Glassman SD, Bridwell K, Dimar JR, Horton W, Berven S, Schwab F. The impact of positive sagittal balance in adult spinal deformity. Spine 2005;30(18):2024–2029
5. Carreon LY, Glassman SD, Lurie J, et al. Cost-effectiveness of operative versus nonoperative treatment of adult symptomatic lumbar scoliosis an intent-to-treat analysis at 5-year follow-up. Spine 2019;44(21):1499–1506
6. Charosky S, Guigui P, Blamoutier A, Roussouly P, Chopin D; Study Group on Scoliosis. Complications and risk factors of primary adult scoliosis surgery: a multicenter study of 306 patients. Spine 2012;37(8):693–700
7. Kim HJ, Iyer S, Zebala LP, et al; International Spine Study Group (ISSG). Perioperative neurologic complications in adult spinal deformity surgery: incidence and risk factors in 564 patients. Spine 2017;42(6):420–427
8. Anand N, Baron EM, Thaiyananthan G, Khalsa K, Goldstein TB. Minimally invasive multilevel percutaneous correction and fusion for adult lumbar degenerative scoliosis: a technique and feasibility study. J Spinal Disord Tech 2008;21(7):459–467
9. Chou D, Mundis G, Wang M, et al; International Spine Study Group. Minimally invasive surgery for mild-to-moderate adult spinal deformities: impact on intensive care unit and hospital stay. World Neurosurg 2019; 127:e649–e655
10. Silva FE, Lenke LG. Adult degenerative scoliosis: evaluation and management. Neurosurg Focus 2010;28(3):E1
11. Mummaneni PV, Shaffrey CI, Lenke LG, et al; Minimally Invasive Surgery Section of the International Spine Study Group. The minimally invasive spinal deformity surgery algorithm: a reproducible rational framework for decision making in minimally invasive spinal deformity surgery. Neurosurg Focus 2014;36(5):E6
12. Saigal R, Mundis GM Jr, Eastlack R, Uribe JS, Phillips FM, Akbarnia BA. Anterior column realignment (ACR) in adult sagittal deformity correction: technique and review of the literature. Spine 2016;41(Suppl 8):S66–S73
13. Choy W, Miller CA, Chan AK, Fu KM, Park P, Mummaneni PV. Evolution of the minimally invasive spinal deformity surgery algorithm: an evidence-based approach to surgical strategies for deformity correction. Neurosurg Clin N Am 2018;29(3):399–406
14. Anand N, Kong C, Fessler RG. A staged protocol for circumferential minimally invasive surgical correction of adult spinal deformity. Neurosurgery 2017;81(5):733–739
15. Kanter AS, Tempel ZJ, Agarwal N, et al. Curve laterality for lateral lumbar interbody fusion in adult scoliosis surgery: the concave versus convex controversy. Neurosurgery 2018;83(6):1219–1225
16. Scheer JK, Khanna R, Lopez AJ, et al. The concave versus convex approach for minimally invasive lateral lumbar interbody fusion for thoracolumbar degenerative scoliosis. J Clin Neurosci 2015;22(10):1588–1593
17. Hijji FY, Narain AS, Bohl DD, et al. Lateral lumbar interbody fusion: a systematic review of complication rates. Spine J 2017; 17(10):1412–1419
18. Minimally invasive scoliosis surgery assisted by O-arm navigation for Lenke Type 5C adolescent idiopathic scoliosis: a comparison with standard open approach spinal instrumentation. J Neurosurg Pediatr 2017; 19(4):472–478
19. Joseph JR, Smith BW, Patel RD, Park P. Use of 3D CT-based navigation in minimally invasive lateral lumbar interbody fusion. J Neurosurg Spine 2016;25(3):339–344
20. Oh T, Park P, Miller CA, Chan AK, Mummaneni PV. Navigation-assisted minimally invasive surgery deformity correction. Neurosurg Clin N Am 2018;29(3):439–451
21. Park P. Three-dimensional computed tomography-based spinal navigation in minimally invasive lateral lumbar interbody fusion: feasibility, technique, and initial results. Neurosurgery 2015;11(Suppl 2): 259–267
22. Bederman SS, Hahn P, Colin V, Kiester PD, Bhatia NN. Robotic guidance for S2-Alar-Iliac

screws in spinal deformity correction. Clin Spine Surg 2017;30(1):E49–E53

23. Du JP, Fan Y, Liu JJ, Zhang JN, Chang Liu S, Hao D. Application of gelatin sponge impregnated with a mixture of 3 drugs to intraoperative nerve root block combined with robot-assisted minimally invasive transforaminal lumbar interbody fusion surgery in the treatment of adult degenerative scoliosis: a clinical observation including 96 patients. World Neurosurg 2017;108:791–797
24. Macke JJ, Woo R, Varich L. Accuracy of robot-assisted pedicle screw placement for adolescent idiopathic scoliosis in the pediatric population. J Robot Surg 2016;10(2):145–150
25. Hawasli AH, Khalifeh JM, Chatrath A, Yarbrough CK, Ray WZ. Minimally invasive transforaminal lumbar interbody fusion with expandable versus static interbody devices: radiographic assessment of sagittal segmental and pelvic parameters. Neurosurg Focus 2017;43(2):E10
26. Overley SC, Cho SK, Mehta AI, Arnold PM. Navigation and robotics in spinal surgery: where are we now? Neurosurgery 2017; 80(3S):S86–S99
27. Bourgeois AC, Faulkner AR, Bradley YC, et al. Improved accuracy of minimally invasive transpedicular screw placement in the lumbar spine with 3-dimensional stereotactic image guidance: a comparative meta-analysis. J Spinal Disord Tech 2015;28(9):324–329
28. Zhang YH, White I, Potts E, Mobasser JP, Chou D. Comparison perioperative factors during minimally invasive pre-psoas lateral interbody fusion of the lumbar spine using either navigation or conventional fluoroscopy. Global Spine J 2017;7(7):657–663
29. DiGiorgio AM, Edwards CS, Virk MS, Mummaneni PV, Chou D. Stereotactic navigation for the prepsoas oblique lateral lumbar interbody fusion: technical note and case series. Neurosurg Focus 2017;43(2):E14
30. Lian X, Navarro-Ramirez R, Berlin C, et al. Total 3D Airo® navigation for minimally invasive transforaminal lumbar interbody fusion. BioMed Res Int 2016;2016:5027340
31. Kirnaz S, et al. Minimally invasive transforaminal lumbar interbody fusion using 3-dimensional total navigation: 2-dimensional operative video. Oper Neurosurg (Hagerstown); 2019
32. Lee JY, Bhowmick DA, Eun DD, Welch WC. Minimally invasive, robot-assisted, anterior lumbar interbody fusion: a technical note. J Neurol Surg A Cent Eur Neurosurg 2013; 74(4):258–261
33. Troude L, Boissonneau S, Malikov S, et al. Robot-assisted multi-level anterior lumbar interbody fusion: an anatomical study. Acta Neurochir (Wien) 2018;160(10):1891–1898
34. Yee TJ, Joseph JR, Terman SW, Park P. Expandable vs static cages in transforaminal lumbar interbody fusion: radiographic comparison of segmental and lumbar sagittal angles. Neurosurgery 2017;81(1):69–74
35. Madhavan K, Kolcun JPG, Chieng LO, Wang MY. Augmented-reality integrated robotics in neurosurgery: are we there yet? Neurosurg Focus 2017;42(5):E3

18 Intraoperative Neurophysiology Monitoring in Deformity Correction Scoliosis Surgeries

Muhammad Tariq Imtiaz and Parmod Kumar Bithal

Introduction

Intraoperative neurophysiology monitoring (IONM) has fast established itself as a major component of care in many spinal surgical procedures. Iatrogenic paraplegia is a devastating yet preventable complication during spinal surgeries. IONM serves to help patients undergoing spinal surgeries resulting in potentially better outcomes by reducing preventable postoperative complications.[1,2] This chapter will focus on IONM in deformity especially scoliosis correction surgeries. Since the practice of IONM is not standardized around the globe and individual variations in application, acquisition, reading, and correlation of IONM modalities exist, a need to review the practice of IONM is warranted. Most common practices are highlighted in this chapter. The current trend in IONM is to prepare a multimodality setup of several tests/modalities.[3–8] Understanding and interpreting data together from these modalities is paramount to achieving successful results. This technology cannot monitor every function of the spinal cord,[7] but it is continuously evolving. Therefore, it is plausible that the significance and utilization of IONM during spinal surgery will increase with more data, awareness, availability, and medicolegal issues related to safety. Although this chapter focuses on scoliosis surgeries, concepts and details discussed here can be considered for other spinal procedures.[9]

Following are the IONM modalities currently in practice in scoliosis surgeries:

- Somatosensory-evoked potentials (SSEP).
- Transcranial motor-evoked potentials (TcMEP).
- Electromyogram (EMG).
- Triggered electromyogram (TEMG).
- Electroencephalogram (EEG).

Pearl

Plan a multimodality setup.

Multimodality Monitoring

All these modalities have considerable importance at various levels in deformity surgeries. Modalities 1 (SSEP) and 2 (TcMEP) are often jointly termed as spinal cord monitoring (SCM) by various groups.[3,4,6,10] Modalities 3 (EMG) and 4 (TEMG) are interlinked and have importance in cervical and lumbar spinal level surgeries, providing nerve root protection.[7] Modality 4 is exclusive to screw stimulation and aims to assist in identification of lateral/medial screw breaches of the spinal canal with presence or absence of data changes in SCM. Last but not least, modality 5 (EEG) is not commonly practiced in scoliosis correction surgeries but is important in identification and maintenance of intravenous anesthetic depth and accurate reading of SCM data,[8] especially during significant spinal manipulation with prevention of false alarms for surgeons. Contribution by the anesthetic team is extremely important in correct acquisition and reading of data.

Pearl

Somatosensory-evoked potentials (SSEP) and transcranial motor-evoked potentials (TcMEP) are major IONM modalities in scoliosis surgeries and often termed together as spinal cord monitoring (SCM).

Methodology of Signal Acquisition and Recommendations

Field of IONM is still evolving; hence, there are many variations and discrepancies currently practiced especially in the methodology and signal acquisition components of IONM. In general, patient's baseline data serves as control in all IONM cases. Baseline signals are acquired for all planned modalities before incision and compared for changes during surgery. All modalities are performed bilaterally from symmetrical stimulation and recording sites.

In almost all IONM modalities (excluding EEG and EMG), two fundamental concepts to understand are "stimulation" and "recording." These two concepts have their own specific parameters. Incorrect use of those parameters with an inexperienced team may significantly and adversely alter results. Stimulation and recordings are performed, leading to acquisition of signals, and these are done by placing electrodes at various anatomical sites on patient's body. Electrodes are usually termed as stimulating or recording electrodes. These can vary by form (sticker or needle) and by size (e.g., needle size). Incorrect or improper use and placements may also affect signal acquisition.

In addition, understanding of various anatomical pathways including dorsal columns, corticospinal tracts, and detailed understanding of myotomal variations is necessary in planning of IONM cases.[3–7] Discussion of these individual pathways is beyond the scope of this chapter since the focus is on methodology and techniques. For example, stimulation electrodes for upper limb SSEP are sticker electrodes, placed on the wrist for median or ulnar nerve anatomical sites,[5] whereas needle electrodes are used at Erb's point (brachial plexus) and corkscrew electrodes on the skull.[5,11] Understanding of Penfield sensory and motor homunculus and 10/20 EEG system is also important, since recording or stimulating electrodes are placed in the skull following the 10/20 EEG system.[5,6] For example, last recording site for an SSEP test will be on the skull, correlating with primary sensory cortex underneath. Similarly, for a motor test (TcMEP) with motor system being a descending pathway, stimulation electrodes are placed on the skull accordingly and presumably on the primary motor cortex while recording signals are acquired in the form of compound muscle action potentials (CAMP) from needle electrodes placed on muscle relevant to the surgical location and instrumentation levels.[4,6,12–17]

Pearls

- Understanding the two concepts, (i.e., stimulation and recording in neurophysiology).
- Results in IONM depend largely on using the correct parameters.
- Data acquired in baseline (whether robust or poor) is what you intend to keep until the end of surgery.

Somatosensory-Evoked Potentials (SSEP) (Fig. 18.1)

Historically, this is the first modality introduced to the spinal operating rooms in late 1970s.[3,5] This is the measure of electrical signals with ascending sensory pathways (dorsal columns) and provides information related to proprioception only.[5] Being an ascending pathway, the point of

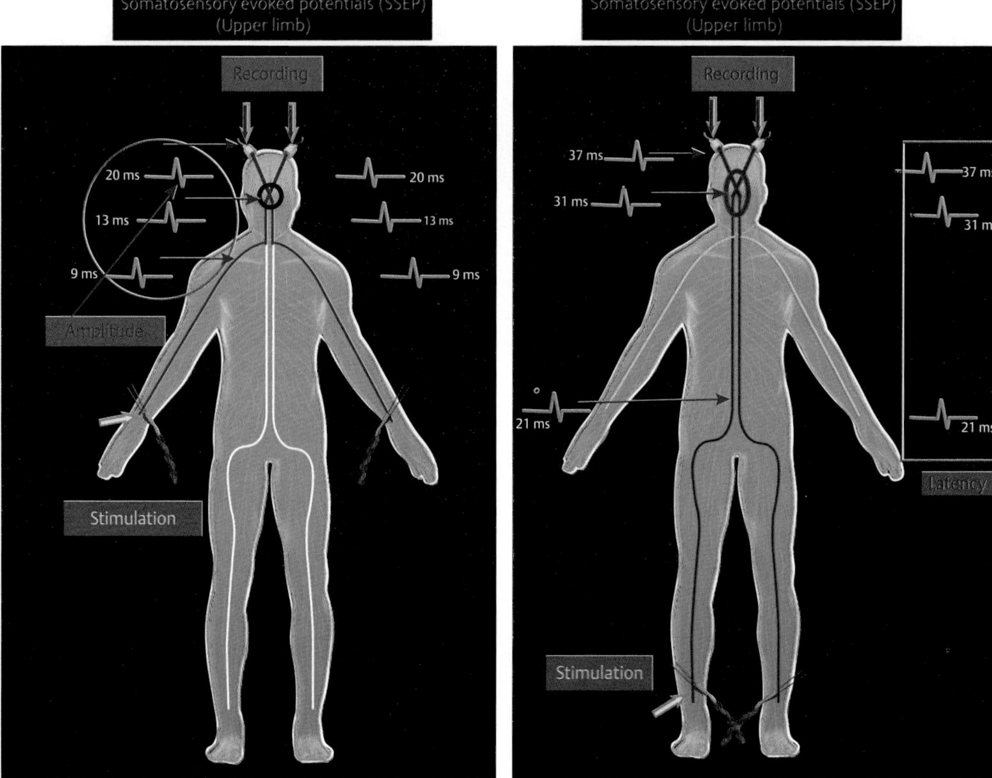

Fig. 18.1 Imtiaz-Bithal pocket review of SSEP data acquisition technique and interpretation.

"stimulation" is a peripheral nerve (median or ulnar in the upper limbs and posterior tibial and/or common peroneal nerves in the lower limbs).[11] Recordings are acquired usually from Erb's point in the upper limbs and popliteal fossa for the lower limbs and from relevant electrodes placed on the skull (described above).[18] Peripheral recordings measure the peripheral conduction time, and recordings from within the central nervous system show the central conduction time. For an adolescent idiopathic scoliosis (AIS) involving thoracic or lumbar levels, use of upper limb SSEP serves as control group and is useful in identifying brachial plexus injury related to positioning changes in the arms. Changes are measured by comparing baselines and looking at amplitude (size or morphology of the waves, measured in microvolts) or latency (conduction time from stimulation site to recording site, measured in milliseconds) and determines an alarm or stoppage.[5,8,12–16]

Significance Criteria

With a drop of more than 50% in amplitude or a latency change of 10% or more, an alarm is communicated to the surgeons.

Pearls

- Normal latency recorded on the scalp for an upper limb SSEP (from median/ulnar/radial nerves simulation at wrist in an average build adult is 20 milliseconds and often termed as N20 (N denotes negative polarity on amplitude).
- Normal latency recorded on the scalp for lower limb SSEP in average build adult is 37 milliseconds and is often termed as 37P (P denotes positive polarity/amplitude).

Transcranial Motor-Evoked Potentials (TcMEP) (Fig. 18.2)

In this test, point of stimulation is scalp electrodes with recording from relevant muscles in the upper limb (at least one upper limb controls muscle bilaterally) and lower limb.[4,6,19] It is desirable to have muscle recordings from muscles at least one or two levels below the last instrumentation spinal level. In addition, muscles showing preexisting weakness ideally be included. For lower limbs, muscles generally used for recording compound muscle action potentials (CMAPs) are quadriceps femoris, tibialis anterior, extensor hallucis longus, gastrocnemius, extensor hallucis brevis, and anal sphincters bilaterally.[11] For surgeries involving all lumbar levels, all the above may be included in the protocol. For surgeries involving predominantly thoracic levels only, general practice is to pick important dorsiflexion muscles bilaterally (tibialis anterior and extensor hallucis longus). Data is compared to baselines acquired before incision. A change in amplitude is identified, compared, and correlated with steps of the surgery, and an alarm is considered accordingly.[4]

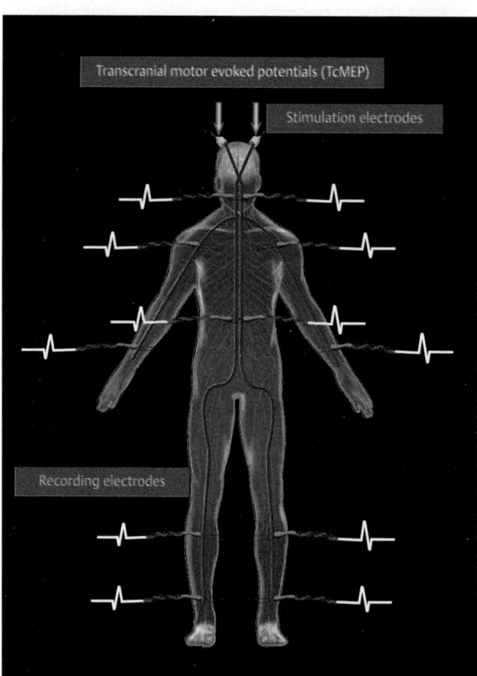

Fig. 18.2 Imtiaz-Bithal pocket review of TcMEP-technique and interpretation.

Why TcMEP Is Superior over SSEP? (Fig. 18.2 and Fig. 18.3)

TcMEP has the advantage of monitoring the spinal cord motor tract instantly without averages; hence, acquisition of data is much faster than SSEP.[20] These signals are exquisitely sensitive to altered spinal cord blood flow due to either hypotension or a mechanical insult,[3,21] thereby facilitating more rapid identification of impending spinal cord injury. Combined TcMEP and SSEP IONM showed a much higher sensitivity of 92.3% and a specificity of 99.6% in the prediction of postoperative neurologic status.[22]

Significance Criteria

A drop of more than 50% in amplitude is considered significant to create an alarm or suggest a momentary pause during surgery. Surgery can be continued with caution with relevant measures taken (e.g., increase in mean arterial pressure),[21,23] until there is a constant deterioration in amplitude. This criteria is applicable to AIS and spine surgeries and not for brain surgeries.

Pearls

- TcMEP is fast to pick a deterioration in signals, compared to SSEP.
- TcMEP is sensitive to surgical manipulations affecting the spinal cord.
- TcMEP demands competence from anesthetic team with the use of total intravenous anesthesia (TIVA with no muscle relaxants).
- All patients with clinical motor power +3 should have robust TcMEP signals under steady-state TIVA.
- A drop in TcMEP does not mean paralysis, instead it is an alarm, and surgeons may continue with caution and with keeping a healthy mean arterial pressure.

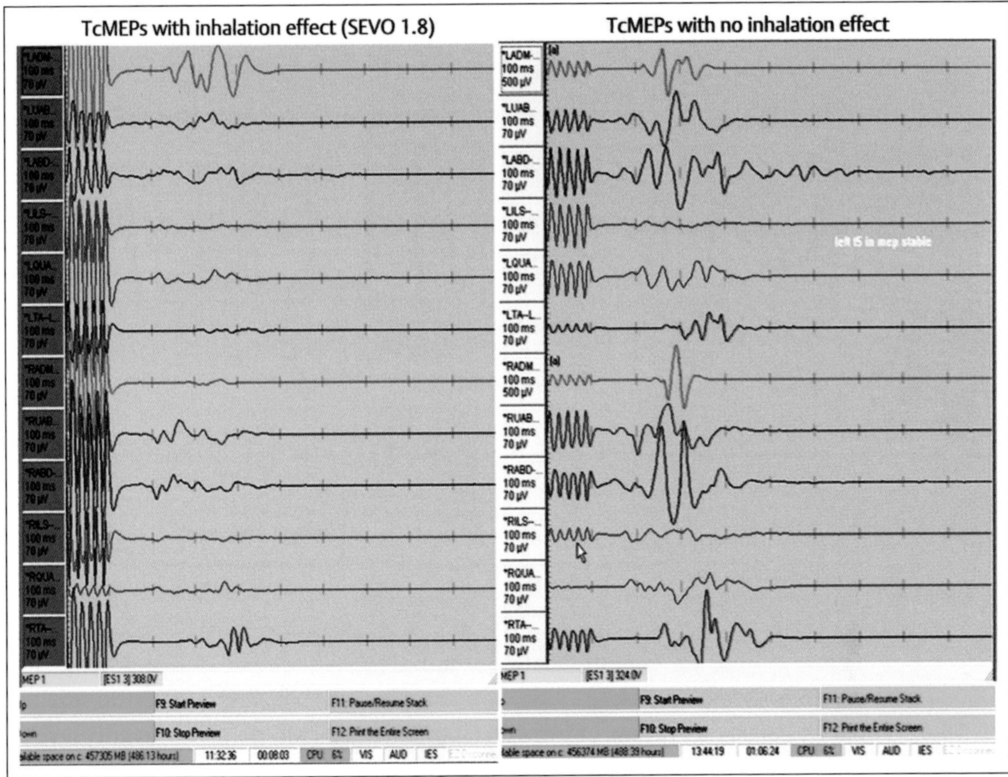

Fig. 18.3 Imtiaz-Bithal Pocket Review of TcMEP technique and interpretation with inhalation effect showing generalised smaller amplitude CMAP with and without inhalational agents.

Electromyograms (EMG)

This test is performed by using the same needle electrodes that are used for recording of TcMEP **(Fig. 18.4)**. This modality serves to protect the nerve roots during various stages of surgery. There is no stimulation performed unlike SSEP and TcMEP; instead, it serves to spontaneously record mechanical manipulations by the surgeon. A minor insult to the nerve root is generally seen as a small fasciculation and mostly no alarm is created.[7] However, if fasciculation leads to stronger irritations with further exaggeration to high-frequency and high-amplitude discharges, immediate caution is suggested to the surgeon with momentary pause and/or use of cold normal saline irrigation. A significant alarm in any muscles is always cross checked with a following TcMEP response for that muscle and an alarm is created accordingly looking at presence or absence of deterioration noticed in TcMEP for that muscle.[2,7,10,24]

Significance Criteria

High-frequency and high-amplitude discharges leading to changes in TcMEP for relevant muscles.

Pearl

EMG has importance in cervical and lumbar pathologies in spine. Instrumentation or work-up at lumbar levels in AIS may show significant EMG irritations. A constant irritation leading to a change in TcMEP for that muscle can be dangerous. Most nerve root EMG irritations will settle down simply by using cold irrigations.

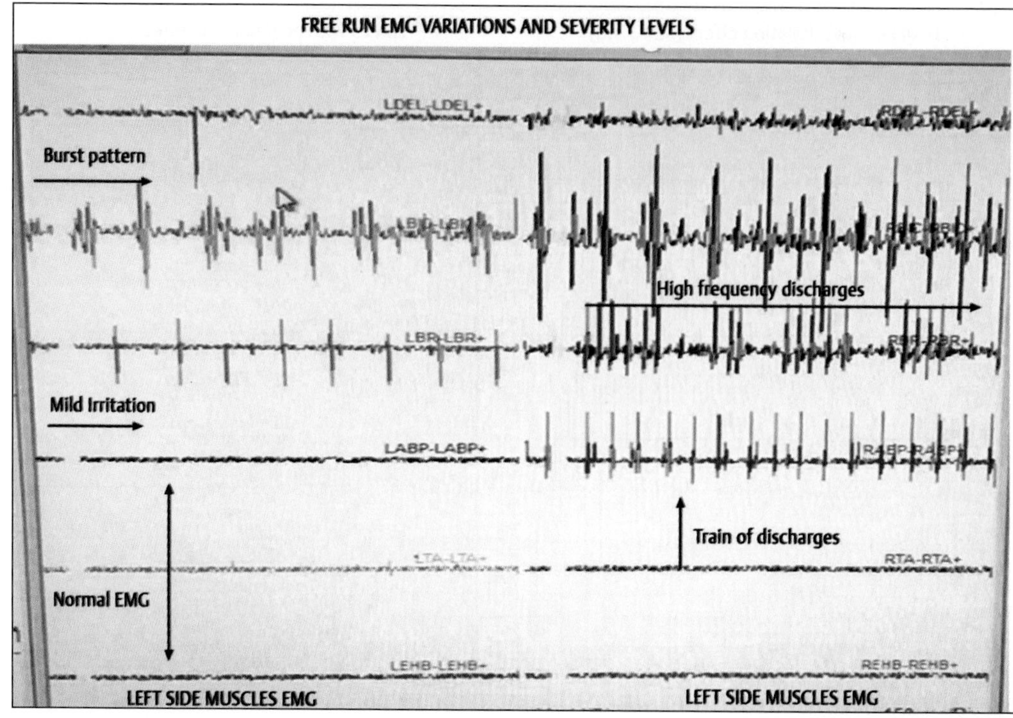

Fig. 18.4 Imtiaz-Bithal pocket review of free-run (spontaneous) EMG data and severity levels.

Triggered Electromyograms (TEMG)

This test is useful in identifying lateral breaches during pedicle holes and screw insertion **(Fig. 18.5)**. This is a modified EMG test where stimulation of a pedicle hole or a screw is performed by the surgeon using a monopolar probe with CMAP recordings from relevant muscle electrodes. The idea is to look for low-intensity current stimulation, producing responses, indicating a breach in pedicle that is providing a passage for current to escape and hit the nearby nerve,[2,7,24,25] which postoperatively may translate into clinical features of radiculopathies or motor deficits.

Significance Criteria

A CMAP acquired with current intensity 10 milli-Amperes (MA) or higher is considered safe for all screws at all spinal levels. A response acquired after current intensity of 8 to 10 MA at lumber-level screws reflects grey area and surgeons generally decide based on purchase they acquire while screw placement. Generally, surgeons keep that screw if there is no resultant EMG activity or TcMEP deterioration in relevant myotome. A response at less than 8 MA or lower for a lumbar-level screw may mean a breach in pedicle. For thoracic screws, there is more debate and controversies and a response acquired at less than 6 MA from relevant rectus abdominus or intercostal muscles is carefully examined.[26]

Pearl

TEMG is extremely sensitive test and has possibilities of false alarms. A very low response (<6 MA) may be considered serious at lumbar levels. For responses above 6 MA, the surgeon generally decides based on the purchase acquired during screw placement. A screw with good purchase can be kept if no TcMEP changes are noticed on relevant muscle groups.

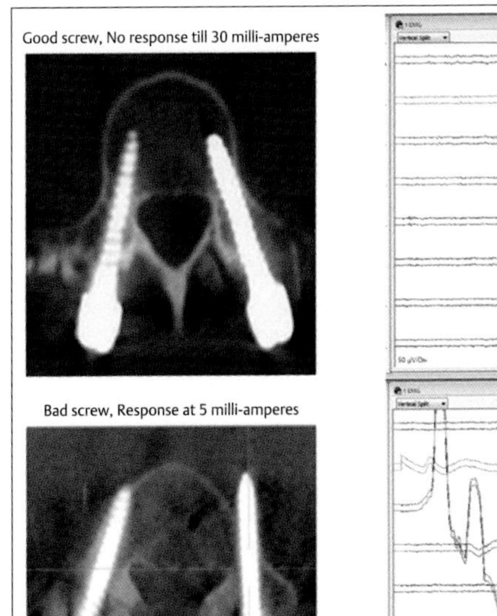

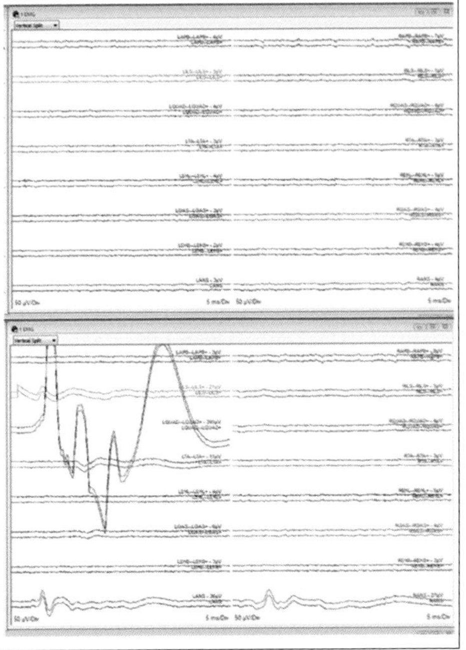

Fig. 18.5 Imtiaz-Bithal pocket review of TEMG data and severity levels.

Electroencephalogram (EEG)

A four-channel EEG is desirable and it is author's practice to use the electrodes already on scalp as SSEP recording electrodes. This test not only helps the anesthetic team with depth of anesthesia information but also helps in titration of anesthetic regimen as surgeon approaches closures and completion of procedure.[8] In addition, this modality helps especially when inadvertent TIVA bolus is administered especially during a critical phase of surgery resulting in deterioration of signals that may not have originated from a surgical insult. Use of anesthetic regimen is extremely important for accurate acquisition of data and correct interpretation of signals. Hence, the following paragraphs are focused anesthesia considerations and practices.

Significance Criteria

Presence of continuous delta waves (frequency 0.5–4 Hz) is desirable for IONM.[8] A burst suppression pattern is ideal for most surgeries showing progressive increase in depth of anesthesia.

Pearl

Recommended modality especially if anesthesia is not used for managing patients under TIVA. TIVA doses can be adjusted based on raw EEG data. Lack of robust TcMEP data in an otherwise healthy patient may be suggestive of deeper than required anesthetic levels.

Anesthetic Considerations and Understanding Anesthetic Variables Affecting IONM Data

Various anesthetic agents to a varying degree influence IONM data (**Tables 18.1** and **18.2**). Anesthetic agents are carefully chosen not to depress the signal acquisition during monitoring. As a rule, IONM is useful with TIVA and no muscle relaxant after intubation. General trend is to use a combination of steady-state infusion of propofol with fentanyl/remifentanil with muscle relaxant reserved only for intubation.[11]

Table 18.1 Imtiaz-Bithal anesthetic agents' effects on IONM data pocket chart

Anesthetic agents	SSEP	TcMEP
Inhalational agents	Suppressed >1 MAC	Suppressed
Propofol[a]	Unchanged on steady state	Unchanged on steady state
Opioids	Unchanged on steady state	Unchanged on steady state
Dexmedetomidinea	Unchanged on moderate doses	Unchanged on moderate doses
Ketamine	Enhanced	Enhanced
Etomidate	Enhanced	Enhanced
Benzodiazepinea	Unchanged on moderate doses	Unchanged on moderate doses
Barbiturates	Unchanged	Suppressed
Muscle relaxants	Unchanged	Suppressed

Abbreviations: IONM, intraoperative neurophysiology monitoring; MAC, monitored anesthesia care; SSEP, somatosensory-evoked potential; TcMEP, transcranial motor-evoked potential.
[a] Depending upon age and presence or absence of adjuvant.

Table 18.2 Imtiaz-Bithal anesthetic agents' dosages pocket chart

Anesthetic agents	Doses
Propofol	80–250 μg/kg/min[a]
Fentanyl	1–2 μg/kg/h
Remifentanil	0.1–0.8 μg/kg/min
Sufentanil	0.3–0.4 μg/kg/h
Ketamine	10–30 μg/kg/min
Etomidate	10–20 μg/kg/min
Lignocaine	1 mg/kg/h
Dexmedetomidine	0.1–1.0 μg/kg/h following bolus dose of 0.5–0.8 μg/kg over 20 min

[a] Depending upon age and presence or absence of adjuvant.

Pearl

Use Total Intravenous Anesthesia (TIVA) and titrate dosage levels, titration for suitable depth with EEG monitoring.

Why not Inhalation Anesthesia?

The impact of inhalation agents on IONM is directly proportional to the number of synapses in the pathway monitored (**Fig. 18.3**). They act mainly by changing the neuronal excitability through changes in synaptic transmission rather than axonal conduction.[8,23,27,28] All halogenated agents result in a dose-dependent increase in latency and decrease in amplitude of the cortical recordings of SSEP.[4,21,29,30] Halogenated volatile anesthetic agents also easily abolish TcMEP.[4] However, recording is possible only at low concentration of 0.2 to 0.5% of halogenated agents in selected patients. Addition of nitrous oxide potentiates the depressant effects of volatile agents. Studies with newer agents like sevoflurane and desflurane suggest that these agents are similar to older agent isoflurane at steady state. However, because of their rapid onset and offset action, they may appear to be more potent during the period when concentration is increasing.[23,27,28]

Pearl

TcMEP can be acquired in some patients with <0.5 MAC inhalation anesthesia but may lead to otherwise preventable false alarms especially if there is a data change noticed.

Total Intravenous Anesthetic (TIVA) Regimen

Intravenous anesthetic agents (**Tables 18.1** and **18.2**) act primarily by enhancing inhibitory functions of gamma amino acid and increase the chloride conduction, membrane hyperpolarization, and produce synaptic inhibition, affecting latency and amplitude of evoked potentials to some extent. Ketamine appears to act by blocking N-methyl-D-aspartate receptors[10,31] leading to reduction of sodium as well as calcium flux inside the cells. Opioids activate Mu (μ), Kappa (κ), and Delta (δ) receptors and their mechanism of action is by increasing inward potassium currents and decreasing outward sodium current. This explains why intravenous anesthetic agents and opioids have very little influence on evoked potentials.

Pearls

- Reading doctor (neurophysiologist) may communicate with anesthesia team and emphasize on the use of TIVA and offer suitable combinations.
- Proper understanding of data variations with anesthetic variables is imperative for thorough surgeries and preventing false alarms.

Why Ketamine and Etomidate Enhance Signal Amplitude?

Effects of anesthetic agents are the result of direct inhibition of synaptic pathways or indirect effect on pathways by altering the balance between inhibitory and excitatory influences.[28] Ketamine and etomidate belong to the latter category. Thus, all other anesthetics depress the amplitude and prolong the latency at various dose levels while ketamine and etomidate increase the amplitude, perhaps by attenuating inhibition.[10]

Since the threshold of anesthesia effects on cortical sensory and peripheral motor responses vary in some patients, any amount of inhalational agent may be inacceptable during IONM, necessitating a TIVA. This is especially important if a patient's neural pathway is compromised due to some pathology (e.g., patients below 2 years of age with immature myelination, patients with preexisting deficits, patients undergoing redo surgeries). In the latter instances, an amplitude-enhancing agent (ketamine or etomidate) may be infused to reduce effects of amplitude deterioration (**Tables 18.1** and **18.2**).

Pearls

- Ketamine is often used at authors' place in patients with poor baseline data. Anesthetist needs to discuss possible postop scenarios related to the use of ketamine and etomidate (i.e., psychosis, adrenal insufficiency).
- In experienced hands, ketamine can be added with propofol and fentanyl without concerns.

Nonanesthetic Intraoperative Factors Affecting Evoked Potentials

Many nonanesthetic intraoperative factors such as blood pressure, hypoxia, carbon dioxide pressure, hypothermia, anemia, etc., may influence IONM responses. Systemic hypotension is the most important factor leading to signal deterioration.[21,29]

Data Changing Scenarios during Surgical Manipulations

There is a threshold relationship between regional blood flow and cortical evoked responses. The cortical SSEP responses are unaffected until blood flow is decreased to 20 to 50 mL/100 g/min. Between 15 and 20 mL/100 g/min blood flow, the SSEPs are affected and finally lost. Like effects of anesthetics, peripheral and subcortical responses seem to have lower sensitivity than cortical ones due to reduced blood flow. Even in the presence of normal systemic blood pressure (BP); local factors may cause regional ischemia. In spinal surgery, the effects of hypotension may get aggravated by spinal distraction[20,32] and osteotomies (**Fig. 18.6**), such that an acceptable limit of systemic hypotension cannot be determined without monitoring IONM. That is why, it is imperative to closely monitor data, especially TcMEP during such manipulations. Similarly, peripheral nerve ischemia can result from positioning (either arms or legs), tourniquet, carotid artery interruption, vertebra-basilar insufficiency aggravated by head extension, cerebral vessel vasospasm, and cerebral ischemia from retraction.[20,32]

Pearl

- In major scoliosis with multiple surgical maneuvers planned (osteotomies, etc.), avoid hypotensive exposures.

Autoregulation and Data Changes

A reduction in BP below autoregulation threshold progressively decreases SSEP and TcMEP amplitude. Such changes may not be reversible depending on the severity of reduction of BP. A rapid decrease in mean arterial pressure within the autoregulatory range is also associated with transient change in EP data. Whenever there is depression or loss of signals, it is recommended to increase the mean arterial pressure greater than 80 mmHg, and if required, add vasopressors. Hemorrhagic hypotension produces greater signal loss compared to similar levels of hypotension from anesthetic agents.[20,21,23,28,29,32]

Pearls

- Try and plan normotensive exposure for a major scoliosis surgery.
- Mean arterial pressure (MAP) >75 mmHg be maintained during instrumentation and manipulation.

Anesthetic Management (Steady-State TIVA) and Use of Muscle Relaxants

Based on details discussed above, create a stable anesthetic environment prior to recording a baseline signal. Preferably, do not alter the anesthetic technique (including depth of anesthesia) throughout the procedure. To maintain a constant depth of anesthesia seems easy, but practically it is extremely difficult to achieve. A satisfactory level of anesthesia in the initial phase of surgery requiring muscle dissection may become insufficient during instrumentation. Therefore, the surgeon may demand muscle relaxant during the dissection phase. Thus, a relaxant may be administered during the dissection phase of surgery. However, make sure that immediately prior to instrumentation the effects of the relaxant have dissipated, and motor signals have returned to baseline.[4,23,28]

Pearls

- Use of muscle relaxants (MR) after intubation is not a desirable practice in multimodality IONM.
- If you must use MR, make sure to ask neurophysiologist if TcMEPs have returned to baseline before you start instrumentation and manipulation.

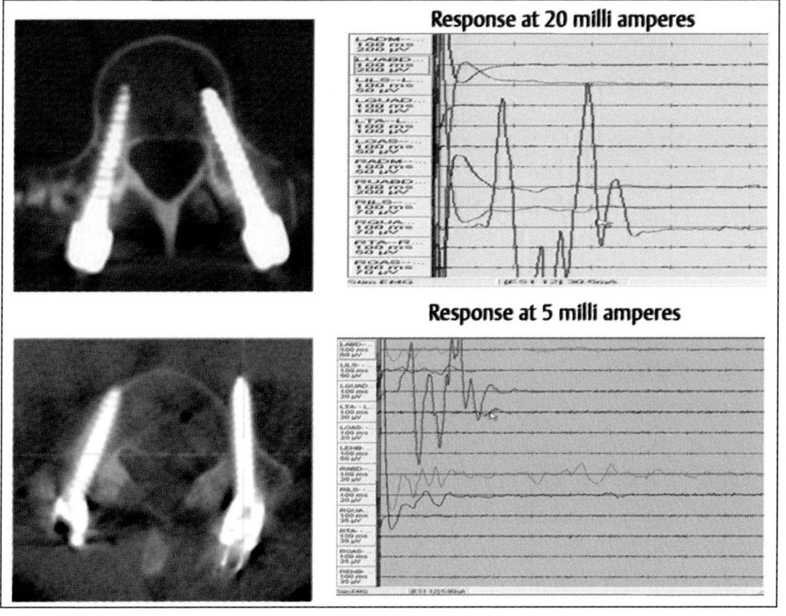

Fig. 18.6 Imtiaz-Bithal pocket review of TcMEP technique and interpretation showing unilateral amplitude drop due to surgical insult and then followed by recovery.

Miscellaneous Factors Affecting Data

Always select an anesthetic agent with rapid onset of action and with minimal effect on evoked responses. A bolus administration of an intravenous anesthetic may lead to complete loss of motor signal. It is advisable to convey to the neurophysiology team of any alteration in anesthetic technique or bolus administration (EEG use justified). One must have understanding that sudden increase in anesthesia depth may result in global signal loss, whereas trauma may be limited to specific surgical areas.

Recovery of lost signals from surgical trauma and anesthetic technique may take 30 minutes or longer in some instances. During this period, absence of signals would predispose a patient to surgical injury without any warning. Additionally, structures with poor baseline signals may be more difficult to monitor because these structures may be more affected by anesthetic regimen. According to some researchers, diabetes, hypertension and anesthetic techniques are the most important risk factors associated with failure to obtain lower extremity TcMEP signals.[1,23,28]

> **Pearl**
>
> Most true data changes can be recovered by keeping healthy and sustained MAP (>75 mmHg).

Reversal of Muscle Relaxants

If there is any suspicion of persistence of residual effect of muscle relaxant (especially, when motor signals are poor/absent), reversal of its effect with combination of neostigmine and glycopyrrolate or sugammadex may be carried out.

Partial Muscle Relaxation

There is growing interest in the use of partial muscle relaxant (pNMB). Sufficient experience with pNMB has demonstrated that this can be used during exposure when the patient otherwise has robust TcMEP muscle responses and the residual muscle response after pNMB is adequate as long as a steady-state degree of relation is maintained.

However, in patients with poor baseline responses it is better to avoid neuromuscular blockade during monitoring.

Effect of Optimum Dose of Various Anesthetic Agents on SSEP and TcMEP

Refer **Table 18.1**.

Recommend Agents and Doses of Anesthetic Agents during Spinal IONM

Refer **Table 18.2**.

Conclusion

SCM is extremely useful and beneficial in deformity correction scoliosis surgeries. Minimum neurophysiology data changes also represent alterations in spinal cord physiology; hence, surgeons and anesthetic teams may be informed of the danger in time to take appropriate corrective actions. Spinal surgeons, in general, understand the concept of monitoring techniques and can correlate their surgical steps and understand dangers associated with risky maneuvers. Substantial body of research has demonstrated that neurophysiologic monitoring can assist in the early detection of complications and possibly prevent postoperative morbidity in patients undergoing spinal surgeries. Also, management of physiologic milieu is significant, as central and peripheral nervous system blood flow, intracranial pressure, temperature, mean arterial pressure, carbon dioxide partial pressure produce alterations in data, which, when detected early, can be reversed and help in improving patient outcomes.

Pearl

Multimodality monitoring in experienced hands and clear communication among all members of involved teams is key to success in surgeries done with IONM.

References

1. Deiner SG, Kwatra SG, Lin H-M, Weisz DJ. Patient characteristics and anesthetic technique are additive but not synergistic predictors of successful motor evoked potential monitoring. Anesth Analg 2010; 111(2):421–425
2. Park J-H, Hyun S-J. Intraoperative neurophysiological monitoring in spinal surgery. World J Clin Cases 2015;3(9):765–773
3. Neuromonitoring Information Statement SRS Information Statement 2019
4. Macdonald DB, Skinner S, Shils J, Yingling C; American Society of Neurophysiological Monitoring. Intraoperative motor evoked potential monitoring: a position statement by the American Society of Neurophysiological Monitoring. Clin Neurophysiol 2013; 124(12):2291–2316
5. Toleikis JR; American Society of Neurophysiological Monitoring. Intraoperative monitoring using somatosensory evoked potentials. A position statement by the American Society of Neurophysiological Monitoring. J Clin Monit Comput 2005; 19(3):241–258
6. Pelosi L, Lamb J, Grevitt M, Mehdian SM, Webb JK, Blumhardt LD. Combined monitoring of motor and somatosensory evoked potentials in orthopaedic spinal surgery. Clin Neurophysiol 2002;113(7):1082–1091
7. Leppanen RE. Intraoperative monitoring of segmental spinal nerve root function with free-run and electrically-triggered electromyography and spinal cord function with reflexes and F-responses. A position statement by the American Society of Neurophysiological Monitoring. J Clin Monit Comput 2005;19(6):437–461
8. Isley MR, Edmonds HL Jr, Stecker M; American Society of Neurophysiological Monitoring. Guidelines for intraoperative neuromonitoring using raw (analog or digital waveforms) and quantitative electroencephalography: a position statement by the American Society of Neurophysiological Monitoring. J Clin Monit Comput 2009;23(6):369–390
9. Li F, Gorji R, Allott G, Modes K, Lunn R, Yang Z-J. The usefulness of intraoperative neurophysiological monitoring in cervical spine surgery: a retrospective analysis of 200 consecutive patients. J Neurosurg Anesthesiol 2012;24(3):185–190
10. Pajewski TN, Arlet V, Phillips LH. Current approach on spinal cord monitoring: the

point of view of the neurologist, the anesthesiologist and the spine surgeon. Eur Spine J 2007; 16(2, Suppl 2):S115–S129
11. Wing-hay HY, Chun-kwong EC. Introduction to Intraoperative Neurophysiological Monitoring for Anaesthetists. World Federation of Societies of Anaesthesiologists. Accessed April 21, 2019
12. Brown RH, Nash CL Jr, Berilla JA, Amaddio MD. Cortical evoked potential monitoring. A system for intraoperative monitoring of spinal cord function. Spine 1984;9(3): 256–261
13. Celesia GG. Somatosensory evoked potentials recorded directly from human thalamus and Sm I cortical area. Arch Neurol 1979; 36(7):399–405
14. Cohen AR, Young W, Ransohoff J. Intraspinal localization of the somatosensory evoked potential. Neurosurgery 1981;9(2):157–162
15. Kelly DL Jr, Goldring S, O'Leary JL. Averaged evoked somatosensory responses from exposed cortex of man. Arch Neurol 1965; 13(1):1–9
16. Larson SJ, Sances A Jr. Evoked potentials in man. Neurosurgical applications. Am J Surg 1966;111(6):857–861
17. MacDonald DB. Individually optimizing posterior tibial somatosensory evoked potential P37 scalp derivations for intraoperative monitoring. J Clin Neurophysiol 2001;18(4):364–371
18. Ghaly RF, Stone JL, Levy WJ. A protocol for intraoperative somatosensory (SEP) and motor evoked potentials (MEP) recordings. J Neurosurg Anesthesiol 1992;4(1):68–69
19. Stecker MM. A review of intraoperative monitoring for spinal surgery. Surg Neurol Int 2012;3(Suppl 3):S174–S187
20. Cheh G, Lenke LG, Padberg AM, et al. Loss of spinal cord monitoring signals in children during thoracic kyphosis correction with spinal osteotomy: why does it occur and what should you do? Spine 2008;33(10): 1093–1099
21. Lieberman JA, Feiner J, Lyon R, Rollins MD. Effect of hemorrhage and hypotension on transcranial motor-evoked potentials in swine. Anesthesiology 2013;119(5): 1109–1119
22. Thirumala PD, Huang J, Thiagarajan K, Cheng H, Balzer J, Crammond DJ. Diagnostic accuracy of combined multimodality somatosensory evoked potential and transcranial motor evoked potential intraoperative monitoring in patients with idiopathic scoliosis. Spine 2016;41(19):E1177–E1184
23. Albin MS. Textbook of neuroanesthesia with neurosurgical and neuroscience perspectives. McGraw-Hill; 1997
24. Gavassi BM, Pratali RR, Barsotti CEG, Ferreira RJR, Santos FPE, Oliveira CEAS. Positioning of pedicle screws in adolescent idiopathic scoliosis using electromyography. Coluna/Columna 2015;14:97–100
25. Hayashi H, Kawaguchi M, Yamamoto Y, et al. Evaluation of reliability of post-tetanic motor-evoked potential monitoring during spinal surgery under general anesthesia. Spine 2008;33(26):E994–E1000
26. Samdani AF, Tantorski M, Cahill PJ, et al. Triggered electromyography for placement of thoracic pedicle screws: is it reliable? Eur Spine J 2011;20(6):869–874
27. Richards CD. Actions of general anaesthetics on synaptic transmission in the CNS. Br J Anaesth 1983;55(3):201–207
28. Sloan TB, Heyer EJ. Anesthesia for intraoperative neurophysiologic monitoring of the spinal cord. J Clin Neurophysiol 2002; 19(5):430–443
29. MacKenzie MA, Vingerhoets DM, Colon EJ, Pinckers AJ, Notermans SL. Effect of steady hypothermia and normothermia on multimodality evoked potentials in human poikilothermia. Arch Neurol 1995;52(1): 52–58
30. Deiner S, Ed. Highlights of anesthetic considerations for intraoperative neuromonitoring. Seminars in cardiothoracic and vascular anesthesia. Los Angeles, CA: SAGE Publications; 2010
31. O'Shaughnessy CT, Lodge D. N-methyl-D-aspartate receptor-mediated increase in intracellular calcium is reduced by ketamine and phencyclidine. Eur J Pharmacol 1988; 153(2-3):201–209
32. Dolan EJ, Transfeldt EE, Tator CH, Simmons EH, Hughes KF. The effect of spinal distraction on regional spinal cord blood flow in cats. J Neurosurg 1980;53(6):756–764

19 Junctional Kyphosis following Spinal Fixation and Scoliosis Corrective Surgery

Amjad Shad, Fardad T. Afshari, Davor Dasic, and Mehmet Zileli

Introduction

Junctional kyphosis is a complication following long-segment spinal fusion which can occur both in the proximal section to fixation or distal segment. In this chapter, we will focus on the proximal junctional kyphosis (PJK) as it is the more common of the two. PJK is a complication following long-segment spinal fusion composed of angulation in the sagittal plane, kyphotic deformity, proximal to the uppermost section of fixation. The junctional kyphosis concept has emerged as one of the complications faced post spinal fixation with the increasing number of cases of degenerative or adolescent-related scoliosis surgery (**Fig. 19.1a, b**).

The proximal kyphotic deformity can range from being asymptomatic and only a radiological finding, to more severe cases associated with significant angulation resulting in pain, neurological compromise, and poor functional outcomes. The latter has been named in the literature as a proximal junctional failure (PJF).[1] There is currently no unified agreement on the exact definition of PJK; however, it is well recognized that this complication is increasingly detected and has attracted attention. The causes of PJK have been postulated to be multifactorial, ranging from patient-related factors, such as alignment of the spine, bone quality, and obesity, to surgical-related factors such as length of fixation, the integrity of ligaments, and method of fixation. Although not every case of PJK requires treatment and surgical intervention, more severe cases and particularly those leading to worsening pain and functional outcome and neurological compromise require revision and further surgical correction of the deformity (**Fig. 19.2a, b** and **Fig. 19.3a–d**). Increasing understanding of this condition and particularly the biomechanics of this complication is of paramount importance in preventing and treating such cases. This chapter will review some of the critical concepts in PJK and pathophysiology behind it.

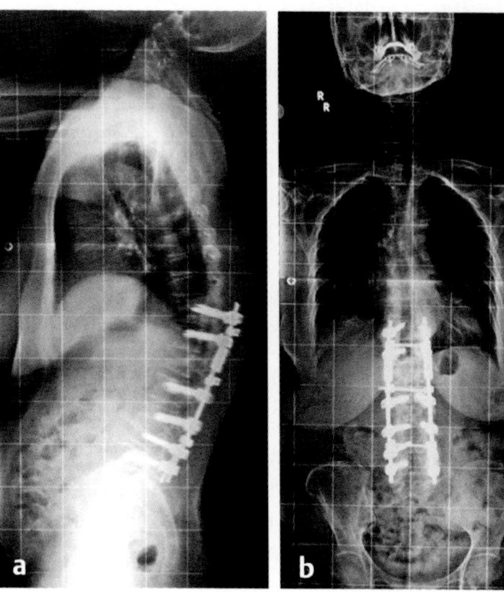

Fig. 19.1 (a, b) Radiological evidence of proximal junctional kyphosis.

Definition

There is currently no agreed, single, unified definition of PJK, with different authors reporting different criteria for the measurement of Cobb's angle in the diagnosis of PJK. Lee et al[1,2] defined PJK as kyphosis of five degrees at the proximal level to instrumented fusion segment in adolescent scoliosis correction. Glattes et al[3] have defined it as a sagittal Cobb's angle between lower end plate of the uppermost instrumented vertebra and upper end plate of two supra adjacent vertebra, 10 degrees higher than preoperative measurement. Hostin et al have further increased this cut-off point to more than 15 degrees angulation at two adjacent vertebrae above the uppermost instrumented vertebrae.[4] Helgeson et al have defined it as more than 15 degrees of angulation at one adjacent vertebra above the uppermost instrumented vertebra rather than two vertebrae.[5] Others, like Bridwell et al, have defined it as more than 20 degrees Cobb's angle at two levels above upper instrumented vertebra (UIV).[6] Various definitions of PJK are listed in **Table 19.1**.

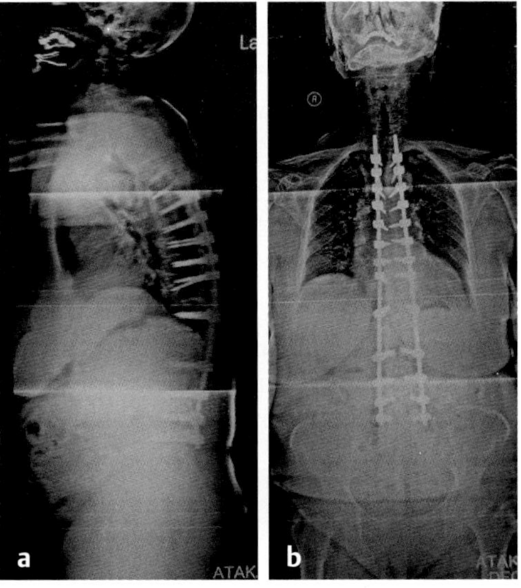

Fig. 19.2 (a, b) Progressive proximal junctional kyphosis eventually leading to multiple revisions and instrumentation extensions.

A survey of the Scoliosis Research Society members found that 86.2% considered PJK as proximal junction angle of ≥20 degrees.[7] Allowing for variation in the diagnostic criteria, based on data on adult and adolescent scoliosis correction surgical cases, overall kyphotic deformity ranging between 10 and 20 degrees proximal to uppermost instrumented vertebrae currently can be qualified as PJK. Consensus on the diagnostic criteria is required to allow unified diagnosis and assessment of such patients and compare studies and outcomes.

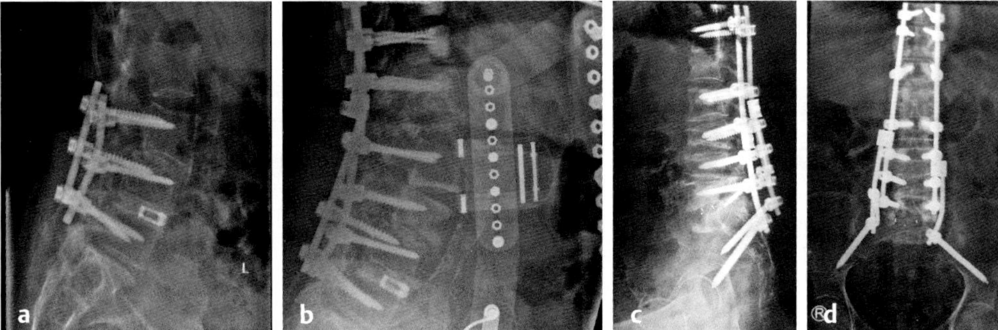

Fig. 19.3 (a–d) Multiple revisions for proximal junctional kyphosis leading to complete thoracolumbosacral segment instrumentation and fusion.

No consensus on criteria for diagnosis of PJK and PJF.

Table 19.1 Definitions of proximal junctional kyphosis

Authors	Publication year	Study population	Definition
Glattes et al[3]	2005	Adult spinal deformity	Cobb angle between the UIV and two supra-adjacent vertebra ≥10 degrees
Helgeson et al[5]	2010	Adolescent idiopathic scoliosis	Cobb angle between the UIV and two supra-adjacent vertebra ≥15 degrees
O'Shaughnessy et al[8]	2012	Adult spinal deformity	Cobb angle between the UIV and two supra-adjacent vertebra ≥20 degrees
Hostin et al[4]	2013	Adult spinal deformity	Cobb angle between the UIV and two supra-adjacent vertebra ≥15 degrees
Bridwell et al[6]	2013	Adult spinal deformity	Cobb angle between the UIV and two supra-adjacent vertebra ≥20 degrees
Lee et al[1]	2016	Adult spinal deformity	Cobb angle between the UIV and two supra-adjacent vertebra ≥5 degrees

Abbreviation: UIV, uppermost instrumented vertebra.

Pearls

- Proximal junctional kyphosis (PJK): ≥10 degrees angulation of proximal junction compared to preoperative measurements.
- Proximal junctional failure (PJF): When there is mechanical failure and/or spinal instability.

PJK and PJF are the most common complications of deformity surgery. The incidence is very low in adolescent scoliosis (7%), while it is more common in adult degenerative scoliosis/kyphosis (approximately 35–45%).

Incidence and Timing of Development

The reported incidence of PJK varies between 6[4] and 41%.[9] The wide variation in the reported incidence of PJK is likely due to different criteria for diagnosis used by various authors. Although the length of fixation, level of fixation, method of fixation, and different lengths of follow-up are likely to play a role in PJK diagnosis, it is evident that most cases of PJK do occur early postfusion (within the first 3 months), with 80% cases of PJK cases declaring clinically or radiologically within the first 18 months postfixation.[10,11]

Pearls

- Incidence of PJK has been reported to be between 6 and 41%.
- Variable diagnostic criteria are likely a factor in wide range of incidence.

Pathogenesis and Risk Factors

The pathogenesis of PJK is not well established. Understanding this condition is hampered by unclear diagnostic criteria, different methodology in studies, length of follow-up, and different outcome measures. The junctional failure mode is most commonly due to fracture, followed by soft tissue failure, adjacent segment degeneration, screw pull-out, and trauma.[4] Biomechanically, junctional failures result from the imbalance in the anterior column compression forces versus the posterior tension band resistance.

The etiology of PJK is likely composed of patient-related and surgical-related factors. Patient-related risk factors have been suggested to involve older age,[6] large abnormal preoperative sagittal parameters such as preoperative thoracic kyphosis angle (T5–T12) >40[12] or <20 degrees,[13] high BMI,[6] and paraspinal muscle size[14] as some of the factors. Surgical-related factors also undoubtedly play a role in this condition. Some authors have suggested extensive muscle dissection[2] and disruption of posterior tension band (posterior ligamental disruption),[15,16] compression fracture at the instrumented vertebrae, proximal instrumentation failure, facet disruption,[3] pedicle screws[5,10] and greater curvature correction,[6,17] length of fixation and level of fixation,[18] fusion to lumbar and sacral region,[19,20] anterior and posterior fixation,[21] and rod stiffness[22] as some of the factors playing a role in the development of PJK. A meta-analysis of over 2,200 patients in 14 studies found that age above 55, fusion to S1, thoracic kyphosis >40 degrees, low bone mineral density, and a sagittal vertical axis (SVA) >5 cm are significant risk factors for PJK. On the other hand, gender, combined anterior–posterior surgery, pedicle screw at the top of the construct, hybrid instrumentation, and thoracoplasty do not significantly affect the risk of developing PJK.[12] **Table 19.2** summarizes some of the factors reported to be associated with PJK.

Pearls

- Risk factors for PJK are composed of patient-related and surgical factors.
- Surgical factors appear to be more detrimental on development of this condition.
- Extensive muscle dissection, disruption of posterior ligaments, pedicle screw use alone, facet disruption, greater curvature correction, fusion to sacrum, length and selection of upper instrumented vertebral level, and density of rod have all been suggested toplay roles in PJK development.

Proximal Junctional Kyphosis Severity Spectrum

PJK severity ranges from a purely radiological finding with no overt symptoms in patients to severe cases impairing patient function and gait disturbance, causing pain and even neurological deficits. Symptomatic PJK is often called PJF. Many studies have compared the outcomes between PJK and non-PJK patients post fusion. Some studies have failed to demonstrate differences in outcomes.[3,11] Others have shown poorer outcomes in the PJK group in terms of pain scores. Notably, Kim et al studied 364 patients and demonstrated that the PJK group had significantly higher pain compared to non-PJK group (29.4 vs. 9%).[23]

Table 19.2 Risk factors associated with proximal junctional kyphosis

Surgical risk factors	Patient risk factors
• Posterior ligamentous injury, facet injury, fracture in noninstrumented level • Fusion including sacrum • Long fixations up to T1–T3 • Overcorrection, increasing lumbar lordosis >30 degrees • Thoracic kyphosis > lumbar lordosis • Lack of sagittal balance	• Age >55 • High body mass index • Osteoporosis • Increased pelvic Incidence • Thoracic kyphosis >40 or <20 degrees • Sagittal vertical axis (SVA) >5 cm

Table 19.3 Classification of the grades and severity of proximal junctional kyphosis/proximal junctional failure by Yagi et al and Complex Spine Study Group[24]

Type	Description
1	Disc and ligamentous failure
2	Bone failure
3	Implant/bone interface failure
Grade	
A	Proximal junctional increase 10–19 degrees
B	Proximal junctional increase 20–29 degrees
C	Proximal junctional increase ≤30 degrees
Spondylolisthesis	
PJF-U	No obvious spondylolisthesis above UIV
PJF-S	Spondylolisthesis above UIV

Abbreviations: PJF, proximal junctional failure; UIV, uppermost instrumented vertebra.

Some of the differences in findings may be explainable by varied diagnostic criteria, the spectrum of severity of this condition and the various outcome measures used in different studies, leading to varied results. What can be agreed on is that severe forms of PJK need specific attention as more data is emerging in this subgroup of patients regarding pain, mobility, and functional outcomes.[24] The classification system by Yagi et al[25] and the Hart-International Spine Study Group PJK severity scale have been described in **Tables 19.3** and **19.4**.

Prevention

Although risk factors associated with PJK are not fully understood, every step must be taken to prevent the development of PJK based on our current knowledge of contributing factors to this complication. Each patient needs to be thoroughly counselled before surgery, and sagittal alignment of the patient needs to be adequately studied.

Length of the construct and the UIV level must be chosen carefully to minimize the PJK due to inadequate length of fixation, or upper instrumented fusion in abnormal vertebrae (**Table 19.5**).

The odontoid hip axis (OD-HA) is a useful measure in studying an individual's overall sagittal balance. The OD-HA is an angle made between the highest point of the odontoid process and the vertical line connecting to the acetabulum center. In asymptomatic patients, the OD-HA ranges between +2 and −5 degrees. If the OD-HA is positive and >+2 degrees the standard value, then it suggests that the patient is out of global balance, and there is an increase in the lever arm on the UIV and thus a risk of junctional breakdown.[27]

The lower instrumented vertebra is also an important consideration. Some studies suggest that fusion to the sacrum is a risk factor for PJK, although avoiding certain vertebral levels might not always be possible.

Simple surgical techniques such as respecting the facet joint capsule, posterior tension band, and interspinous ligament[28] will likely reduce risk of PJK. PJK has been suggested to be minimized by vertebroplasty in UIV. Some authors suggest that augmentation in UIV to prevent compression fractures can reduce risk of PJK.[29] The concept of augmentation at this site is controversial, and some suggest that this may lead to further change in load transfer and risk of adjacent vertebral fractures.

Table 19.4 PJK severity scale

Parameter	Qualifier	Severity scale
Neurologic deficit	None	0
	Radicular pain	2
	Myelopathy/motor deficit	4
Focal pain	None	0
	VAS ≤4	1
	VAS ≥5	3
Instrumentation problem	None	0
	Partial fixation loss	1
	Prominence	1
	Complete fixation loss	2
Change in kyphosis/PLC integrity	0–10 degrees	0
	10–20 degrees	1
	>20 degrees	2
	PLC failure	2
UIV/UIV+1 fracture	None	0
	Compression fracture	1
	Burst/chance fracture	2
	Translation	3
Level of UIV	Thoracolumbar junction	0
	Upper thoracic spine	1

Abbreviations: PJK, proximal junctional kyphosis; PLC, posterior ligamentous complex; UIV, uppermost instrumented vertebra; VAS, visual analog scale.
The Hart-International Spine Study Group proximal junctional kyphosis severity scale. Any patient having ≥7 scale will need a surgery. From Hart et al.[26]

Table 19.5 Some preventive measures for proximal junctional kyphosis

1. • Achieve a good sagittal balance
   • Distal osteotomy
2. • Decrease loads on upper instrumented vertebra (UIV)
   • Use hook, polyethylene junctional tethers at the UIV
   • Cement augmentation at UIV and noninstrumented levels (prophylactic vertebroplasty)
   • Multilevel stabilization (longer instrument design)
   • Proximal transition rods of reduced diameter
3. • Decrease instrument rigidity, use hybrid systems
   • Use composite metal in long fixations (Co-Chr)
   • Protect soft tissue on UIV

Others have explored the use of hybrid systems or transverse process hooks and have demonstrated a reduction in PJK when hooks are used with pedicle screws for fixation.[5,30]

Computer simulation is being developed and could play a role in preoperative planning. It estimates the maximum bending moment location in the spine (M_{max}). Thus, the fusion constructs are avoided from stopping at the level of M_{max} to prevent junctional overstress.[31] In fact, in their study of pre- and postoperative imaging in 12 patients with PJK, Faundez et al found that most occurred at or one level away from the M_{max}.

Pearls

- Appropriate length of construct and position of uppermost and lowermost of instrumented vertebrae are likely to play important role in prevention of PJK.
- Use of hooks in addition to pedicle screws has been shown to be effective in reducing PJK.

Treatment

In severe cases of PJK, surgical intervention may be required. Depending on the clinical presentation of the patient, the management differs. In cases of myelopathy or neural compression, patients will require decompression with extension or realignment of instrumentation. In revision cases, the instrumentation needs to be either extended (**Fig. 19.4a–j**) to suitable proximal level or whole sagittal alignment may need to be revised using an osteotomy technique (**Fig. 19.5a–h**).

It has been suggested that treatment depends on the flexibility of the spine. In cases of a harmonious kyphotic and flexible spine, an extension of the instrumentation can suffice alone or together with a Smith-Petersen osteotomy. However, in either a localized angular kyphosis or ankylosed rigid segments, the extension of the instrumentation together with three-column pedicle subtraction osteotomies will likely be required.[32] The rate of recurrence for PJK

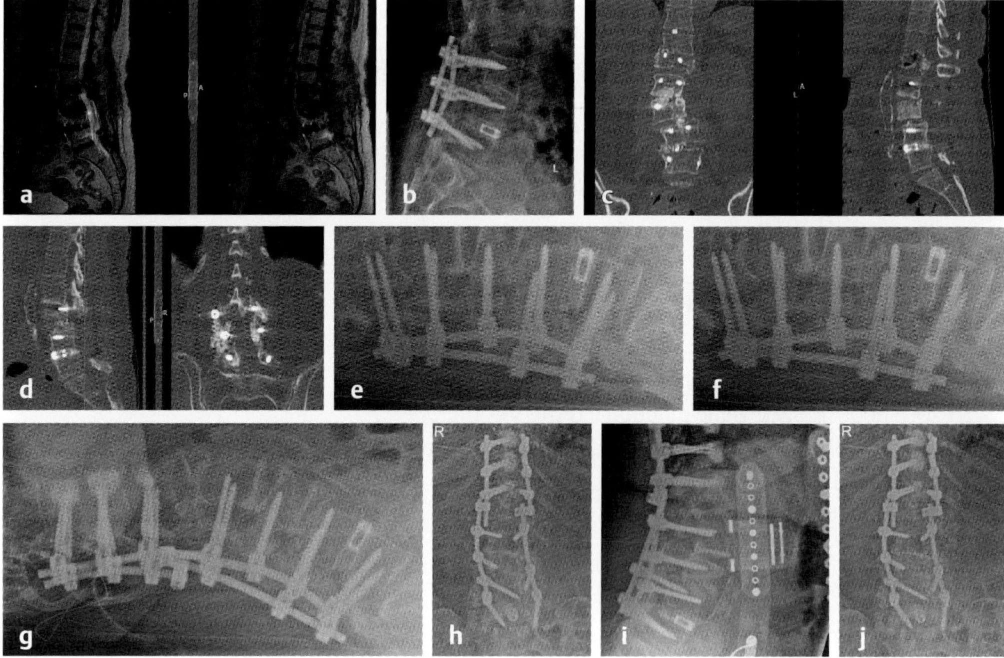

Fig. 19.4 (a–j) Gradual extension of instrumentation following development of proximal junctional kyphosis.

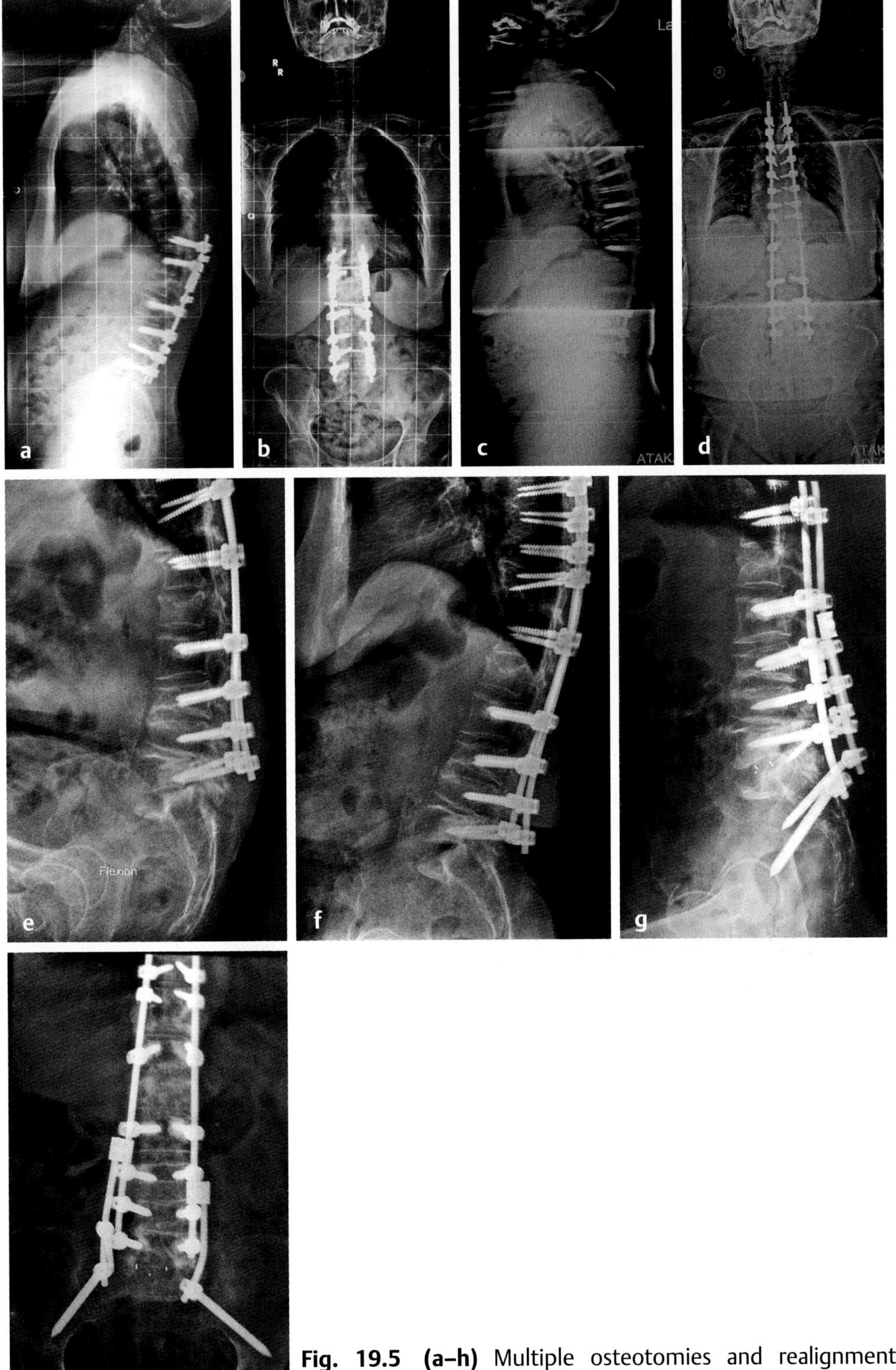

Fig. 19.5 (a–h) Multiple osteotomies and realignment of thoracolumbosacral spine for initially thoracic proximal junctional kyphosis.

is as high as 44%.[33] High recurrence rate after revision surgery further confirms the fact that our understanding of biomechanics and etiology for PJK remains in its infancy and needs more attention. More unified diagnostic criteria and outcome measure assessments will allow studies to be comparable with more meaningful conclusions in the study of this debilitating complication.

A revision surgery is more necessary if there is a traumatic etiology, the proximal junctional angle is high, the sagittal vertical axis is high, the primary surgery is a combined approach, and the patients are female.[34]

During a revision surgery for PJK, the following additions to surgery will be helpful:

- The instrumentation should almost always be lengthened. If it is ending at L2 level, lengthening may be up to T10. If it is ending at T10 level, lengthening may be up to T2–T5.
- Adding vertebroplasty to UIV and noninstrumented will be helpful.
- Using hooks at the upper level.
- Making decompression at the kyphotic level.
- Sagittal balance must be corrected.
- Interbody fusion should be added to the upper level.
- An osteotomy can be added.

Pearls

- Asymptomatic PJK cases may not require treatment.
- Severe cases of PJK with progression or neurological compromise need surgical correction.
- Surgical correction may require decompression, extension of proximal level, or whole sagittal alignment or osteotomies.

Conclusion

PJK presents a significant challenge in spinal surgery. Due to the use of long constructs in spinal instrumentation, especially in scoliosis and deformity surgery, patients with PJK present more often than ever. Thus, the PJK is not an infrequent radiographic finding after long spinal fusion. Many studies on the causes, risk factors, prevention, and treatment of PJK have been conducted and presented. It often presents as a pathological development at the adjacent segment after a spinal fusion and is not an instantaneous symptom but is considered as one of the various ongoing adjacent segmental problems. The authors know that some patients with this condition may display no symptoms. However, some other patients develop pain, walking difficulties, and neurological deficits. This group of patients can be challenging to treat; they often require revision surgery, an extension of the instrumentation, and ultimately further difficulties, even clinical and radiological failure. We need to invest more time and effort in understanding this condition, above all, how to prevent it and avoid it. Equally, we need a better understanding of how to stop its progression and treat it effectively once it develops.

References

1. Lee J, Park YS. Proximal junctional kyphosis: diagnosis, pathogenesis, and treatment. Asian Spine J 2016;10(3):593–600
2. Lee GA, Betz RR, Clements DH III, Huss GK. Proximal kyphosis after posterior spinal fusion in patients with idiopathic scoliosis. Spine 1999;24(8):795–799
3. Glattes RC, Bridwell KH, Lenke LG, Kim YJ, Rinella A, Edwards C II. Proximal junctional kyphosis in adult spinal deformity following long instrumented posterior spinal fusion: incidence, outcomes, and risk factor analysis. Spine 2005;30(14):1643–1649
4. Hostin R, McCarthy I, O'Brien M, et al; International Spine Study Group. Incidence, mode, and location of acute proximal junctional failures after surgical treatment of adult spinal deformity. Spine 2013;38(12):1008–1015
5. Helgeson MD, Shah SA, Newton PO, et al; Harms Study Group. Evaluation of proximal junctional kyphosis in adolescent idiopathic scoliosis following pedicle screw,

hook, or hybrid instrumentation. Spine 2010;35(2):177–181

6. Bridwell KH, Lenke LG, Cho SK, et al. Proximal junctional kyphosis in primary adult deformity: evaluation of 20 degrees as a critical angle. Neurosurgery 2013;72: 899–906
7. Scheer JK, Fakurnejad S, Lau D, et al; SRS Adult Spinal Deformity Committee. Results of the 2014 SRS Survey on PJK/PJF: a report on variation of select SRS member practice patterns, treatment indications, and opinions on classification development. Spine 2015; 40(11):829–840
8. O'Shaughnessy BA, Bridwell KH, Lenke LG, et al. Does a long-fusion "T3-sacrum" portend a worse outcome than a short-fusion "T10-sacrum" in primary surgery for adult scoliosis? Spine (Phila Pa 1976) 2012;37:884-90
9. Maruo K, Ha Y, Inoue S, et al. Predictive factors for proximal junctional kyphosis in long fusions to the sacrum in adult spinal deformity. Spine 2013;38(23):E1469–E1476
10 Wang J, Zhao Y, Shen B, Wang C, Li M. Risk factor analysis of proximal junctional kyphosis after posterior fusion in patients with idiopathic scoliosis. Injury 2010;41(4): 415–420
11. Yagi M, King AB, Boachie-Adjei O. Incidence, risk factors, and natural course of proximal junctional kyphosis: surgical outcomes review of adult idiopathic scoliosis. Minimum 5 years of follow-up. Spine 2012;37(17):1479–1489
12. Liu FY, Wang T, Yang SD, Wang H, Yang DL, Ding WY. Incidence and risk factors for proximal junctional kyphosis: a meta-analysis. Eur Spine J 2016;25(8):2376–2383
13. Oe S, Togawa D, Hasegawa T, et al. The risk of proximal junctional kyphosis decreases in patients with optimal thoracic kyphosis. Spine Deform 2019;7(5):759–770
14. Pennington Z, Cottrill E, Ahmed AK, et al. Paraspinal muscle size as an independent risk factor for proximal junctional kyphosis in patients undergoing thoracolumbar fusion. J Neurosurg Spine 2019;31(3):380–388
15. Kim YJ, Bridwell KH, Lenke LG, Glattes CR, Rhim S, Cheh G. Proximal junctional kyphosis in adult spinal deformity after segmental posterior spinal instrumentation and fusion: minimum five-year follow-up. Spine 2008;33(20):2179–2184
16. Kim HJ, Bridwell KH, Lenke LG, et al. Patients with proximal junctional kyphosis requiring revision surgery have higher postoperative lumbar lordosis and larger sagittal balance corrections. Spine 2014;39(9):E576–E580
17. Kim YJ, Bridwell KH, Lenke LG, Rhim S, Kim YW. Is the T9, T11, or L1 the more reliable proximal level after adult lumbar or lumbosacral instrumented fusion to L5 or S1? Spine 2007;32(24):2653–2661
18. Fu X, Sun XL, Harris JA, et al. Long fusion correction of degenerative adult spinal deformity and the selection of the upper or lower thoracic region as the site of proximal instrumentation: a systematic review and meta-analysis. BMJ Open 2016;6(11): e012103
19. Yagi M, Akilah KB, Boachie-Adjei O. Incidence, risk factors and classification of proximal junctional kyphosis: surgical outcomes review of adult idiopathic scoliosis. Spine 2011;36(1):E60–E68
20. Mendoza-Lattes S, Ries Z, Gao Y, Weinstein SL. Proximal junctional kyphosis in adult reconstructive spine surgery results from incomplete restoration of the lumbar lordosis relative to the magnitude of the thoracic kyphosis. IOWA Orthop J 2011;31:199–206
21. Kim HJ, Yagi M, Nyugen J, Cunningham ME, Boachie-Adjei O. Combined anterior-posterior surgery is the most important risk factor for developing proximal junctional kyphosis in idiopathic scoliosis. Clin Orthop Relat Res 2012;470(6):1633–1639
22. Han S, Hyun SJ, Kim KJ, Jahng TA, Lee S, Rhim SC. Rod stiffness as a risk factor of proximal junctional kyphosis after adult spinal deformity surgery: comparative study between cobalt chrome multiple-rod constructs and titanium alloy two-rod constructs. Spine J 2017;17(7):962–968
23. Kim HJ, Bridwell KH, Lenke LG, et al. Proximal junctional kyphosis results in inferior SRS pain subscores in adult deformity patients. Spine 2013;38(11):896–901
24. Smith MW, Annis P, Lawrence BD, Daubs MD, Brodke DS. Early proximal junctional failure in patients with preoperative sagittal imbalance. Evid Based Spine Care J 2013; 4(2):163–164
25. Yagi M, Rahm M, Gaines R, et al; Complex Spine Study Group. Characterization and surgical outcomes of proximal junctional failure in surgically treated patients with adult spinal deformity. Spine 2014;39(10): E607–E614
26. Hart R, McCarthy I, O'Brien M, et al; International Spine Study Group. Identification of decision criteria for revision surgery among

patients with proximal junctional failure after surgical treatment of spinal deformity. Spine 2013;38(19):E1223–E1227

27. Le Huec JC, Thompson W, Mohsinaly Y, |Barrey C, Faundez A. Sagittal balance of the spine. Eur Spine J 2019;28(9):1889–1905
28. Cammarata M, Aubin CE, Wang X, Mac-Thiong JM. Biomechanical risk factors for proximal junctional kyphosis: a detailed numerical analysis of surgical instrumentation variables. Spine 2014;39(8):E500–E507
29. Hart RA, Prendergast MA, Roberts WG, Nesbit GM, Barnwell SL. Proximal junctional acute collapse cranial to multi-level lumbar fusion: a cost analysis of prophylactic vertebral augmentation. Spine J 2008;8(6):875–881
30. Hassanzadeh H, Gupta S, Jain A, El Dafrawy MH, Skolasky RL, Kebaish KM. Type of anchor at the proximal fusion level has a significant effect on the incidence of proximal junctional kyphosis and outcome in adults after long posterior spinal fusion. Spine Deform 2013; 1(4):299–305
31. Faundez AA, Richards J, Maxy P, Price R, Léglise A, Le Huec J-C. The mechanism in junctional failure of thoraco-lumbar fusions. Part II: Analysis of a series of PJK after thoraco-lumbar fusion to determine parameters allowing to predict the risk of junctional breakdown. Eur Spine J 2018;27(Suppl 1): 139–148
32. Le Huec J-C, Richards J, Tsoupras A, Price R, Léglise A, Faundez AA. The mechanism in junctional failure of thoraco-lumbar fusions. Part I: Biomechanical analysis of mechanisms responsible of vertebral overstress and description of the cervical inclination angle (CIA). Eur Spine J 2018;27(Suppl 1):129–138
33. Kim HJ, Wang SJ, Lafage R, et al; International Spine Study Group. Recurrent proximal junctional kyphosis: incidence, risk factors, revision rates and outcomes at 2 year minimum follow up. Spine 2019;45(1):E18–E24
34. Zileli M, Dursun E. How to improve outcomes of spine surgery in geriatric patients. World Neurosurg 2020;140:519–526

20 Craniofemoral Traction in Severe Rigid Scoliosis

Arvind G. Kulkarni and Sameer Ruparel

Introduction

The word "scoliosis" is derived from Greek word meaning "crooked." According to Scoliosis Research Society (SRS), it is defined as lateral curvature of spine greater than or equal to 10 degrees Cobb with rotation on standing anteroposterior (AP) radiograph. Scoliosis is a deformity affecting the spinal column in all three planes—coronal, sagittal, and axial with varied etiologies.

But, how do we define "severe" and "rigid" scoliotic curves. Ambiguity in literature further complicates this definition. O' Brien et al[1] defined it as a Cobb angle more than 70 degrees; later, Tokunaga et al[2] defined it as a scoliotic deformity more than 80 degrees. Greiner[3] reported that adolescent idiopathic scoliosis (AIS) patients did not exhibit clinically significant respiratory symptoms until their curves were 60 to 100 degrees, thus defining severe scoliosis as Cobb angle of more than 60 degrees. On the other hand, definition of "rigid" scoliosis is based on flexibility index (FI). Greiner[3] defined rigid curves as a coronal deformity with less than 40% FI on bending films. For the sake of discussion, authors usually consider curves more than 80 degrees as "severe" ones and those with FI less than or equal to 0.5 as "rigid" curves.

Management

Management of scoliosis mainly depends on two factors: type based on classification and curve flexibility. Thus, it is very necessary to define "severe" and "rigid" curves. High correction rates and successful outcomes have been reported in adolescent scoliotic patients with curves between 40 and 70 degrees.[4] Such flexible curves are easily treated with either anterior or posterior approaches.[5–7] However, simple methods of correction have limited potential in deformities which are rigid and of high magnitude. These usually require staged corrections which have a profound impact on patient outcomes. The various treatment options available include:

- Anterior Release + Anterior/Posterior Instrumentation.
- Anterior Release + Posterior Instrumentation.
- Anterior Release + Halo Gravity Traction + Posterior Instrumented fusion.
- Posterior Spinal Osteotomy (Ponte's) + Posterior Instrumented fusion.
- Vertebral Column Resection + Posterior Instrumented fusion.

Curves more than 80 degrees that do not reduce to 50 to 55 degrees on bending radiographs often require an anterior release.[8] A combined anterior and posterior approach was postulated for treating severe rigid scoliosis.[9,10] However, anterior approach has its own complications in the form of increased morbidity, increased blood loss, operative time, and pulmonary complications.[11] With the advent of pedicle screw system, there has been an increased interest in posterior-only surgery. Posterior-only surgery reduces hospital stay, costs, and blood loss.[12,13] It is cosmetically more appealing, as it obviates the need of a second incision without affecting clinical and radiological outcomes.[12,14,15] Vertebral column resection and multilevel osteotomies are excellent options.[16] However, these are associated with significant morbidity.[17]

Pearls

- Scoliosis curves more than 80 degrees are usually regarded as "severe" ones and those with FI less than or equal to 0.5 as "rigid" curves.
- Simple methods of correction have limited potential in correction of such deformities.

Skeletal Traction for Treatment of Scoliosis

Traction as a modality of treatment for treating scoliosis has been used since a long time. The development of the halo opened a new era in the surgical treatment of severe scoliosis in terms of spinal traction. With halo-femoral traction, Kane et al[18] reported in 1967 their series of 30 scoliotic patients. The average original curve measured 112 degrees and reduced to 58 degrees after final correction. However, these require extended periods of bed rest[18,19] and were associated with several long-term complications.[20] With the advent of surgical methods to treat scoliosis, a three-stage procedure of anterior release traction and posterior instrumented fusion came into vogue. This was based on the premise that correction of scoliotic curves under traction is accomplished through two mechanisms.[21] The initial correction is due to the elastic properties (stiffness) of tissues. Since tissues exhibit viscoelastic properties, the initial elastic deformation is followed by a creep phase where most of the correction is achieved. There is a period of primary creep for about 2 to 4 hours, in which the correction is relatively important. A secondary creep period allows a more gradual reduction of the spinal deformity, such that near maximal curve correction can be obtained after about 10 to 12 days.[22] Thus, traction was implemented for 14 to 21 days between stages. However, these were also not spared of complications. Issues like pin site infections,[23] brain abscesses,[24] avascular necrosis of odontoid, and cervical spondylosis[25–28] were documented.

To avoid complications related to anterior approaches and prolonged traction, an all-posterior deformity correction approach aided with intraoperative traction and neuromonitoring was evolved. This chapter focuses on this efficacious technique in detail.

Indications

As described above, this powerful technique of scoliosis correction is indicated in patients with severe and rigid scoliosis. However, there is no contraindication of using this technique in routine scoliosis cases if difficulty is expected in getting correction. With regard to etiologies, numerous papers describing its efficacy in idiopathic scoliosis,[29–31] AIS,[32] neuromuscular scoliosis,[33] and congenital scoliosis have been documented. To improve its safety, surgeons have shown excellent results with the aid of neuromonitoring[34] and navigation systems.[35]

Pearl

This technique of an all-posterior deformity correction approach aided with intraoperative traction and neuromonitoring is used in severe and rigid curves, which is advantageous in comparison to other techniques.

Contraindications

This technique is contraindicated in patients having cervical and upper cervical instabilities. It is expected that with the cranial traction applied these might worsen. Similarly, traction is contraindicated in patients with spinal cord pathologies. Therefore, it is extremely necessary to get upper cervical radiological examination and magnetic resonance imaging (MRI) in all patients where this technique is contemplated. In addition to these, local conditions which preclude the use of cranial/femoral traction like infections, skin abnormalities, fracture/trauma, and osteoporotic bones serve as contraindications. Relative contraindications would be patients with severe acute curves in which better correction would be achieved with osteotomies. Nonavailability of neuromonitoring is also a contraindication which serves as a guide to prevent neurological complications.

Pearl

Upper cervical instabilities and spinal cord pathologies serve as contraindications to the technique.

Approach to a Case with Severe and Rigid Scoliosis

The basic approach to a patient with scoliosis with regard to clinical and radiological examination, preoperative planning, intraoperative execution, and postoperative management protocols fairly remains the same. Only salient features are different, and some of these features that need attention are described here.

Symptoms, Signs, and Clinical Examination

Apart from cosmetic deformity and associated pain, a patient with severe rigid scoliosis may complain of inability to sit, stand, and walk without support. This is particularly seen in neglected cases of AIS. Functional disability is also a common feature in patients with neuromuscular scoliosis who find it difficult to sit due to severe pelvic obliquity. Special attention must be given to breathing difficulties and related fatigue due to pulmonary dysfunction. The magnitude of the curve is clearly appreciated on inspection. A fair idea of flexibility can be made by asking the patient to side bend/applying manual traction or suspension. Adams forward bending gives an estimate of rotational component. In patients with neuromuscular scoliosis it is necessary to pay attention to upper/lower limbs as they may have concomitant dislocations which need treatment. Secondary features of scoliosis are usually present like rib humps, abnormal skin creases, and loin prominences. Shoulder levels and pelvic obliquity needs to be noted. As with every patient, thorough neurological examination needs to be done.

Radiological Examination

A 14 × 36 inches standing full-length AP and lateral full-spine scanograms (from C1 to pelvis) need to be taken. To assess the flexibility and differentiate structural and nonstructural curves, supine right and left side-bending X-rays are taken. Traction films are required in addition to severe rigid curves. Cobb angle measurement and classification of curves are done routinely. It is essential to find out the FI of the deformity. FI is calculated by subtracting the magnitude of the side bend/traction Cobb angle from the magnitude of the preoperative upright coronal Cobb angle, and then dividing it by the preoperative upright coronal Cobb angle.[32]

$$\text{Flexibility Index (FI)} = \frac{\text{Erect Cobb} - \text{Traction/Side-Bending Cobb}}{\text{Erect Cobb}}$$

It is very essential to measure FI of the deformity to plan corrective surgery. As described above, curves >60 degrees Cobb and FI <0.5 need more than routine techniques of correction.

Similarly, an estimate of correction that can be achieved is better assessed with traction films rather than side-bending films for larger curves. Past literature has strongly suggested that side-bending radiographs demonstrate flexibility in curves less than 60 degrees and in curves more than 60 degrees, and the true flexibility of the deformity is assessed more accurately with traction radiographs.[36–39] It has also been seen that postoperative correction of high-magnitude curves best matches the preoperative magnitude in traction.[40]

MRI examination and upper cervical radiology are must to rule out any pathologies there in, since they serve as strict contraindications to application of traction, as mentioned above.

Pearls

- An estimate of correction that can be achieved is better assessed with traction films rather than side-bending films for larger curves.
- In curves more than 60 degrees, the true flexibility of the deformity is assessed more accurately with traction radiographs.

Typical Case to Start/Avoid in the Beginning

As with all surgical techniques, application of intraoperative traction as a method for a correction of scoliosis has a definite learning curve. It is very necessary to be wise and choose an ideal case during this period to avoid complications. Before venturing into a case with severe and rigid deformities, the surgeon must have gathered adequate experience in correction of flexible curves <60 degrees. He/she must be well versed with all techniques of deformity correction like rod translation, rod rotation, derotation maneuvers along with anterior releases and posterior osteotomies. This is particularly important if the correction expected on table is not achieved or in case of an unforeseen hurdle; the surgeon must be confident enough to change the plan and provide optimum results. As described by Erdem et al,[29] high correction rates and excellent outcomes have been reported for curves between 40 and 70 degrees.[4] However, curves >90 degrees are usually difficult to correct and require additional techniques for satisfactory outcomes.[41–43] They describe curves between 70 and 90 degrees as "gray zone" curves. In this chapter, the authors considered curves with Cobb more than 60 degrees and FI <0.5 as rigid. We advise to initially employ this technique in "gray zone" curves. A deformity with Cobb between 60 and 70 degrees and FI between 0.5 and 0.4 with idiopathic etiology would be ideal. Similarly, a curve more than 100 degrees and FI equal to or less than 0.2 should be strictly avoided. Once the surgeon has operated on a few ideal cases, he may venture to operate on curves with greater severity and rigidity gradually in a stepwise fashion.

Pearl

Typically start with a case in the "gray zone"—deformity with Cobb between 60 and 70 degrees and flexibility index between 0.5 and 0.4 with idiopathic etiology.

Positioning

Once preoperative planning is complete, the next step is execution of surgery. With the patient in the operating room, there should be good understanding between the surgeon, anesthetist, and neurophysicist. The anesthetist and surgeon should keep in mind the poor pulmonary reserve of the patient. Also anesthetic requirements from neuromonitoring perspective should be conveyed. Once intubated, application of craniofemoral traction is undertaken (**Fig. 20.1, Fig. 20.2,** and **Fig. 20.3**). Gardner-Wells tongs and supracondylar femoral pins are used. The patient

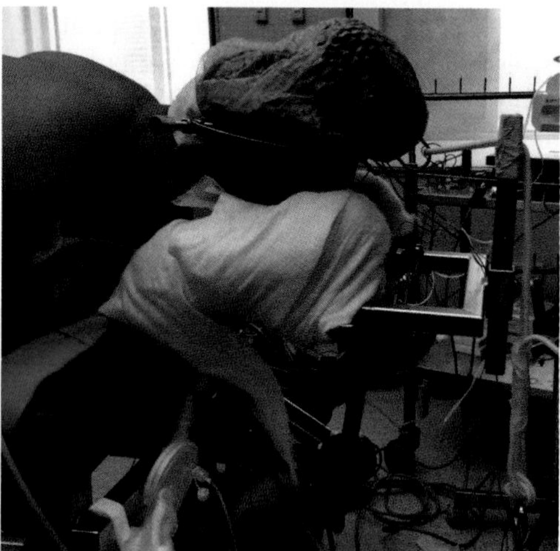

Fig. 20.1 Intraoperative C-arm image after application of traction.

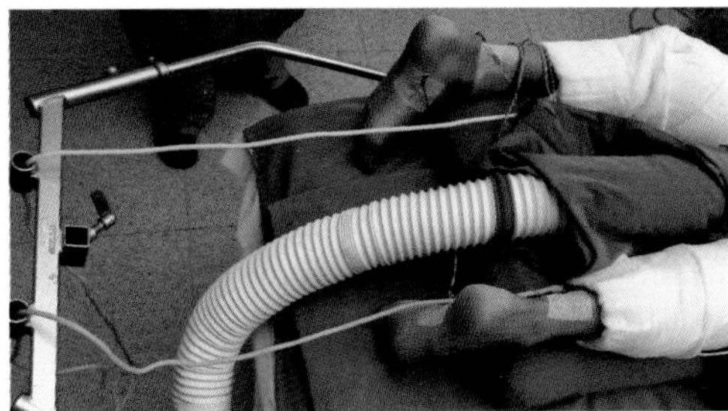

Fig. 20.2 Preoperative images anteroposterior and lateral.

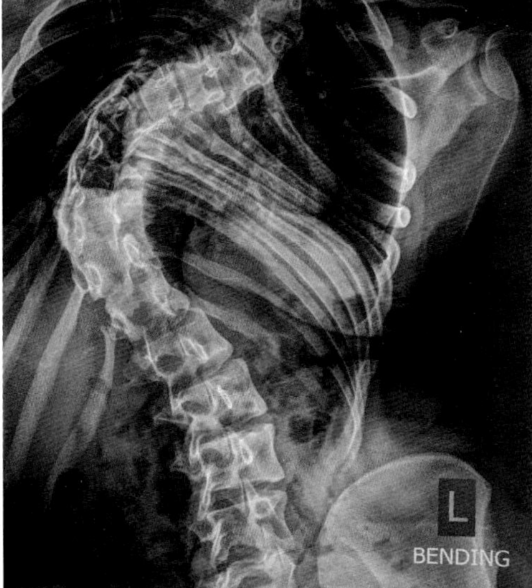

Fig. 20.3 Right-bending film.

is positioned prone on the operating table. Traction weight (50% of body weight) is suspended on the lower limbs (divided between the two lower limbs) and countertraction of one-third of body weight is suspended on the skull.

There are numerous methods of application of cranial traction. One study has also used a head-halter and skin traction.[44] However, most studies in the literature have used percutaneous skeletal traction with a distal femoral traction pin and a halo or Gardner-Wells skull tongs.[34,45,46] The application of skeletal traction also serves as a secure positioning device for the patient during the surgery. The authors prefer the use of Gardner-Wells skull tongs because of the ability of the tongs to provide sufficient support to the skull while not causing visible forehead scars as compared to the use of halo.[47] The amount of weights used for traction also varies in the literature. Lewis et al[34] used a standard protocol for intraoperative traction of approximately 20% of body weight (to a maximum of 15 lb) through the Gardner-Wells tongs and 50% of body weight (to a maximum of 65 lb) evenly distributed between the bilateral femurs. Keeler et al[13] used 15 lbs of traction on the halo and 15 to 35 lbs distally. Hamzaoglu et al[31] started with 12 kg (6 kg on the head, 3 kg on each leg). Weights are gradually (1 kg/h) and equally added to a total of 12 kg on each end. The total weight did not exceed 30 to 50% of the total body weight. Jhaveri et al[45] used traction with approximately 50% of body weight through the limbs and applied countertraction with 20 to 25% of body weight through the skull, a protocol that we also follow in our patients.

In patients with neuromuscular scoliosis and pelvic obliquity, application of craniofemoral traction has an added advantage. By applying unilateral traction to lower limb with higher pelvis, traction efficiently balances the pelvis in them. Neutralizing pelvic obliquity goes a long way in achieving sitting balance in such patients.

Pearls

- Craniofemoral traction with Gardner-Wells tongs and supracondylar pins is ideal.
- Traction is applied with approximately 50% of body weight through the limbs and countertraction with 20 to 25% of body weight through the skull.
- In cases with pelvic obliquity, unilateral traction to high-riding pelvis is applied.

Procedure: Tips and Tricks

With regard to surgical execution, most of the steps are similar to routine scoliosis surgery, except that with adequate correction achieved, additional steps can be omitted.

This significantly reduces the operative time and blood loss and improves the operative parameters. Al Sayegh et al[46] found that the mean blood loss (2,083 vs. 1.485 mL), blood transfusions (64% vs. 33%) and operative time (447.6 vs. 375.6 min) was significantly less when traction was used, compared to a group in which traction was not used.

Once the traction is applied, the dramatic correction can be easily appreciated in C-arm images (**Fig. 20.4** and **Fig. 20.5**) (As it can be seen, these are images of the same patient before application of traction and then.) With the placement of pedicle screws and posterior release with adequate facet resections, further traction weight can be applied (within permissible limits as mentioned above) under neuromonitoring, which further aids correction.

Traction indirectly helps in numerous surgical steps. Skeletal traction leads to apical vertebral derotation.[45] This derotation of the spine facilitates surgical exposure, screw and rod insertion, thus minimizing the need for multiple techniques of deformity correction.[13,34,45] It elongates not only the spinal column, but also the thoracic cavity, improving the compromised pulmonary function[31] and avoiding an anterior surgery,[13,34,45] thereby reducing the hospital stay and cost.

Postoperative Care and Follow-up

These patients need more than usual care and comfort in postoperative period. Apart from paying attention that the pin sites heal adequately (which is usually the case) aggressive medical management with physiotherapy and rehabilitation is necessary. Every attempt must be made that these patients attain a functional state of living.

Complications

As described by LaMothe et al,[48] complications related to intraoperative traction are rare. Since the use of traction is limited for a short period of time, complications related to pin sites are unusual. The only reported traction-related complication was one anterosuperior iliac spine skin pressure sore from head halter skin traction.[44] Since head halter relies on skin traction and has been found to be ineffective, it is not usually used now as a modality of curve correction. In a meta-analysis conducted by LaMothe et al,[48] they found no major complications related to the use of intraoperative traction.

However, the complication rate was 13% including intraoperative + motor-evoked

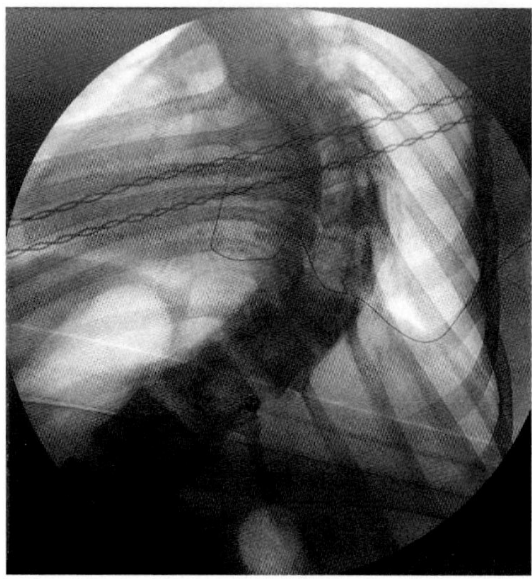

Fig. 20.4 Left-bending film.

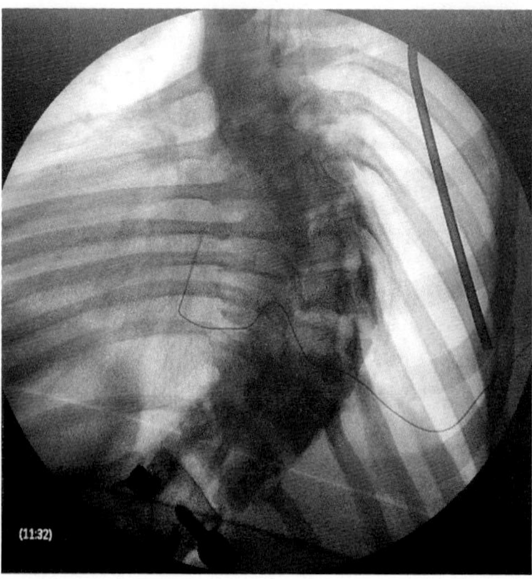

Fig. 20.5 Traction film.

potential (MEP) changes without postoperative neurologic sequelae. Intraoperatively, the application of traction led to changes in MEP in more severe and stiff curves.[34] In these patients, MEP changes responded immediately by decreasing or removing the traction weight and as a result there was no long-term permanent neurologic damage.

Pearl

No major complications have been described with this technique in literature.

Tips to Avoid Complications

Lewis et al[34] conducted a study monitoring neurophysiological changes in AIS patients corrected with the help of intraoperative traction. They recommended intraoperative traction should not be used in the absence of MEP monitoring. Somatosensory-evoked potentials (SSEP) as the sole means of monitoring is strongly discouraged. They also found that thoracic location of the major curve, mean Cobb angle of 86 degrees or more, and increased rigidity (low traction and FI) are risk factors for changes in MEP monitoring with traction. Most of the neurophysiological changes reversed completely with one or more of the maneuvers of reduction of traction, complete removal of traction, and rod loosening while optimizing cord perfusion and oxygenation. Keeping note of contraindications and ideal cases to start with during the learning curve (as mentioned above) will greatly help to avoid complications.

Pearl

Use of neuromonitoring is recommended which greatly enhances the safety of the technique.

Case Example

A 16-year-old girl came to us with severe scoliosis as depicted in **Fig. 20.6**. She complained of back pain and cosmetic deformity with no neurological signs and symptoms. Her main thoracic curve on standing AP radiograph measured 85 degrees, whereas thoracolumbar curve measured 54 degrees. The main thoracic curve measured 68 degrees on bending films (**Fig. 20.7** and **Fig. 20.8**). The FI calculated for side-bending images was 0.36. Considering the

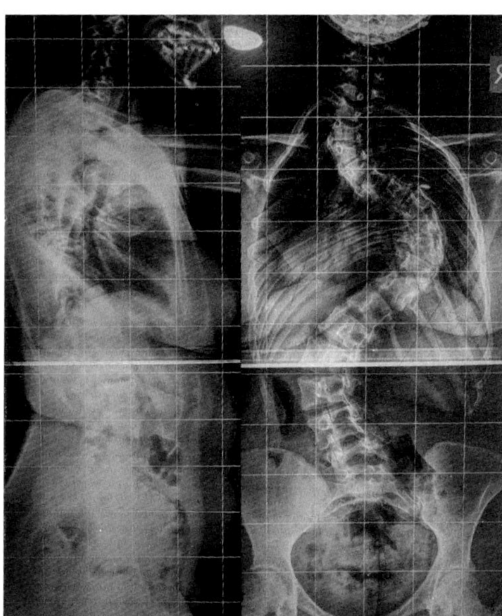

Fig. 20.6 Application of cranial traction.

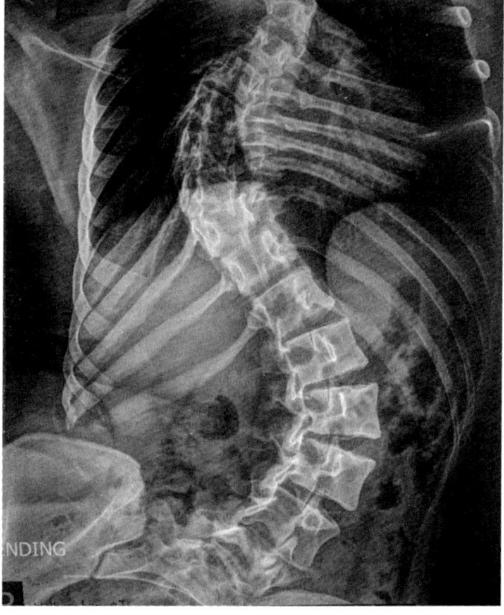

Fig. 20.7 Application of femoral traction.

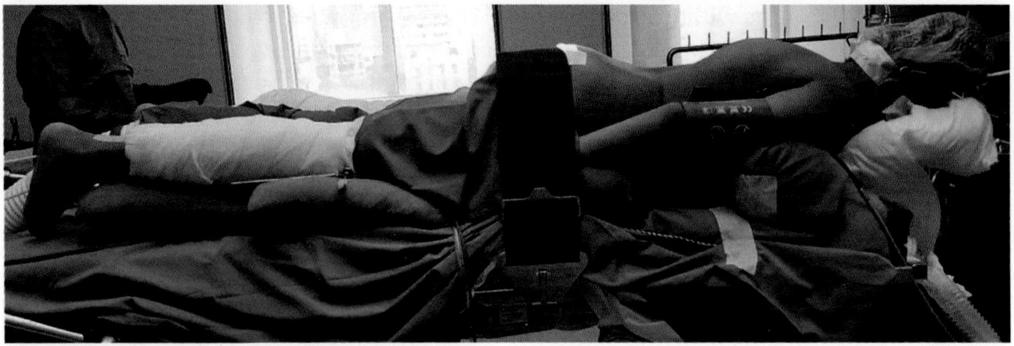

Fig. 20.8 Positioning of patient.

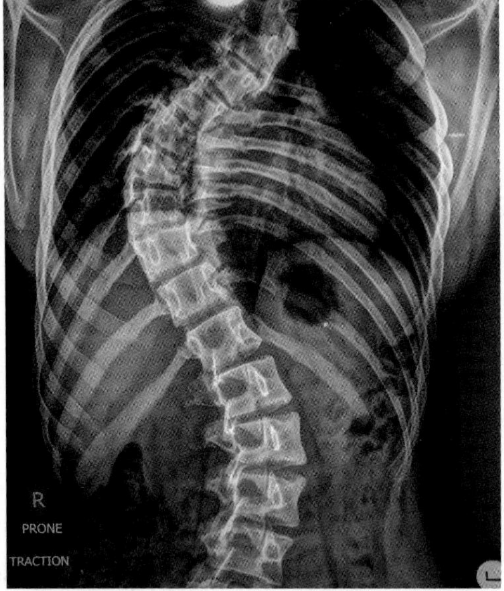

Fig. 20.9 Intraoperative C-arm image before application of traction.

above values, the curve falls within the criteria of a severe and rigid deformity. On traction films (**Fig. 20.9**), the curve showed marginal correction to 57 degrees with FI of 0.33. The surgery was planned and we decided to correct the curve using the technique of an all-posterior deformity correction with intraoperative skeletal traction and neuromonitoring. The craniofemoral traction was applied as shown in **Fig. 20.1** and **Fig. 20.2** and the patient was positioned (**Fig. 20.3**). The dramatic correction of scoliosis can be appreciated on intraoperative C-arm images (**Fig. 20.4** and **Fig. 20.5**). Additional correction was then achieved with posterior facet releases. The follow-up images (**Fig. 20.10** and **Fig. 20.11**) showed well-balanced sagittal and coronal profiles with significant correction of main thoracic curve to 48 degrees. As it can be appreciated, the postoperative correction values are much closer to preoperative values on traction films. Postoperatively, the patient maintained the neurological status and is subjectively happy with the surgery.

Authors' Experience

The primary author has vast experience in treating severe rigid deformities over the years and finds the above-described technique extremely efficacious. This principle stems from a biomechanical study by White and Panjabi[49] which proved that large curves corrected better with axial traction rather than translational maneuvers. Presently, he has operated over 28 patients having such deformities. In his study[32] published in 2012 with a cohort of 10 patients (8 with neglected AIS and 2 with neuromuscular scoliosis), the mean age of patients was 27.4 years (19–36 y). This number is greater than that provided by most studies in literature. The osteoligamentous structures and the musculature are stiff and do not easily yield to manipulation. The Cobb angle improved from a mean of 89.35 degrees preoperatively to 40.25 degrees postoperatively, giving a mean correction of 55.29%. Apical vertebral rotation (Nash

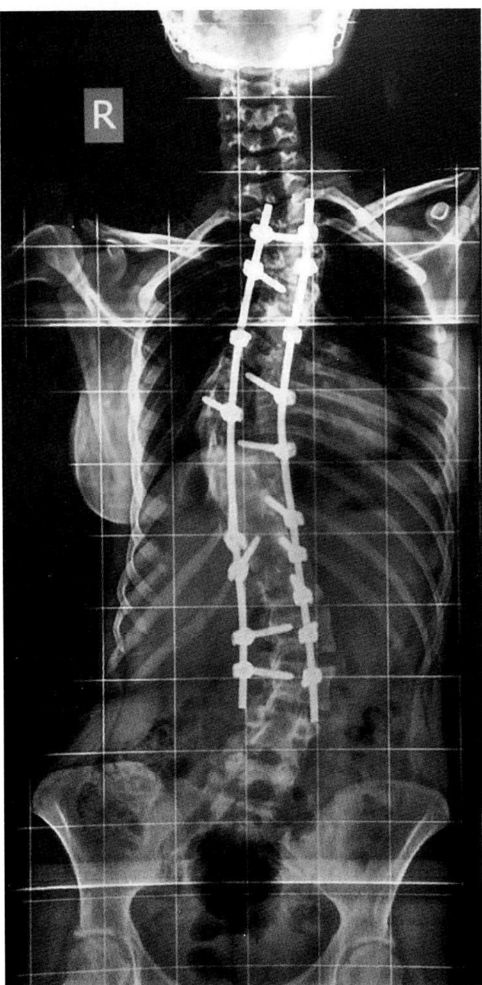

Fig. 20.10 Final correction. Postoperative X-ray anteroposterior.

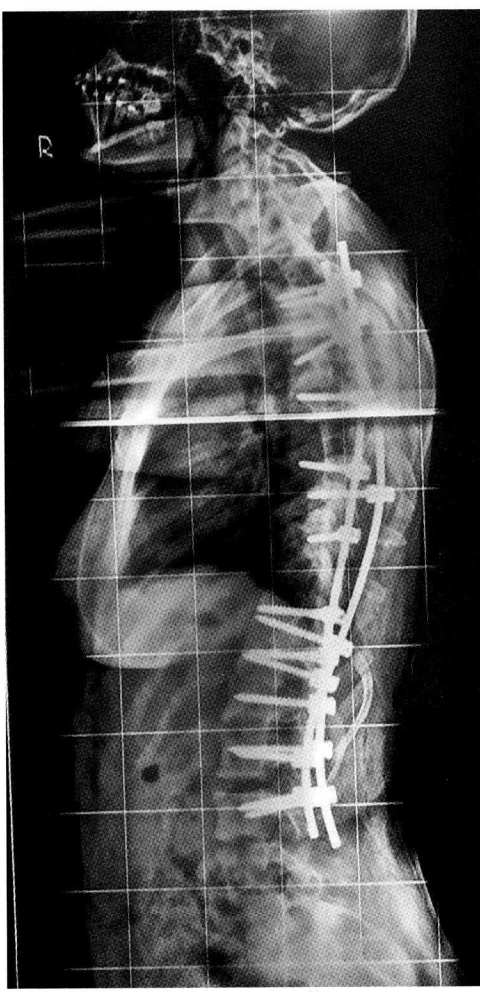

Fig. 20.11 Final correction. Postoperative X-ray lateral.

and Moe[49]) improved from a mean of grade 3(2–4) to a mean of grade 2(1–3). Apical vertebral translation improved from a mean of 2.19 cm preoperatively to 0.98 cm postoperatively (55.41% correction). There were no intraoperative adverse events or postoperative complications. All patients had good shoulder balance and were satisfied with the correction achieved. The same results are seen in patients being operated over the years and no significant loss of correction at follow-up.

Conclusion

Intraoperative skull-femoral traction can be a safe-and-effective method to assist correction of severe and rigid scoliosis. It facilitates surgical exposure and pedicle screw insertion. It obviates the need of an anterior release surgery and associated morbidity, thus reducing the hospital stay and costs. It provides a much simpler way to correct the sagittal and coronal imbalance, as well as the pelvic obliquity.

References

1. O'Brien MF, Lenke LG, Bridwell KH, Blanke K, Baldus C. Preoperative spinal canal investigation in adolescent idiopathic scoliosis curves > or = 70 degrees. Spine 1994;19(14): 1606–1610
2. Tokunaga M, Minami S, Kitahara H, Isobe K, Nakata Y, Moriya H. Vertebral decancellation for severe scoliosis. Spine 2000;25(4): 469–474
3. Greiner KA. Adolescent idiopathic scoliosis: radiologic decision-making. Am Fam Physician 2002;65(9):1817–1822
4. Suk SI, Kim JH, Kim SS, Lim DJ. Pedicle screw instrumentation in adolescent idiopathic scoliosis (AIS). Eur Spine J 2012;21(1):13–22
5. Wang Y, Fei Q, Qiu G, et al. Anterior spinal fusion versus posterior spinal fusion for moderate lumbar/thoracolumbar adolescent idiopathic scoliosis: a prospective study. Spine 2008;33(20):2166–2172
6. Tis JE, O'Brien MF, Newton PO, et al. Adolescent idiopathic scoliosis treated with open instrumented anterior spinal fusion: five-year follow-up. Spine 2010;35(1):64–70
7. Norton RP, Patel D, Kurd MF, Picetti GD, Vaccaro AR. The use of thoracoscopy in the management of adolescent idiopathic scoliosis. Spine 2007;32(24):2777–2785
8. Rinella A, Lenke L, Whitaker C, et al. Perioperative halo-gravity traction in the treatment of severe scoliosis and kyphosis. Spine 2005;30(4):475–482
9. King AG, Mills TE, Loe WA Jr, Chutkan NB, Revels TS. Video-assisted thoracoscopic surgery in the prone position. Spine 2000; 25(18):2403–2406
10. Niemeyer T, Freeman BJ, Grevitt MP, Webb JK. Anterior thoracoscopic surgery followed by posterior instrumentation and fusion in spinal deformity. Eur Spine J 2000;9(6): 499–504
11. Kim YJ, Lenke LG, Bridwell KH, Kim KL, Steger-May K. Pulmonary function in adolescent idiopathic scoliosis relative to the surgical procedure. J Bone Joint Surg Am 2005;87(7):1534–1541
12. Good CR, Lenke LG, Bridwell KH, et al. Can posterior-only surgery provide similar radiographic and clinical results as combined anterior (thoracotomy/thoracoabdominal)/ posterior approaches for adult scoliosis? Spine 2010;35(2):210–218
13. Keeler KA, Lenke LG, Good CR, Bridwell KH, Sides B, Luhmann SJ. Spinal fusion for spastic neuromuscular scoliosis: is anterior releasing necessary when intraoperative halo-femoral traction is used? Spine 2010;35(10):E427–E433
14. Kim YB, Lenke LG, Kim YJ, Kim YW, Bridwell KH, Stobbs G. Surgical treatment of adult scoliosis: is anterior apical release and fusion necessary for the lumbar curve? Spine 2008; 33(10):1125–1132
15. Dobbs MB, Lenke LG, Kim YJ, Luhmann SJ, Bridwell KH. Anterior/posterior spinal instrumentation versus posterior instrumentation alone for the treatment of adolescent idiopathic scoliotic curves more than 90°. Spine 2006;31(20):2386–2391
16. Lenke LG, Sides BA, Koester LA, Hensley M, Blanke KM. Vertebral column resection for the treatment of severe spinal deformity. Clin Orthop Relat Res 2010;468(3):687–699
17. Bradford DS, Tribus CB. Vertebral column resection for the treatment of rigid coronal decompensation. Spine 1997;22(14): 1590–1599
18. Kane WJ, Moe JH, Lai CC. Halo-femoral pin distraction in the treatment of scoliosis. J Bone Joint Surg Am 1967;49:1018–1019
19. Schmidt AC. Halo-tibial traction combined with the Milwaukee Brace. Clin Orthop Relat Res 1971;77(77):73–83
20. Edgar MA, Chapman RH, Glasgow MM. Pre-operative correction in adolescent idiopathic scoliosis. J Bone Joint Surg Br 1982; 64(5):530–535
21. Koptan W, ElMiligui Y. Three-staged correction of severe rigid idiopathic scoliosis using limited halo-gravity traction. Eur Spine J 2012;21(6):1091–1098
22. Clark JA, Hsu LCS, Yau AC. Viscoelastic behaviour of deformed spines under correction with halo pelvic distraction. Clin Orthop Relat Res 1975; (110):90–111
23. Sink EL, Karol LA, Sanders J, Birch JG, Johnston CE, Herring JA. Efficacy of perioperative halo-gravity traction in the treatment of severe scoliosis in children. J Pediatr Orthop 2001;21(4):519–524
24. Victor DI, Bresnan MJ, Keller RB. Brain abscess complicating the use of halo traction. J Bone Joint Surg Am 1973;55(3):635–639
25. Dove J, Hsu LC, Yau AC. The cervical spine after halo-pelvic traction. An analysis of the complications of 83 patients. J Bone Joint Surg Br 1980;62-B(2):158–161
26. Kalamchi A, Yau AC, O'Brien JP, Hodgson AR. Halo-pelvic distraction apparatus. An analysis

of one hundred and fifty consecutive patients. J Bone Joint Surg Am 1976;58(8):1119–1125
27. O'Brien JP, Yau AC, Hodgson AR. Halo pelvic traction: a technic for severe spinal deformities. Clin Orthop Relat Res 1973; (93): 179–190
28. Ransford AO, Manning CW. Complications of halo-pelvic distraction for scoliosis. J Bone Joint Surg Br 1975;57(2):131–137
29. Erdem MN, Oltulu I, Karaca S, Sari S, Aydogan M. Intraoperative halo-femoral traction in surgical treatment of adolescent idiopathic scoliosis curves between 70° and 90°: Is it effective? Asian Spine J 2018;12(4):678–685
30. Bacon S, Sharma O, Jhaveri S, Hedden D, Howard A, Halpern E, Lewis S. Combined anterior/posterior spinal fusion compared to posterior fusion with intra-operative traction in the correction of scoliosis curves greater than 75 Degrees. The Spine Journal 2009;9(10)
31. Hamzaoglu A, Ozturk C, Aydogan M, Tezer M, Aksu N, Bruno MB. Posterior only pedicle screw instrumentation with intraoperative halo-femoral traction in the surgical treatment of severe scoliosis (>100°). Spine 2008; 33(9):979–983
32. Kulkarni AG, Shah SP. Intraoperative skull-femoral (skeletal) traction in surgical correction of severe scoliosis (>80°) in adult neglected scoliosis. Spine 2013;38(8): 659–664
33. Takeshita K, Lenke LG, Bridwell KH, Kim YJ, Sides B, Hensley M. Analysis of patients with nonambulatory neuromuscular scoliosis surgically treated to the pelvis with intraoperative halo-femoral traction. Spine 2006;31(20):2381–2385
34. Lewis SJ, Gray R, Holmes LM, et al. Neurophysiological changes in deformity correction of adolescent idiopathic scoliosis with intraoperative skull-femoral traction. Spine 2011;36(20):1627–1638
35. Bourget-Murray J, Brown GE, Peiro-Garcia A, Earp MA, Parsons DL, Ferri-de-Barros F. Quality, safety and value of innovating classic operative techniques in scoliosis surgery: intraoperative traction and navigated sequential drilling. Spine Deform 2019; 7(4):588–595
36. Polly DW Jr, Sturm PF. Traction versus supine side bending. Which technique best determines curve flexibility? Spine 1998; 23(7):804–808
37. Watanabe K, Kawakami N, Nishiwaki Y, et al. Traction versus supine side-bending radiographs in determining flexibility: what factors influence these techniques? Spine 2007;32(23):2604–2609
38. Liu RW, Teng AL, Armstrong DG, Poe-Kochert C, Son-Hing JP, Thompson GH. Comparison of supine bending, push-prone, and traction under general anesthesia radiographs in predicting curve flexibility and postoperative correction in adolescent idiopathic scoliosis. Spine 2010;35(4):416–422
39. Vaughan JJ, Winter RB, Lonstein JE. Comparison of the use of supine bending and traction radiographs in the selection of the fusion area in adolescent idiopathic scoliosis. Spine 1996;21(21):2469–2473
40. Hamzaoglu A, Talu U, Tezer M, Mirzanli C, Domanic U, Goksan SB. Assessment of curve flexibility in adolescent idiopathic scoliosis. Spine 2005;30(14):1637–1642
41. Suk SI, Chung ER, Kim JH, Kim SS, Lee JS, Choi WK. Posterior vertebral column resection for severe rigid scoliosis. Spine 2005;30(14):1682–1687
42. Zhou C, Liu L, Song Y, et al. Anterior and posterior vertebral column resection for severe and rigid idiopathic scoliosis. Eur Spine J 2011;20(10):1728–1734
43. Zhou C, Liu L, Song Y, et al. Anterior release internal distraction and posterior spinal fusion for severe and rigid scoliosis. Spine 2013;38(22):E1411–E1417
44. Mac-Thiong JM, Labelle H, Poitras B, Rivard CH, Joncas J. The effect of intraoperative traction during posterior spinal instrumentation and fusion for adolescent idiopathic scoliosis. Spine 2004;29(14):1549–1554
45. Jhaveri SN, Zeller R, Miller S, Lewis SJ. The effect of intra-operative skeletal (skull femoral) traction on apical vertebral rotation. Eur Spine J 2009;18(3):352–356
46. Al Sayegh S, LaMothe J, Letal M. Intraoperative Skull Femoral Traction (ISFT) in posterior instrumentation for adolescent idiopathic scoliosis: safety and effect on perioperative care. Can J Surg 2013;56:S54–S55
47. Limpaphayom N, Skaggs DL, McComb G, Krieger M, Tolo VT. Complications of halo use in children. Spine 2009;34(8):779–784
48. LaMothe JM, Al Sayegh S, Parsons DL, Ferri-de-Barros F. The use of intraoperative traction in pediatric scoliosis surgery: a systematic review. Spine Deform 2015;3(1): 45–51
49. Nash CL Jr, Moe JH. A study of vertebral rotation. J Bone Joint Surg Am 1969;51(2): 223–229

21 Dynamic Stabilization and Deformity Surgery

Ali Fahir Ozer and Murat Korkmaz

History

The concept of dynamic stabilization started with Henry Graf.[1] Graf stated that the main cause of pain in degenerative instabilities is abnormal mobility and suggested that patients will benefit from abnormal mobility being controlled.

Graf noted that fusion surgery is an overtreatment for these types of problems. Thus, Graf discovered new ligament that was later named after him and tried to prevent abnormal movement by attaching these ligaments to the heads of pedicular screws. Although favorable results have been obtained from the surgery with Graf ligaments, the surgery has not been widely supported for some important reasons.[2]

The critics focused mainly on two points. First, the system preventing hyperextension was weak, and the ligaments were relaxed. The second ligament was placed with two pedicular screws under tension, decreasing the volume of the foramen and increasing the irritation of the root, and was passed through the degenerative foramen. These deficiencies have been overcome by the development of the Dynesys system. Dubois has contributed to the development of this new system considerably and has published successful results.[3]

A spacer was placed between two pedicular screws to prevent foraminal stenosis. In addition, the tension in the ligament used as a rod was standardized (**Fig. 21.1**). Despite successful results in Europe, the FDA did not approve this system as a dynamic system, and the biggest criticism was that the screws loosened.[4]

Despite all sorts of criticism, this system continues to be used across the world, except in the United States, and favorable results continue to be shared.

In the meantime, there has been another development in dynamic systems. In a study conducted in South Africa, Strempel et al placed a hinge between the screw body and the head to increase the load on the bone graft placed between two vertebral bodies; thus, the authors of the study aimed to provide better fusion outcomes.[5]

The clinical results showed that although some of the patients developed pseudarthrosis, these patients did not have any complaints or signs of loosening in the screws. In subsequent clinical trials, the authors tried using this system without bone grafting, that is, without fusion, and achieved successful results. They developed the cosmic system and led it to the market (**Fig. 21.2**).

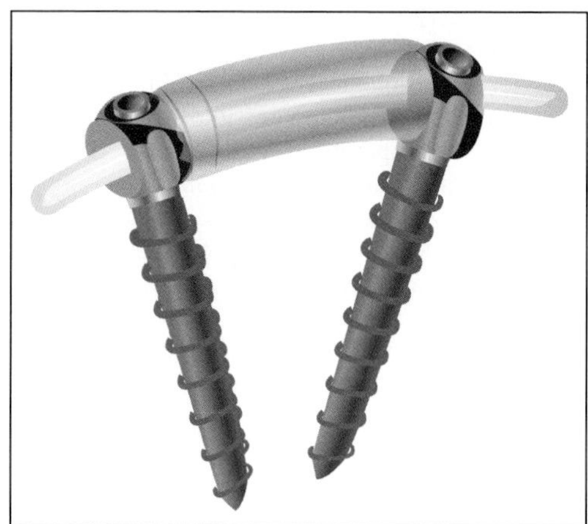

Fig. 21.1 Dynesys dynamic stabilization system.

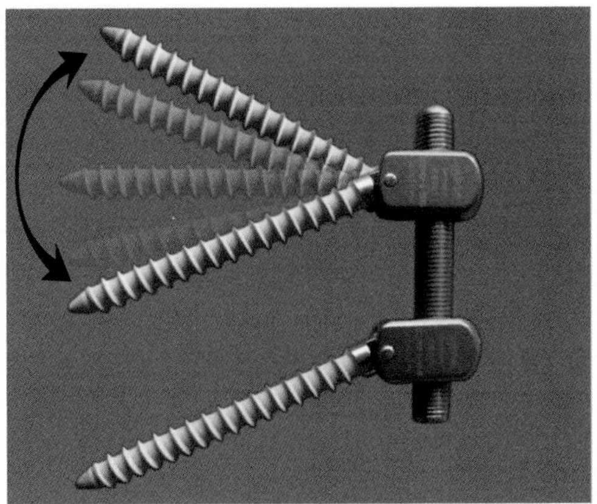

Fig. 21.2 Cosmic dynamic stabilization system.

Thus, a new dynamic approach was added to the dynamic rod concept, and the dynamic screw concept was born. This system has received considerable criticism, especially when used over two distances, and it has been stated that the system becomes more rigid because it naturally increases the rigidity of the posterior column; therefore, its use above two levels is not recommended. This system cannot be used in dynamic uses according to the FDA in the United States and is approved for use in fusion surgery.[6]

In the meantime, there has been another development that has gone unnoticed. Dynamic screws have been used with more flexible peek rods to increase the dynamism of the system. The outcomes of this approach were reported to be better.[7,8] Even compared with the use of rods that are more flexible than the peek rod, which will be discussed later, it has been shown that this approach yields more favorable biomechanical results. A classification system of dynamic stabilization systems, including the use of this combination approach, was created by Kaner et al in 2010.[9]

Again, it is a fact that many disc nucleus supporters using stand-alone fusion become frustrated. Dynamic screws have been used together with a prosthetic disc nucleus by one of the nucleus supporters, but the results were not favorable. The problem was not in the dynamic screw system but rather in the prosthetic disc nucleus, as it did not gain the required flexibility in a sufficient amount of time.[10]

Pearl

The dynamic system has been developed to avoid the negative effects of fusion, just like lumbar disc prostheses.

Biomechanical Aspect

In many biomechanical studies, it has been reported that the Dynesys system restores abnormal movement in the distorted neutral zone (NZ) and improves load distribution.[11] However, the most remarkable study within the biomechanical studies involving Dynesys is the work by Kiapour et al.[12]

Partial facetectomy had a minimal effect on range of motion (ROM) in the segment where the Dynesys was applied, whereas total facetectomy increased movement by 40% in flexion and 200% in axial rotation. The authors stated that the Dynesys screw failed against the high stress caused by the generic rigid screw under specific loads. Niosi et al showed that when the standard length was used in intact and injured segments, ROM significantly decreased, and the smallest amount of change was observed in axial rotation.[13]

The authors reported that when the Dynesys was applied to the impaired NZ, it restored the impaired NZ, but the strength was weak compared to that of the intact mobile segment. The Dynesys showed a significant posterior shift in the helical axis of motion (HAM) in flexion, extension, and axial rotation. The authors also claimed that the length of the spacer seriously affected the ROM. They noted that the long spacer caused excessive ROM mobilization in all directions, which was not related to the preload period.

The largest changes in ROM were in axial rotation. Increasing the spacer's length by 4 mm increased intersegmental mobility by 30% in axial rotation, 23% in extension, 14% in flexion, and 11% in lateral bending. However, spacers of different lengths do not affect NZ. Typically, a short spacer leads to a larger shift and larger changes in the HAM orientation. A long spacer leads to an ROM and movement pattern close to those of a normal mobile segment, which is repressed by the HAM. This study showed that the Dynesys spacer length disrupts the segmental position and thus affects kinematic behavior.

The first of the biomechanical studies on the dynamic screw system is the finite element study by Erbulut et al.[14] Since the system was designed for fusion, hinged screws provide a very favorable environment for the graft placed in the space between the vertebrae. The authors showed that in a finite element model, the system supports the destabilized motion segment without revealing rotational instability, but the hinged screw carries more load than the nucleus portion on which the graft is placed, which is located in the space between the vertebrae. They stated that the hinged dynamic screw is suitable for increasing the fusion rate.

After this finite element study, a cadaver study related to dynamic screws was carried out by Schmoelz et al in 2009.[15] In this study, the authors showed that ROM was decreased in all three planes to that of a monosegmentally stabilized intact segment with hinged screws. The authors stated that when an additional motion segment was added to the system, the ROM was further reduced in the whole system. They also stated that ROM was increased when the motion segment was destabilized, especially in axial rotation, and ROM normalized to that of an intact segment after hinged screw stabilization.[15]

A similar study was then carried out with Safinas dynamic screws.[16] This study was performed in a single motion segment, and it was shown that a higher level of stabilization was achieved near the intact spine with a dynamic screw than with a rigid system. The authors showed that the dynamic screw system was subjected to less load and less stress, but the kinematics were disrupted in both systems.

For the first time in the literature, Erbulut and Oktenoglu answered the question of how the combined use of a dynamic screw and a dynamic rod will affect the NZ in a disrupted motion segment. They used the spiral dynamic rod, which they called the Talin rod, for both cadaver and finite element studies.[14]

In the finite element study, talin rod and hinged screw (dynamic combination), rigid rod and hinged screw (semirigid combination), rigid rod and rigid screw (rigid combination) systems were compared in terms of the stress values of ROM, facet joint loading, intradiscal pressure, and screws. The biomechanical results of this study support the hypothesis that dynamic screw and dynamic rod constructs as a posterior stabilization system provide a stabilizing function, and this approach may address the problems of adjacent segment degeneration and implant failure better than rigid or semirigid constructs. A long-term clinical investigation is necessary for evaluating the functionality of these constructs. The authors stated that laboratory results should be evaluated with clinical results with long follow-up times.

Erbulut and Oktenoglu performed the same study in cadavers with the same combinations and showed that in all three combinations, the spine was stabilized, but the dynamic rod and dynamic screw combination stabilized the spine with values close to those of the normal motion segment.[14] There is no significant similar biomechanical study on this topic in the literature.

Pearl

Pedicular dynamic system stabilizes the neutral zone, which is impaired in segmental instability.

Clinical Applications

Today, dynamic systems are applied by spine surgeons who believe in this system in every country in the world, except in the United

States. Why are surgeons hoping for dynamic systems? The answer to this question lies in the fusion system, which is currently accepted as the gold standard.

Upon further examination, fusion surgery is a risky surgery, and as the level of fusion increases, the complication rate increases. In terms of complications, pseudarthrosis, blood loss, infection, and pain are the most concerning issues that persist even when the fusion surgery is successful. For example, you perform fusion surgery on a degenerative spondylolisthesis patient, and the patient comes to you on foot and complains of low back pain only. Imagine 3 months after the surgery; if pseudarthrosis develops, this patient will no longer come to you on foot. You will need to perform a more involved surgery to enable the patient to stand on his or her feet.

The situation is different when an infection is encountered. Even in patients with degenerative kyphosis or scoliosis whose pelvic parameters are not considerably impaired, the mortality and morbidity rates of fusion surgery of four or more segments are very high. As a result, fusion surgery has been performed for 100 years, and there are no alternatives, except for minimally invasive methods, have been developed for better clinical outcomes or to find various bioactive materials for better fusion results. There is also a problem with the dynamic systems; has been performed for a century. Except for Minimally invasive method, there were no alternative available. Dynamic stabilization was introduced for better clinical outcomes and for better fusion results using bioactive materials.

Today, whether you use the semirigid combination, dynamic combination, or another system in single-level stabilizations, the results are consistent with the single-level results of fusion. In addition, these systems should be considered serious alternatives to fusion in resolving chronic instabilities.[7,17–20]

In authors' opinion, the problem is currently in long segment stabilization. Very well-known problems encountered in lumbosacral fixation in fusion surgery are also encountered in dynamic systems. Anterior support is important, especially when the L5–S1 level is attached to a long instrumentation segment in fusion surgery. An anterior support (bone graft or cancellous grafts with cages) is placed between the L5 and S1 vertebral bodies to reduce load on S1 screws. If S1 screws are insufficient in carrying load, the other recommended solutions are the following: the use of S2 screws, attaching a hook system to the S2 foramen to decrease the load on the S1 screws, and finally, use of the iliac screws, which has been accepted as the classic solution. Often, combinations of these solutions are applied together in long segment fusion and instrumentation. In the long segment, the problem is seen especially at the lumbosacral or thoracolumbar junction. In particular, screw loosening in dynamic systems is observed in these regions (**Fig. 21.3**). In authors' opinion, the proposed solutions for fusion should be followed in dynamic systems. Incomplete but promising clinical trial results will be published in the near future.

Putzier was the first surgeon to use the hinged screw in conjunction with Discectomy to prevent instability after lumbar Discectomy. He stated that "the applied dynamic stabilization system is useful to prevent progression of lumbar spinal segments after nucleotomy." Many articles supporting the dynamic system have been published in the literature.[6,19,21] Favorable results have been published in a 2-year international joint study on the cosmic system involving one and two levels.[22]

In 2013, Canbay et al reported that they achieved good results with a hinged screw in the surgical treatment of degenerative disc disease.[21] In 2016, Yang et al used the cosmic system, a dynamic rod and an articulated screw known as bioflex in single-distance degenerative spondylolisthesis, and concluded that "lumbar dynamic stabilizations, using pedicle screws with Nitinol spring rod system and a hinged screw head

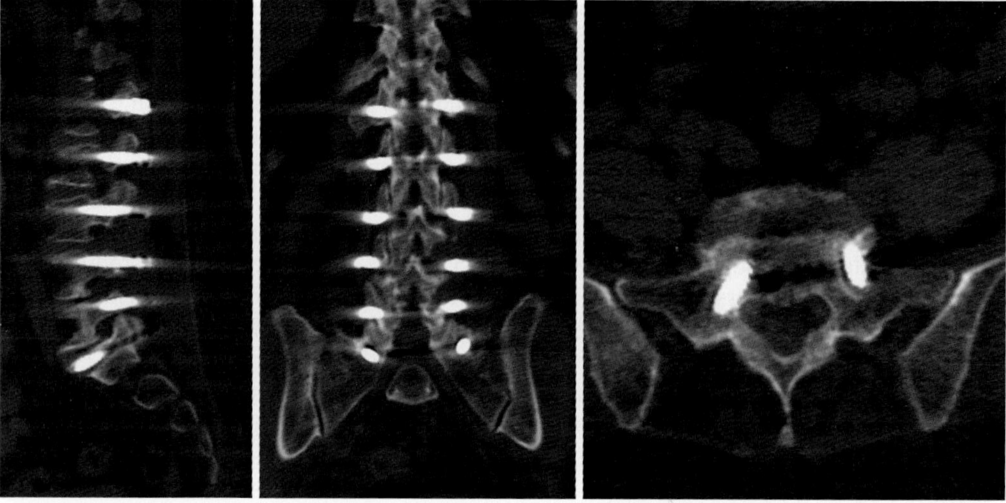

Fig. 21.3 Screw loosening in long-level stabilization with Dynesys system.

system, may control the motion of instability level, and both device systems may maintain the ROM of adjacent segments. These outcomes may play a role in decreasing the risk of Adjacent Segment Disease (ASD) after dynamic stabilization, at least 2 years after surgery."[23] Dynamic stabilization has been used to protect the degenerate adjacent segment.[24] Afterwards, hybrid use of the adjacent fusion level in particular has become very common.[25–28]

Pearl

Dynamic stabilization gives equivalent results to fusion surgery in monosegmental instability.

Studies Opposed to the Pedicular Dynamic System

Many articles that are not in favor of dynamic systems have been published. Since it is the most widely used system in the market, the Dynesys system has the highest number of related publications. In 2011, Kim et al used a single and multilevel Dynesys system and stated that it had no positive effects on the adjacent segment and that the system was more rigid than necessary.[29]

When other publications were reviewed, screw loosening and infection became prominent.[30] Other criticisms are that stabilization by the dynamic system is not superior to that by fusion. Some authors published a comparison of the results of dynamic stabilization and fusion groups in their articles. There were no differences in the clinical outcomes and, in particular, no advantages when using the Dynesys system.[31–35]

Putzier et al stated that the dynamic systems used to protect the adjacent segment in hybrid systems do not work.[36]

Landi stated that all existing dynamic systems will always be unsuccessful, as they ignore the elastic resistance of the spine.[37] He mentioned the existing dynamic systems in the article, but he did not examine the dynamic rod and dynamic screw combination in his article.

In addition, there is no ideal elastic rod, which the authors have repeatedly emphasized in this study. It is certain that this problem will be overcome with technological developments. Nevertheless, based on authors' own experience and the results of other publications, single-distance stabilization is highly acceptable. When they consider the process as a simple stabilization system, beyond protecting movement, it is still not wrong to think that it is preferable to fusion.

In their comprehensive literature review in 2015, Pham et al concluded that "the Dynesys system was developed as an alternative to rigid instrumentation and fusion constructs. A review of complications associated with this system found similar infection rates and reoperation rates when compared with published literature on lumbar fusion."[38]

This conclusion is based on the finding that dynamic systems are superior to fusion when used appropriately. The answer to the question, "why should dynamic systems be preferable?" can be many, such as a smaller amount of anatomical damage, a smaller amount of blood loss, a shorter duration of surgery, and a shorter time to participation in social life. If there are no differences between the results, the choice of a safer treatment for the patient may not be wrong.

Pearl

Although there is a screw loosening problem in the long segment, it has good results in multilevel instability.

Dynamic Systems and Deformity Surgery

The use of dynamic systems in multilevel instabilities started in 2009 with Park et al when they used a bioflex system.[39] They explained that patients using the bioflex system for two or three levels improved ROM, prevented ASD and clinically benefited patients.

It was 2010 when dynamic systems were first used in scoliosis surgery by Di Silvestre.[40] In that paper, he reported favorable results in the clinic using a dynamic stabilization system. He concluded that "dynamic stabilization with pedicle screws in addition to decompressive laminectomy resulted in a safe procedure in elderly patients with degenerative lumbar scoliosis; it was able to maintain enough stability to prevent progression of scoliosis and instability, enabling a wide laminectomy in cases of associated lumbar stenosis. This nonfusion stabilization technique was less aggressive than instrumented fusion and obtained a statistically significant improvement of the clinical outcome at last follow-up."

Di Silvestre then compared the scoliosis surgeries that he had performed using the Dynesys system in 2014 with those he performed using the rigid fusion system.[41] In this article, he stated that he achieved better results with rigid systems in the correction of scoliosis, but a shorter duration of surgery and fewer undesirable results were observed with the dynamic system, even though fewer scoliosis corrections were performed with the dynamic system. Importantly, there was no difference between the fusion system and the dynamic system when the 5-year follow-up periods were compared.

Di Silvestre also published midterm results in 2013 in a group of patients who did not undergo fusion.[42] He concluded that "in elderly patients with mild degenerative lumbar scoliosis without sagittal imbalance, pedicle screw-based dynamic stabilization is an effective option, with low complications incidence, granting curve stabilization during time and satisfying clinical results."

In 2014, Lee et al stabilized 21 patients with lumbar stenosis and degenerative scoliosis using the Dynesys system and followed up with them for 2 years.[43] They concluded that "adding nonfusion stabilization after decompressive surgery resulted in a safe and effective procedure for elderly patients with lumbar stenosis with a mild to moderate scoliosis angle (<30°). Statistically significant improvement of the clinical outcome was obtained at the last follow-up evaluation with no progression of the degenerative scoliosis".

Although there are many publications on the use of the dynamic system in conjunction with rigid instrumentation, one example is a publication by Oktenoglu and Ozer[44] in 2014;

in their articles, they performed fusion, and rigid instrumentation continued to upper and lower levels with the hybrid dynamic system for the first time in deformity surgery (**Fig. 21.4**).

Pearl

Dynamic systems restore spinal imbalance in mobile deformities.

Indication of Dynamic Systems in Deformity

Based on the experience of Di Sivestre, Lee, and authors, patients with a scoliosis angle of more than 30 degrees and pelvic parameters within the boundary of compensation are not suitable for treatment with a pure dynamic system. In both cases, continuity of the levels outside the osteotomy level(s) can be achieved with the dynamic system. There are cases where we use this treatment method and obtain good results. Attempting to reach an ideal spine alignment in degenerative scoliosis in patients with low Cobb angles is an unnecessary effort. On the other hand, patient's quality of life should not be compromised in patients with additional medical problems.

It is a correct approach to use a pure dynamic system in deformity correction of the spine in compensated cases (**Fig. 21.5**).

The expectation of these patients is to attain a painless spine that allows them to live their daily life comfortably. These patients do not want to win any athletic competitions. Therefore, this condition should be kept in mind during surgery. These patients should be given an ideal position of the spine with the help of the operating table and supporting pillows. Rigid screws should be placed on the osteotomy level, and dynamic screws should be placed on other levels. Smith-Paterson osteotomy or pedicular osteotomy should be performed to the degree that is necessary in patients requiring

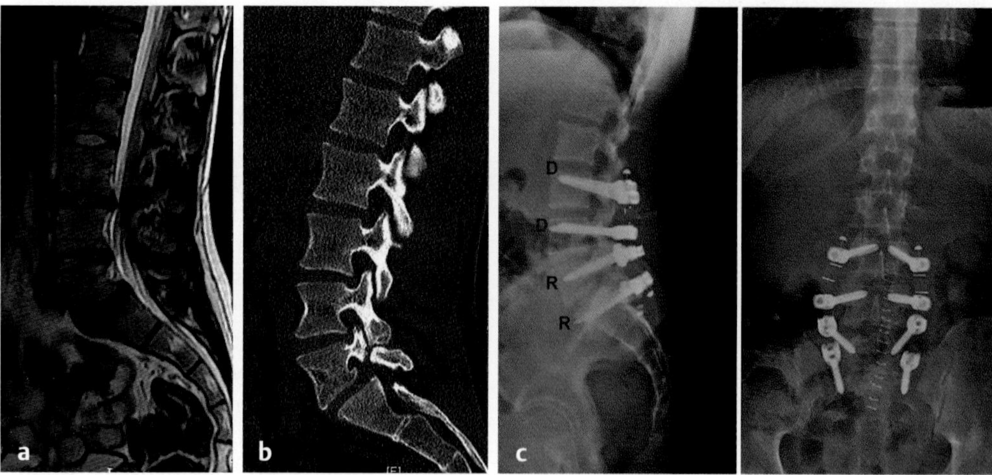

Fig. 21.4 **(a)** L5–S1 spondylolisthesis, L3–L4 bulging [sagittal magnetic resonance (MR) T2], **(b)** L5–S1 isthmic defect [sagittal computed tomography (CT)], and **(c)** a patient stabilized with the hybrid system. Fusion with rigid fixation to the L5–S1 level and dynamic stabilization to the L3–L4 and L4–L5 levels were used due to early degenerative disc disease. The flexible part of the dynamic rod was placed at the L3–L4 level (*arrow*). The moving part of the balance C rod is brought to the L3–L4 level. The L3 and L4 transpedicular screws are dynamic. The distance between L3 and L4 is the most mobile part of the entire system. Balance rods are no longer available in the market.

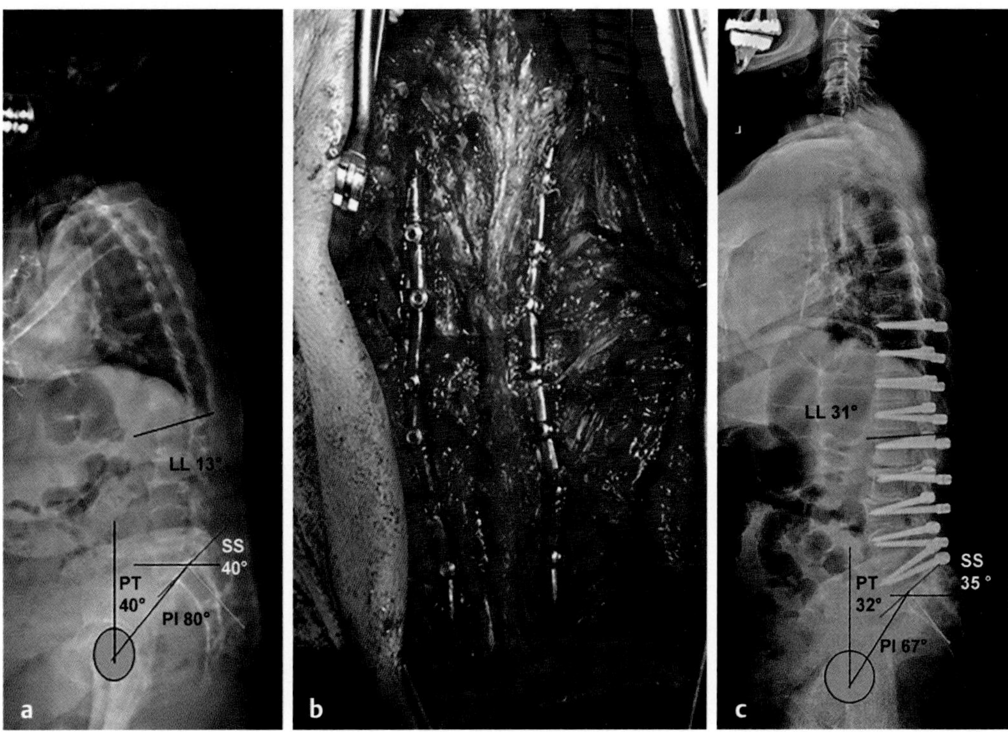

Fig. 21.5 **(a)** There is an imbalance in the sagittal plane. The distance from the vertebral axis to the pelvis is increased, and the pelvic incidence (PI) and pelvic tilt (PT) are also increased. **(b)** The placement of the Dynesys system. **(c)** The pelvic parameters are restored after surgery.

corrections. Then, osteotomy and correction maneuvers should be performed. Dynamic system rods should be placed after rigid rods are placed (**Fig. 21.6**).

The greatest problem in these patients is the low bone stock due to osteoporosis, which is the main cause of screw loosening. We perform two-stage surgery in these patients. If the patient has no neurological deficits other than tolerable pain, we first place the pedicular screws percutaneously under spinal anesthesia. We implant the rods after the patient has passed the average period of osteosynthesis of 4 or 6 months. With this method, their results are very good, and although it may appear as two operations for patients, we actually achieve better clinical results with two less risky surgeries (**Fig. 21.7**).

We also reduced the stress on the S1 screw for the first time in the literature by moving the screw to the iliac wings, especially in the long segment stabilization ending in S1. Thus, we tried to prevent the loosening of the S1 screw, which is particularly at risk of loosening, and achieved good radiological and clinical results.

The first concept in dynamic stabilization is the dynamic rod. However, the idea of placing a hinge between the screw head and the body is a secondary yet important milestone in dynamic systems. In this way, as mentioned in the biomechanics section, the stress shielding on the screws was reduced, but the control of the movement segment passed through the rods to the posterior column. Imagine that you produce a dynamic rod that limits movements to only four degrees of flexion and extension and two degrees of axial rotation in the degenerated NZ of a motion segment. In this way, you have achieved an intact mobile segment.

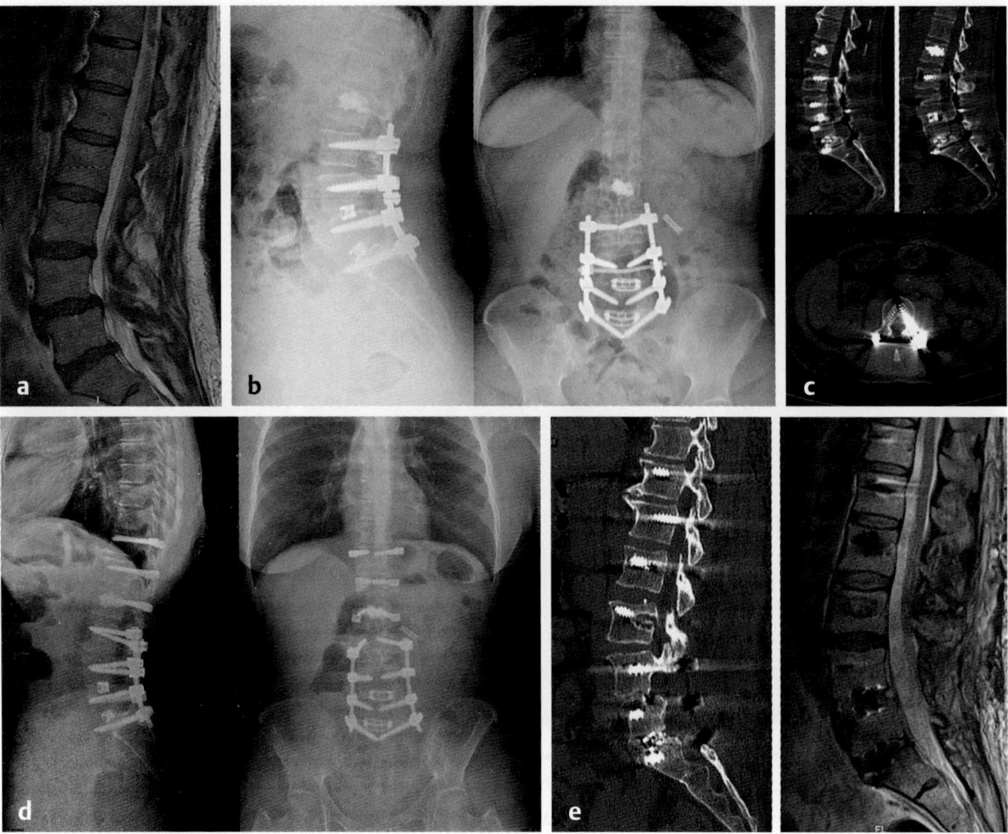

Fig. 21.6 A 57-year-old female: **(a)** A magnetic resonance imaging (MRI) scan showed L4–L5 spondylolisthesis with L3–L4 and L5–S1 degenerative disc disease; **(b)** she was operated on in a spine center 1 year ago, and L5–S1 and L4–L5 fusion and interbody cage procedures were performed. **(c)** L3–L4 was added to a rigid system without a cage, and vertebroplasty was performed on L2 a year after operation. The patient had increasing back pain when she was admitted to authors' department, and she had a very restrictive lifestyle. In her control examination, both screws in L3 were loose. **(d)** and **(e)** The authors did dynamic stabilization as a continuation of the rigid system and fusion system combined with the Dynesys system for the T12 vertebra.

Is there such a rod for this case? Of course not. Does each segment move the same according to age? The answer to this question is also no. With the technology that is currently available, an average dynamic rod can be standardized relative to an average mobile human lumbar spine, but for the time being, rods will continue to be produced as custom-made rods.

A good dynamic system that is close to an ideal system should consist of both dynamic screws and dynamic rods. In authors' single-level instability study, their clinical results were excellent with Balance C rods and Safinas dynamic screws, but now Balance C rods are commercially unavailable. A Dynesys system that is currently used as a dynamic system is accused of being rigid. It is true that it is rigid, and it is difficult to say that the Dynesys system is fully dynamic. It is a semirigid system and is allowed in the United States as a fusion system. When the

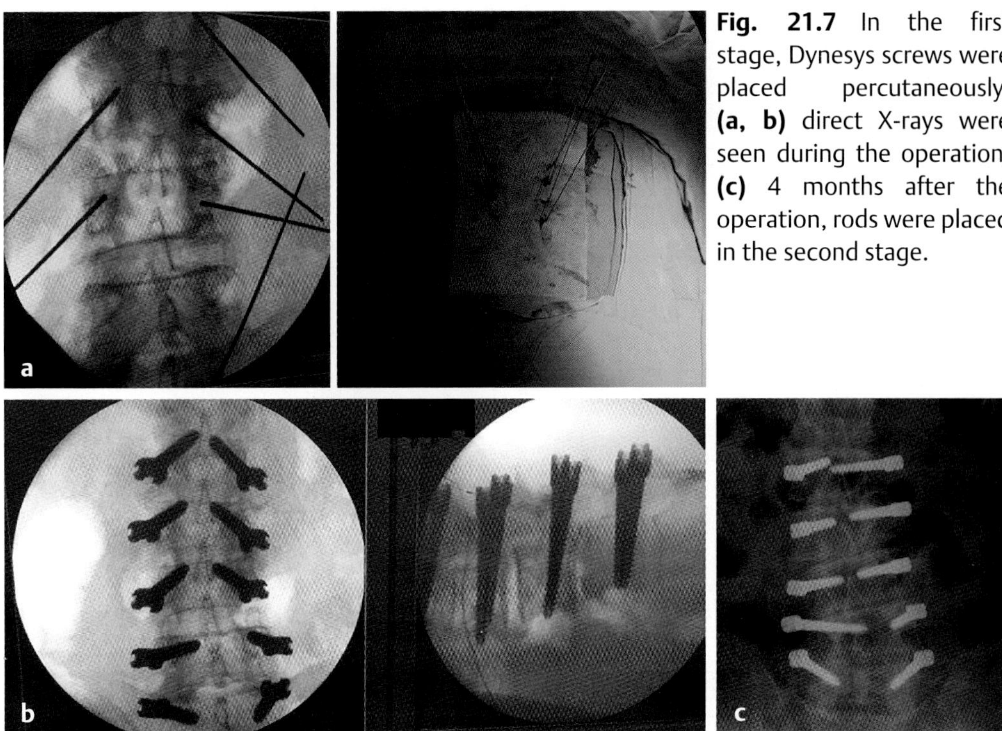

Fig. 21.7 In the first stage, Dynesys screws were placed percutaneously; **(a, b)** direct X-rays were seen during the operation; **(c)** 4 months after the operation, rods were placed in the second stage.

Cosmic dynamic screws or Safinas dynamic screws are used with the rigid rod, can we say that this system is fully dynamic? No; even at one level, it is a semirigid system. There is no chance of applying this system to multilevel instabilities such as degenerative scoliosis. As the rigid rod on both sides posteriorly connects every segment, the system will become increasingly rigid. Alternatively, the PEEK (polyether ether ketone) rod can be used repeatedly, but it is far from eliciting the expected amount of flexibility. In other words, there is no real dynamic rod on the market.

Pearl

Dynamic systems restore the impaired neutral zone, so they can be used in the surgical treatment of all types of chronic instability.

Orthrus Dynamic System

When authors reviewed their own clinical results and those in the literature, they found that the clinical outcomes of single-level dynamic stabilization were satisfactory and complication rates were equivalent to those of fusion. Therefore, they routinely use dynamic systems in our clinic, especially in routine single-level instabilities. This finding gave them the idea for the stabilization of multilevel instabilities. The authors designed and produced a new stabilization system that individually stabilizes each level. They developed this system by splitting the screw heads into two parts and reducing the rod diameter from 6 to 5 mm (**Fig. 21.8**).

Biomechanical tests were performed at the University of Toledo. Because of the positive biomechanical results, they also used this system in their patients (**Fig. 21.9**).

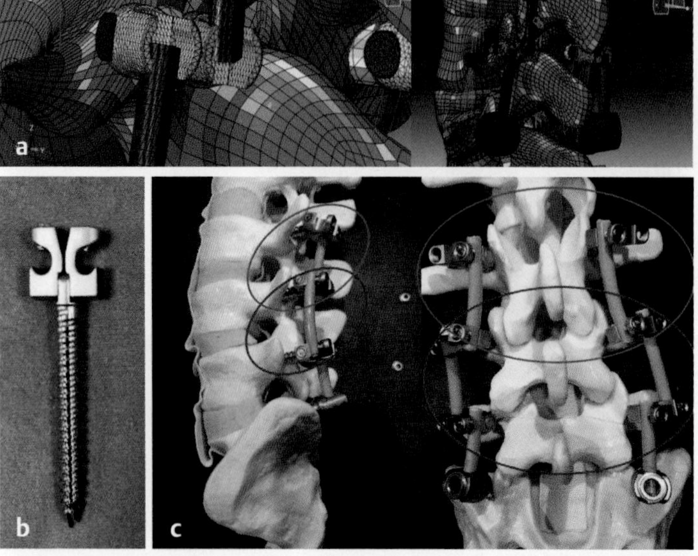

Fig. 21.8 (a) Biomechanic studies showed Orthrus system restored impaired neutral zone; (b) double headed screw (Orthrus). (c) Orthrus is a modular system: double head screws ensure that each level is stabilized like a single level.

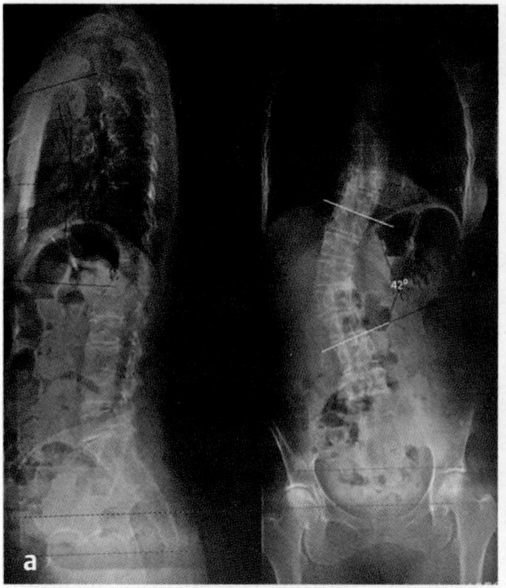

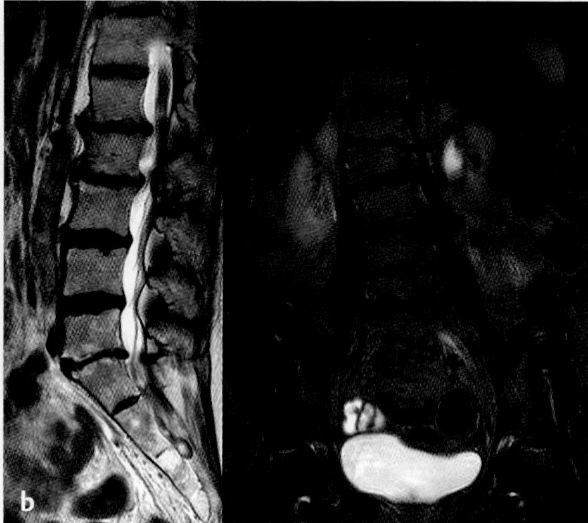

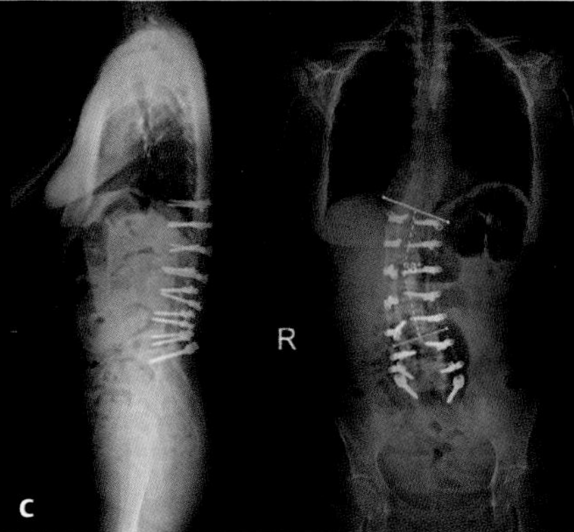

Fig. 21.9 **(a)** A 61-year-old female. She had a spinal deformity until her childhood. In the last 2 years, she had increasing severe back pain. **(b)** In her magnetic resonance imaging (MRI) scan, L5–S1 had spontaneous fusion, and there was no significant problem at L3, but L1–L2 and L2–3 had severe degenerative changes in instability, just dome of the scoliosis. **(c)** Dynamic stabilization with the Orthrus system covered the upper and lower levels. In the preoperative and postoperative X-rays, scoliosis angles were observed to be 42 degrees and 38 degrees.

The system is named "Orthrus." Their early results were quite satisfactory.[45] In the future, new ideas and designs with new technologies will be developed, and they will see many new dynamic systems providing physiological back movements.

Pearl

Since the Orthus dynamic system is a modular system, when there is a problem in long segment stabilization, only the revision of the problematic segment is sufficient and there is no need to disassemble the entire system.

Conclusion

Within the last 10 years, dynamic systems have become much better. Dynamic systems are routinely used for chronic instabilities, single-level instabilities, and two-level instabilities in authors' clinic. Technological advances, diversity in material usage and different designs will increase the use of dynamic systems in patients with multilevel instabilities and deformity surgery.

Pearl

Dynamic stabilization is a newly developing technology and better developments and indications will emerge in the future.

References

1. Graf H. Lumbar instability. Surgical treatment without fusion. Rachis 1992;412:123–137
2. Kanayama M, Hashimoto T, Shigenobu K, Togawa D, Oha F. A minimum 10-year follow-up of posterior dynamic stabilization using Graf artificial ligament. Spine 2007;32(18):1992–1996, discussion 1997
3. Dubois G, de Germay B, Schaerer NS, Fennema P. Dynamic neutralization: a new concept for restabilization of the spine. In: Szpalski M, Gunzburg R, Pope MH, eds. Lumbar segmental instability. Philadelphia, PA: Lippincott Williams and Wilkins; 1999:233–240
4. FDA.gov. FDA Executive Summary for Zimmer Spine's Dynesys Spinal System; 2009. http://www.fda.gov/downloads/advisorycommittees/committeesmeetingmaterials/medicaldevices/medicaldevicesadvisorycommittee/orthopaedicandrehabilitationdevicespanel/ucm188734.pd
5. von Strempel A, Moosmann D, Stoss C, et al. Stabilization of the degenerated lumbar spine in the nonfusion technique with Cosmic posterior dynamic system. WSJ 2006;1(1):40–47
6. Sengupta DK, Herkowitz HN. Pedicle screw-based posterior dynamic stabilization: literature review. Adv Orthop 2012;2012:424268
7. Ozer AF, Oktenoglu T, Egemen E, et al. Lumbar single-level dynamic stabilization with semi-rigid and full dynamic systems: a retrospective clinical and radiological analysis of 71 patients. Clin Orthop Surg 2017;9(3):310–316
8. Oktenoglu T, Erbulut DU, Kiapour A, et al. Pedicle screw-based posterior dynamic stabilisation of the lumbar spine: in vitro cadaver investigation and a finite element study. Comput Methods Biomech Biomed Engin 2015;18(11):1252–1261
9. Kaner T, Sasani M, Oktenoglu T, Ozer AF. Dynamic stabilization of the spine: a new classification system. Turk Neurosurg 2010;20(2):205–215
10. Sasani M, Aydin AL, Oktenoglu T, et al. The combined use of a posterior dynamic transpedicular stabilization system and a prosthetic disc nucleus device in treating lumbar degenerative disc disease with disc herniations. SAS J 2008;2(3):130–136
11. Schmoelz W, Huber JF, Nydegger T, Dipl-Ing, Claes L, Wilke HJ. Dynamic stabilization of the lumbar spine and its effects on adjacent segments: an in vitro experiment. J Spinal Disord Tech 2003;16(4):418–423
12. Kiapour A, Ambati D, Hoy RW, Goel VK. Effect of graded facetectomy on biomechanics of Dynesys dynamic stabilization system. Spine 2012;37(10):E581–E589
13. Niosi CA, Zhu QA, Wilson DC, Keynan O, Wilson DR, Oxland TR. Biomechanical characterization of the three-dimensional kinematic behaviour of the Dynesys dynamic stabilization system: an in vitro study. Eur Spine J 2006;15(6):913–922
14. Erbulut DU, Kiapour A, Oktenoglu T, Ozer AF, Goel VK. A computational biomechanical investigation of posterior dynamic instrumentation: combination of dynamic rod and hinged (dynamic) screw. J Biomech Eng 2014;136(5):051007

15. Schmoelz W, Onder U, Martin A, von Strempel A. Non-fusion instrumentation of the lumbar spine with a hinged pedicle screw rod system: an in vitro experiment. Eur Spine J 2009;18(10):1478–1485
16. Bozkuş H, Senoğlu M, Baek S, et al. Dynamic lumbar pedicle screw-rod stabilization: in vitro biomechanical comparison with standard rigid pedicle screw-rod stabilization. J Neurosurg Spine 2010;12(2):183–189
17. Schaeren S, Broger I, Jeanneret B. Minimum four-year follow-up of spinal stenosis with degenerative spondylolisthesis treated with decompression and dynamic stabilization. Spine 2008;33(18):E636–E642
18. Kuo CH, Chang PY, Wu JC, et al. Dynamic stabilization for L4–5 spondylolisthesis: comparison with minimally invasive transforaminal lumbar interbody fusion with more than 2 years of follow-up. Neurosurg Focus 2016;40(1):E3
19. Yang M, Li C, Chen Z, Bai Y, Li M. Short-term outcome of posterior dynamic stabilization system in degenerative lumbar diseases. Indian J Orthop 2014;48(6):574–581
20. Huang YJ, Zhao SJ, Zhang Q, Nong LM, Xu NW. Comparison of lumbar pedicular dynamic stabilisation systems versus fusion for the treatment of lumbar degenerative disc disease: a meta-analysis. Acta Orthop Belg 2017;83(1):180–193
21. Canbay S, Aydin AL, Aktas E, et al. Posterior dynamic stabilization for the treatment of patients with lumbar degenerative disc disease: long-term clinical and radiological results. Turk Neurosurg 2013;23(2):188–197
22. Maleci A, Sambale RD, Schiavone M, Lamp F, Özer F, von Strempel A. Nonfusion stabilization of the degenerative lumbar spine. J Neurosurg Spine 2011;15(2):151–158
23. Yang JS, Cho YJ, Kang SH, Choi HJ. Dynamic radiographic results of different semi-rigid fusion devices for degenerative lumbar spondylolisthesis: "dynamic rod" versus "dynamic screw head". Turk Neurosurg 2016; 26(2):268–273
24. Maserati MB, Tormenti MJ, Panczykowski DM, Bonfield CM, Gerszten PC. The use of a hybrid dynamic stabilization and fusion system in the lumbar spine: preliminary experience. Neurosurg Focus 2010;28(6):E2
25. Kashkoush A, Agarwal N, Paschel E, Goldschmidt E, Gerszten PC. Evaluation of a hybrid dynamic stabilization and fusion system in the lumbar spine: a 10 year experience. Cureus 2016;8(6):e637
26. Mashaly H, Paschel EE, Khattar NK, Goldschmidt E, Gerszten PC. Posterior lumbar dynamic stabilization instead of arthrodesis for symptomatic adjacent-segment degenerative stenosis: description of a novel technique. Neurosurg Focus 2016;40(1):E5
27. Fay LY, Chang CC, Chang HK, et al. A hybrid dynamic stabilization and fusion system in multilevel lumbar spondylosis. Neurospine 2018;15(3):231–241
28. Herren C, Sobottke R, Pishnamaz M, et al. The use of the DTO™ hybrid dynamic device: a clinical outcome- and radiological-based prospective clinical trial. BMC Musculoskelet Disord 2018;19(1):199
29. Kim CH, Chung CK, Jahng TA. Comparisons of outcomes after single or multilevel dynamic stabilization: effects on adjacent segment. J Spinal Disord Tech 2011;24(1):60–67
30. Akyoldas G, Yilmaz A, Aydin AL, et al. High infection rates in patients with long-segment Dynesys system. World Neurosurg 2018;119:e403–e406
31. Cakir B, Ulmar B, Koepp H, Huch K, Puhl W, Richter M. Posterior dynamic stabilization as an alternative for dorso-ventral fusion in spinal stenosis with degenerative instability. Z Orthop Ihre Grenzgeb 2003;141(4):418–424
32. Grob D, Benini A, Junge A, Mannion AF. Clinical experience with the Dynesys semirigid fixation system for the lumbar spine: surgical and patient-oriented outcome in 50 cases after an average of 2 years. Spine 2005;30(3):324–331
33. Haddad B, Makki D, Konan S, Park D, Khan W, Okafor B. Dynesys dynamic stabilization: less good outcome than lumbar fusion at 4-year follow-up. Acta Orthop Belg 2013;79(1): 97–103
34. Würgler-Hauri CC, Kalbarczyk A, Wiesli M, Landolt H, Fandino J. Dynamic neutralization of the lumbar spine after microsurgical decompression in acquired lumbar spinal stenosis and segmental instability. Spine 2008;33(3):E66–E72
35. Ciplak NM, Suzer T, Senturk S, et al. Complications of 2-level dynamic stabilization: a correlative clinical and radiological analysis at two-year follow-up on 103 patients. Turk Neurosurg 2018;28(5): 756–762
36. Putzier M, Hoff E, Tohtz S, Gross C, Perka C, Strube P. Dynamic stabilization adjacent to single-level fusion: part II. No clinical benefit for asymptomatic, initially degenerated

adjacent segments after 6 years follow-up. Eur Spine J 2010;19(12):2181–2189

37. Landi A. Elastic resistance of the spine: why does motion preservation surgery almost fail? World J Clin Cases 2013;1(4):134–139
38. Pham MH, Mehta VA, Patel NN, et al. Complications associated with the Dynesys dynamic stabilization system: a comprehensive review of the literature. Neurosurg Focus 2016;40(1):E2
39. Park H, Zhang HY, Cho BY, Park JY. Change of lumbar motion after multi-level posterior dynamic stabilization with bioflex system: 1 year follow up. J Korean Neurosurg Soc 2009;46(4):285–291
40. Di Silvestre M, Lolli F, Bakaloudis G, Parisini P. Dynamic stabilization for degenerative lumbar scoliosis in elderly patients. Spine 2010;35(2):227–234
41. Di Silvestre M, Lolli F, Bakaloudis G. Degenerative lumbar scoliosis in elderly patients: dynamic stabilization without fusion versus posterior instrumented fusion. Spine J 2014;14(1):1–10
42. Di Silvestre M, Lolli F, Greggi T, Vommaro F, Baioni A. Adult's degenerative scoliosis: midterm results of dynamic stabilization without fusion in elderly patients—is it effective? Adv Orthop 2013;2013:365059
43. Lee SE, Jahng TA, Kim HJ. Decompression and nonfusion dynamic stabilization for spinal stenosis with degenerative lumbar scoliosis: Clinical article. J Neurosurg Spine 2014;21(4):585–594
44. Oktenoglu T, Ozer AF. Dynamic and dynamic-hybrid instrumentation in deformity surgery. Turk Neurosurg 2014;24(Suppl 1):84–97
45. Ozer AF, Cevik OM, Erbulut DU, et al. A novel modular dynamic stabilization system for the treatment of degenerative spinal pathologies. Turk Neurosurg 2019;29(1):115–120

22 Innovative Techniques for Treating Scoliosis

Yousuf Shaikh, Onur Yaman, and Salman Sharif

Introduction

Traditional scoliosis surgery has evolved over the past few decades. Paul Harrington introduced spinal instrumentation to treat scoliosis in 1960 (1). As technology advanced with our understanding, more sophisticated techniques were developed to address scoliosis surgery including pedicle screws and neuromonitoring. As scoliosis surgery has its share of complications, some less invasive methods have been devised to address deformity correction.

Magnetically Controlled Growing Rods (MCGR)

This represents one of the most advanced and less invasive techniques employed to treat early-onset scoliosis (EOS). A remotely distracting magnetic rod is used to allow frequent distractions in outpatients. Theoretically, it reduces the number of surgical procedures as well as the burden of repeated surgeries in patients with EOS. Clinical and radiological results of these surgeries have also shown promising results.[2–4]

The system consists of a distracting titanium rod with a slightly dilated chamber in the middle. This expansion chamber houses the lengthening mechanism. Whether to use one rod or two depends on the patients' clinical and radiological factors and surgeons' preference. The rod's size depends on the patient's height and anticipated distraction that may be required over time.

The procedure is carried out under general anesthesia, and like any other form of correction, prone positioning is done on a radiolucent spinal table. Two small incisions are given at the cranial and caudal most levels of scoliosis that require fixation with pedicle screws. Four pedicle screws are then placed at the proximal and distal end of scoliosis using standard techniques. This can be achieved by intraoperative use of fluoroscopy or with the help of intraoperative computed tomography (CT). A surgeon must try to use the largest screw possible to achieve a good purchase. The rod of the desired length is then passed subfacially and connected to proximal and distal anchors. In circumstances where two rods are being used, a standard rod is used on one side and an offset rod on the other side. It is important to keep the lengthening mechanism of the offset rod in the opposite direction to that of the standard rod. This helps prevent the rod controlling mechanism of one rod from interfering with the other and allows easy independent control. The fixation points are well fused by decorticating the transverse processes and placing bone graft or substitute. Postprocedure, the patient is generally kept in the brace for 3 to 4 months. Postprocedure distractions vary depending on the degree of scoliosis, height growth rate, and degree of correction required. In most circumstances, distractions are carried out on a monthly basis. The brace is removed during distractions and reapplied after. However, there are no uniform criteria for the lengthening procedure. But a generally acceptable method is to lengthen the rod as per normal spinal growth rates of healthy children of comparable age. The frequency of distractions may vary from every month to once every 3 months, followed both clinically and radiologically. Important radiological parameters to be followed include the Cobb's angle, initial and distracted rod length, T1 to T12, and T1 to S1 spinal height. Generally, it is recommended that a single surgeon on every visit does lengthening, but two independent consultants should do a radiological assessment to reduce bias.

Cheung et al in 2012 published one of the earliest results of MCGR in two patients with EOS who were followed for 24 months.[3] His patients had syndromic scoliosis and significantly improved major spinal curves postop (mean angle 57 degrees). One patient had to undergo revision surgery attributed to device malfunction leading to loss of distraction. The same patient also suffered from a wound infection which was treated medically. In 2013, Dannawi et al published his series of 34 patients. He followed them for 12 months and reported a mean spinal correction of 41%.[5] However, eight of his patients developed complications, out of which six required revision due to loss of distraction, rod fracture, or hook pullout. Similar results were achieved by Akbarnia et al in 2013. He followed 14 patients for 10 months with an average spinal correction of 48%.[4] Ridderbusch et al reported better results in 24 patients with a mean follow-up of 12 months.[6] He reported a mean spinal correction up to 50%, which was higher than most previously published studies. His better radiological outcomes was attributed to the fact that all patients were treated with dual rods and all curves were flexible. These results were also comparable to those described for conventional growing rods techniques.[7]

Physiologically, Noordeen et al[8] demonstrated that the force required to achieve progressive rod distraction does not remain constant in the traditional growing rod (TGR) technique and therefore tends to increase after repeated lengthening. The length obtained at each procedure has a decreasing tendency. Sankar and colleagues proposed a law of diminishing returns whereby the average T1–S1 gain achieved by one surgical lengthening decreases substantially with repeated distractions.[9] Therefore, if we apply the same principle to MCGR, the inability to recognize this limitation and attempting to distract beyond what the spine would tolerate would result in trauma or, more likely, implant failure. The exact cause for such phenomenon is not known but one possible explanation is the progressive stiffness of the immature spine with age and long-term instrumentation which lead to decrease in length gain over time. This phenomenon has been referred to as autofusion. Therefore, frequent distractions of smaller size is likely to avoid these complications, whereas infrequent distractions of larger size can cause sudden instrument failure or spinal fracture. However, the available literature shows no difference in outcome between monthly small distractions over 2 to 3 monthly slightly higher distractions.[4,5,10]

One of the main advantages of MCGR systems is cost-effectiveness. Although the initial implant cost of the magnetic rod is much higher than conventional rods, there are significant cost savings in repeated hospital admissions and surgery costs.[11] Furthermore, less frequent hospital admissions will also have a lesser psychological impact on children and their parents. In terms of complications, Kwan et al, in a systemic review, quoted a complication rate of 46.7% with MCGR,[12] whereas Bess et al[13] reported a complication rate of 58% with TGR. Overall, the number of unplanned revision surgeries remain more or less the same for both MCGR group and TGR technique.[14] Proximal junctional kyphosis (PJK) is another common complication seen using MCGR systems.[15] PJK is a serious complication that can have a significant impact on patients' quality of life and overall clinical outcome. In most circumstances, PJK requires a revision surgery to be addressed.[16] An estimated 56% incidence of PJK has been reported by Lee et al in a series of 32 children with standard growing rods with a minimum follow-up of 24 months.[17]

One of the factors which could possibly contribute to PJK is the inability to appropriately correct the sagittal contour with magnetically growing rods. The position and length of the magnetic actuator limits the amount of sagittal contour correction which can be achieved, particularly if it is not located at the thoracolumbar area. Furthermore, the actuator may occasionally lie at the apex of scoliosis, where bending the rod is not possible. This, in turn, affects the sagittal alignment and leads to PJK. Hypothetically, developing a new rod system with a smaller actuator may solve the issue in the coming future. Still, until now, all cases of PJK following placement of MCGR require revision surgery with some form of osteotomy and proximal level instrumentation. Another concern that needs attention is the ability to decide whether one or two MCGR are required. In the TGR technique, dual rods have been shown to provide better stable construct than the single rod, with more stability and better spine control,[18] but until now, no consensus has been devised indicating superiority of one method over the other. However, because of the relatively superficial placement of these large bulky rods, single rods are preferred in thin, lean individuals to avoid significant discomfort.

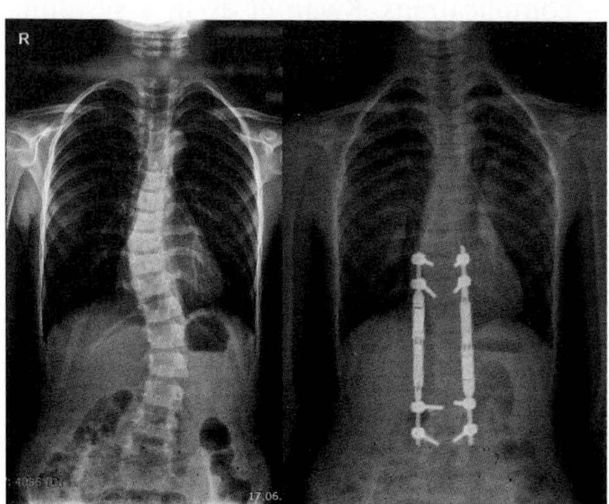

Fig. 22.1 (a) Preoperative scoliosis radiograph and (b) first-year control scoliosis radiograph.

Another significant concern about the use of MCGR is the amount of radiation exposure. Every patient distraction is followed by an X-ray as there are unexplainable disparities between the actual and predicted distraction lengths. Once such factors have been eliminated, radiation exposure can be significantly minimized. Recently a new method utilizing ultrasound waves have been developed to control rod lengthening, thereby reducing the risk of radiation-induced diseases.[19]

In conclusion, the use of MCGR allows less invasive, cheap, and good correction of EOS while reducing the number of surgeries with comparable complications to that of TGR. MCGR can be safely done as primary or revision surgery. Although the technique is still at its primitive stage, provisional results seem to be promising. Since the procedure comes at its learning curve, we postulate that with time, MCGR will become a much safer and better alternative to TGR.

Case Examples

Case 1

A patient with progressive scoliosis diagnosed with Marfan syndrome (**Fig. 22.1a, b**).

Case 2

Applying a growing rod in a patient with unilateral block vertebrae (**Fig. 22.2a, b**).

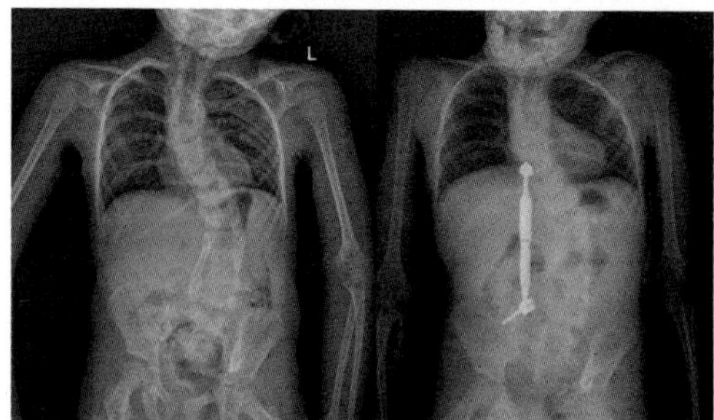

Fig. 22.2 (a) Preoperative scoliosis radiograph and (b) sixth-month control scoliosis radiograph.

Pearls

- Theoretically, MCGR reduces the number of surgical procedures and lessens the burden of repeated surgeries in patients with EOS.
- Less invasive, cheap, and good correction.
- Reduces the number of surgeries.

Vertebral Body Tethering (VBT)

Scoliosis remains a common disease in pediatric patients. Posterior spinal fusion has been the primary surgical treatment option with proven long-term successful outcomes for many years. Adolescent spinal fusion has drawbacks such as restricted growth and mobility and an increased chance of early neighboring segment disease. Also, the need for growth and motion sparing strategies to address EOS has led to the introduction of many successful nonfusion methods. One such effective method is known as VBT, which was first studied in animal models by Newton et al.[20] He observed that a unilateral tether in porcine could induce a curve in the growing spine while retaining flexibility. Similar results were also shown by Braun et al[21] in a goat spine, indicating the safety and reproducibility of this procedure in humans. VBT was created to control spinal growth by inhibiting unilateral growth plates using the Hueter-Volkmann principle.[22,23] Manual full curve correction, occasionally also referred to as nonfusion anterior scoliosis correction, can be performed in patients approaching skeletal maturity.

The procedure is carried out under complete anesthesia, and the patient is positioned laterally with the curved side up. During the entire procedure, sensory- and motor-evoked potentials (IONM) are monitored. Single lung ventilation is carried out, and bolsters are placed to reduce the curve during positioning (**Fig. 22.3**). The majority of surgeons from this point perform the procedure thoracoscopically using three small ports. However, a minithoracotomy can also be done for the placement of bicortical screws. Another possible approach is to give a 10 cm flank incision to access retroperitoneal area in order to address thoracolumbar and lumbar curves. Three 5 mm working ports are created mimicking the shape of a triangle with the apex located at the fifth intercostal space in the anterior axillary line and the base formed from two ports in the midaxillary line, one in the third intercostal space, and the other in the eighth intercostal space (**Fig. 22.4**). A 30 degree camera is passed through one port, a harmonic scalpel in the second, and an endoscopic peanut in the final port. The spine is marked under thoracoscopic imaging, and an AP image is obtained to confirm the desired spinal level. Segmental vessels are coagulated while following any changes observed in neuromonitoring. The parietal pleura is then incised over the vertebral bodies just anterior to the rib head along the length of

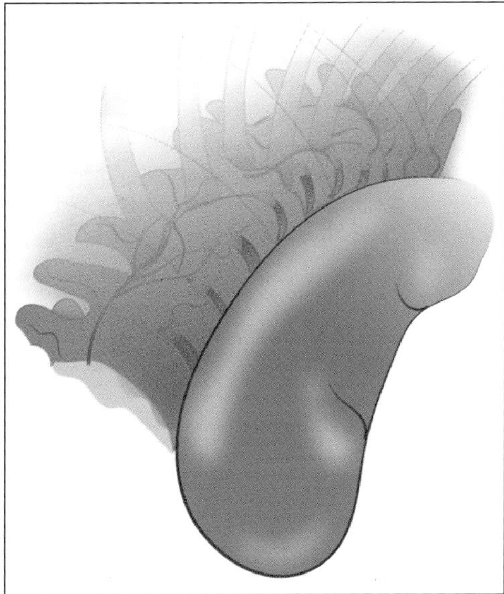

Fig. 22.3 The lung on the convex side of the curvature of the spine is deflated.

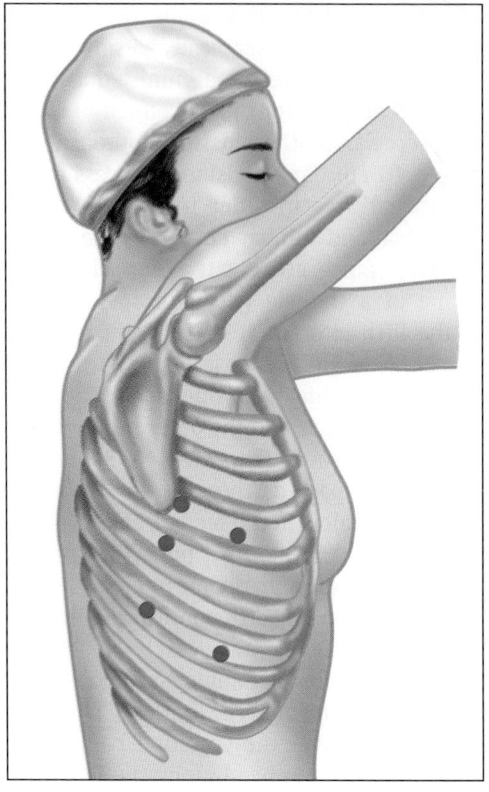

Fig. 22.4 Lateral decubitus position and incision points.

the curve. Extreme care is taken to protect the disc spaces. Positioning of the patient and the number of vertebras requiring fixation are then checked with the fluoroscope.

A straight blunt pedicle finder is advanced through the vertebral body under biplanar fluoroscopic guidance and across the contralateral cortex. A screw hole is then tapped while aiming for the contralateral rib head. After determining the desired screw length, a screw is placed, and the final position is confirmed again with a fluoroscope. The screw is put in a bicortical fashion, with no more than 2- to 3-mm protrusion allowed. Subsequent screws are placed in a similar fashion (**Fig. 22.5a, b**). Sometimes an additional port needs to be created if the surgeon is working on a longer construct. But generally speaking, a port in one intercostal space can be effectively used to place three screws. Once all the screws are in place, a tether is then passed through the tulips of the screws, starting from the most inferior screw and proceeding proximally. The tether, which is usually made up of polyethylene terephthalate, is then subsequently tightened, starting from the apex of the curve in

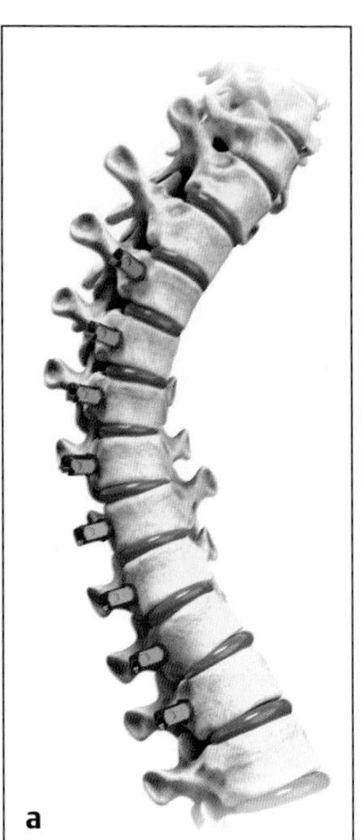

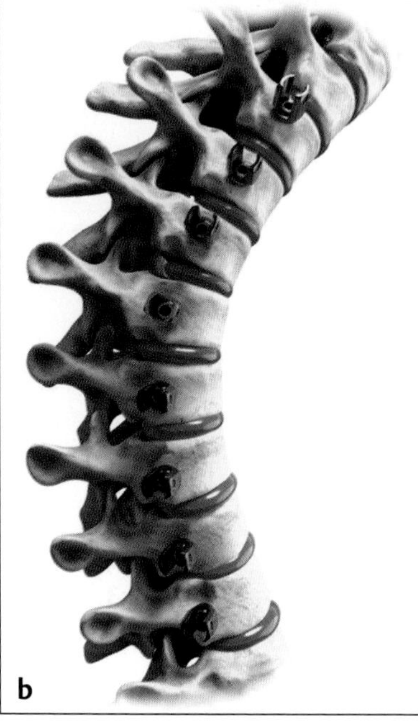

Fig. 22.5 **(a, b)** Screws are placed sequentially from the convex side at the midpoint of the vertebral corpus. **(a)** Front view; **(b)** lateral view.

a way that deformity is gradually corrected (**Fig. 22.6**). Adequate correction of the curve is confirmed in a coronal place under a fluoroscope (**Fig. 22.7a, b**). Once the screws are parallel and deformity is corrected, set screws are placed to lock the tether in the desired position. The tether is then cut at the proximal and distal end, leaving just about 2 to 3 cm residual to allow subsequent adjustment when needed. The thorax is irrigated with saline, and a chest tube is left in place. Occasionally some surgeons would approximate the parietal pleura, but this is usually difficult and not required. The lung is then expanded, and ports are closed in layers. Postoperatively, patients are often kept in the brace for 3 to 6 months.

Crawford and Lenke performed the first case of anterior vertebral body tethering (AVBT) in 2010 in a child who failed brace therapy.[24] Samdani et al was one of the first to present his case series of 11 patients who underwent AVBT.[25] His patients had an average of 31-degree postoperative correction at 2-year follow-up. Similarly, Newton et al published 2 years results of his 17 patients who demonstrated comparable improvements.[26] However, both these studies were performed for thoracic curves only. They did not take into consideration thoracolumbar curves. Hoernschemeyer et al did a retrospective review of 29 patients who underwent AVBT.[27] He categorized his patients into five different categories depending on the location of the curve. The structural curve and both compensatory curves demonstrated continued postoperative correction at follow-up. Patients with a thoracic tether and a lumbar brace also showed similar improvements postoperatively in both thoracic and lumbar curves. Somewhat similar trends were observed in patients with left thoracolumbar curves and large main thoracic and lumbar curves treated with a thoracic and lumbar tether. Patients with long thoracic curves represent a slightly different entity. These individuals require a longer tether. Newton had to add

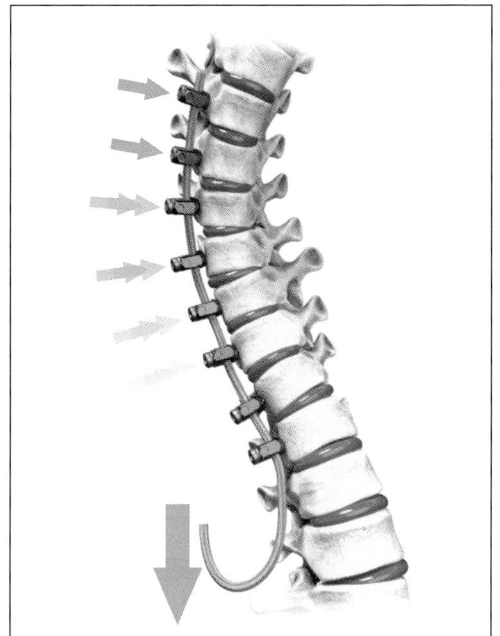

Fig. 22.6 The tension from the cord straightens the patient's spine.

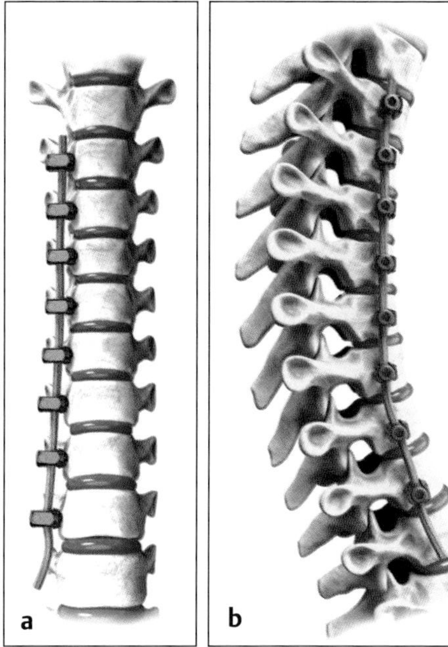

Fig. 22.7 **(a, b)** After the patient's spine is straightened. **(a)** Front view; **(b)** lateral view.

an additional level of tethering to one of his patients with long thoracic curve.[26] One of the largest studies was conducted by Miyanji et al in 2020.[28] Fifty-six of his patients with idiopathic scoliosis underwent AVBT, of which 16 developed complications and 8 required revision surgery. Patients continued to demonstrate progressive curve correction in the follow-up period, establishing that the growth is modified. This technique is an effective technique to address immature skeletons. Animal studies have shown that physeal growth arrests due to compressive forces and accelerates due to distractive forces acting across a growth plate.[29] Stokes also proved on rat tail with asymmetric loading indicating that there is no injury to healthy discs with tethering.[30]

As stated before, AVBT continues to correct deformity with progressive growth of the child. Samdani, in his first series of 11 patients,[25] achieved a mean improvement in coronal deformity from 40.9 to 20.1 degrees postoperatively. At 2-year follow-up, a further correction of 13.5 degrees was achieved. In another study by the same author, he achieved a mean 66 degree correction in 25 patients.[31] The progressive corrective nature of a tether is not always beneficial for the patient. With time, overcorrection can occur, which may require revision surgery. Samdani had an overcorrection in 2 of his 11 patients, which required revision surgery.[25] One of the factors that was retrospectively identified to prevent overcorrection in the future was to perform undercorrection in the immediate postop phase. Because it was not postulated to what extent the immature spine will grow, good corrections achieved immediate postop continued to correct and eventually progressed to overcorrection. Accurate prediction of spine correction remains a difficult task, but in general, young patients with significant growth potential should undergo less correction. Overcorrection of more than 10 degrees is considered as an arbitrary limit beyond which revision surgery is indicated. A broken tether is another complication that needs to be identified as tethers are not routinely picked up on radiographs. Most broken tethers are identified with progressive loss of correction. Baroncini et al were the first to analyze AVBT and address the learning curve associated with it.[32] He reported significant improvement in screw placement time, blood loss per screw, and surgery time between the first 20 and last 20 patients. Although the final results were not different from the first and last 20 patients, the authors believed that the surgical technique and patient selection procedure became much more refined, resulting in a reduced number of complications.

AVBT has gained significant attention because of its good corrective properties. However, more specific patient selection is required. Currently, AVBT is indicated in patients with the immature spine with thoracic curves ranging between 35 and 60 degrees.[25] Skeletal maturity is usually assessed by means of various grades, with Riser sign (≤2) and Sanders score (≤4) being the most commonly used ones. Although these are general guidelines, exceptions can occur subjective to different ages, races, and heights. Absolute contradiction to AVBT include thoracic hyperkyphosis exceeding 40 degrees and a rotational prominence more than 20 degrees.[25]

In conclusion, tethering is best suited for patients who are in or just after the curve acceleration phase of growth. Thoracic curves have shown better outcomes and more predictability than patients with relatively more immature spine with lumbar curves. Furthermore, since the majority of curve correction is achieved intraoperatively, it creates a difficult task of postulating postoperative growth modulation over time. AVBT represents an innovative and effective new technology for correcting EOS that can fill a niche for patients with adolescent idiopathic scoliosis (AIS) seeking fusionless correction of their curves.

Case Example

An 11-year-old girl with progressive AIS (**Fig. 22.8a, b**).

Pearls

- VBT was created to control spinal growth by inhibiting unilateral growth plates using the Hueter-Volkmann principle.
- The main benefit is that it has a logic that allows for flexible movements without fusing.
- Long-term effects have yet to be characterized, making optimal patient selection critical.

Vertebral Body Stapling (VBS)

VBS is a procedure that involves placement of C-shaped Nitinol staples to compress one side of the disc space achieving correction in the coronal plane. The technique works similarly to that of VBT.

The technique involves lateral positioning of the patient with the convex side up after general anesthesia. Various bolsters are used to correct the deformity as much as possible. Single lung ventilation is carried out, and thoracoscopic ports are generally created in the anterior axillary line. After confirming the level under a fluoroscope, a trial staple is used and placed across the disc space involving the upper and lower end plate. The staple should be placed anterior to the rib head. Once the trial staple size is confirmed, it is used to make pilot holes and then removed. Then a permanent staple is used to compress the ipsilateral end plates. The staple can also be pushed to get a better purchase while simultaneously correcting the deformity and locking it in place. The optimal position is again confirmed fluoroscopically, and staple is impacted into the vertebral body. If the staple is not flush with disc space, then it is impacted further until it does. If VBS extends to involve the lumbar levels, then a retroperitoneal approach is indicated for staple placement. Postoperatively these patients are kept in a brace for 6 weeks. VBS is effective in scoliotic curves only up to 35 degrees. Beyond this arbitrary division, VBT is the recommended procedure. The procedure was first proposed in 1951, but the results were quite disappointing.[33]

Since then, various changes have been made, and the recent introduction of Nitinol staples has significantly improved the safety and efficacy of VBS. The staples are strong and provide effective compression of the

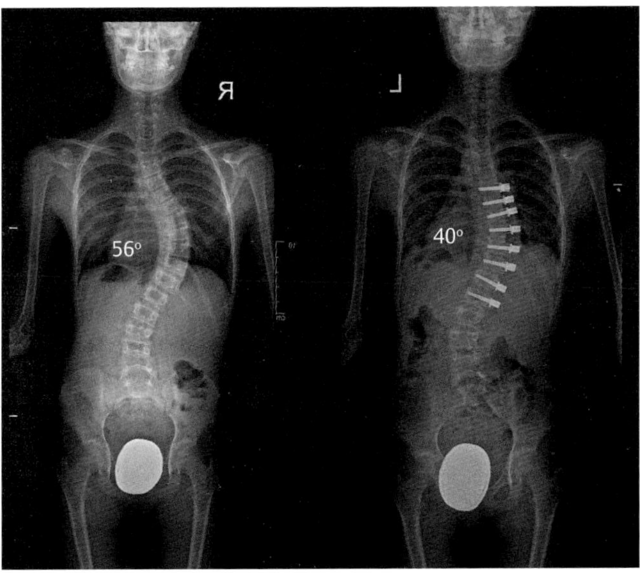

Fig. 22.8 **(a)** Preoperative scoliosis radiograph and **(b)** early control scoliosis radiograph.

ipsilateral growth plate while resisting breakage and pullout. Betz et al have demonstrated the Nitinol staples' feasibility, safety, and utility in AIS.[34] In another study, Betz et al published his results of VBS in 39 patients, of whom 87% demonstrated significant coronal stability at 1-year follow-up.[35] Cuddihy et al prospectively followed 42 patients treated with VBS and compared them to traditional brace therapy.[36] His results showed that patients with VBS achieved 81% correction compared to 61% of brace therapy. Based on his observations, he concluded that suitable candidates for VBS included girls less than 13 years and boys less than 15 years, Sanders score less than 5, and thoracic curves less than 35 degrees. Murray et al performed VBS in seven patients and followed them for 7 years to assess curve correction, progression, and growth across the stapled and nonstapled vertebra.[37] His results showed no difference in growth between the stapled and nonstapled vertebral bodies. The development of the instrumented vertebral bodies has also been compared with the growth of adjacent vertebral bodies. These statements contradict the growth-modulating effect on the spine after fixation as proposed by Stokes.[30] Because the sample size in this particular study was small and VBS represents a relatively new technique, the cause leading to such a phenomenon cannot be explained entirely; however, some theories have been proposed.

In conclusion, the results of VBS are comparable to brace therapy. However, larger studies are required to validate the long-term safety and efficacy of VBS.

Pearls

- VBS is a procedure that involves the placement of C-shaped Nitinol staples to compress one side of the disc space achieving.
- The technique works in a similar fashion to that of VBT.

Conclusion

As technological advancements drive us toward less invasive techniques, we should appreciate the struggles of our predecessors and utilize the basic principles to build upon existing techniques of instrumentation and scoliosis correction. Since the last decade has shown tremendous innovation in scoliosis correction, we can only postulate what the future holds.

The innovations have already been there, starting from the ancient Indian times when traction was applied to correct deformities to the AVCENNA (SINA 980–1037 AD), who is known as one of the first doctors who developed instruments to correct spinal deformity, to nonoperative bracing casting and traction of the modern era, to present day innovation of thoracoscopic and minimally invasive surgery to correct deformity

References

1. Dickson JH, Harrington PR. The evolution of the Harrington instrumentation technique in scoliosis. J Bone Joint Surg Am 1973;55(5): 993–1002
2. Akbarnia BA, Cheung K, Noordeen H, et al. Next generation of growth-sparing techniques: preliminary clinical results of a magnetically controlled growing rod in 14 patients with early-onset scoliosis. Spine 2013;38(8): 665–670
3. Cheung KM-C, Cheung JP-Y, Samartzis D, et al. Magnetically controlled growing rods for severe spinal curvature in young children: a prospective case series. Lancet 2012; 379(9830):1967–1974
4. Akbarnia BA, Mundis GM Jr, Salari P, Yaszay B, Pawelek JB. Innovation in growing rod technique: a study of safety and efficacy of a magnetically controlled growing rod in a porcine model. Spine 2012;37(13):1109–1114
5. Dannawi Z, Altaf F, Harshavardhana NS, El Sebaie H, Noordeen H. Early results of a remotely-operated magnetic growth rod in early-onset scoliosis. Bone Joint J 2013; 95-B(1):75–80

6. Ridderbusch K, Rupprecht M, Kunkel P, Hagemann C, Stücker R. Preliminary results of magnetically controlled growing rods for early-onset scoliosis. J Pediatr Orthop 2017;37(8):e575–e580
7. Akbarnia BA, Marks DS, Boachie-Adjei O, Thompson AG, Asher MA. Dual growing rod technique for the treatment of progressive early-onset scoliosis: a multicenter study. Spine 2005; 30(17, Suppl):S46–S57
8. Noordeen HM, Shah SA, Elsebaie HB, Garrido E, Farooq N, Al-Mukhtar M. In vivo distraction force and length measurements of growing rods: which factors influence the ability to lengthen? Spine 2011;36(26):2299–2303
9. Sankar WN, Skaggs DL, Yazici M, et al. Lengthening of dual growing rods and the law of diminishing returns. Spine 2011; 36(10):806–809
10. Hickey BA, Towriss C, Baxter G, et al. Early experience of MAGEC magnetic growing rods in the treatment of early onset scoliosis. Eur Spine J 2014; 23(1, Suppl 1):S61–S65
11. Rolton D, Richards J, Nnadi C. Magnetic controlled growth rods versus conventional growing rod systems in the treatment of early onset scoliosis: a cost comparison. Eur Spine J 2015;24(7):1457–1461
12. Kwan KYH, Alanay A, Yazici M, et al. Unplanned reoperations in magnetically controlled growing rod surgery for early onset scoliosis with a minimum of two-year follow-up. Spine 2017;42(24):E1410–E1414
13. Bess S, Akbarnia BA, Thompson GH, et al. Complications of growing-rod treatment for early-onset scoliosis: analysis of one hundred and forty patients. J Bone Joint Surg Am 2010;92(15):2533–2543
14. Akbarnia BA, Pawelek JB, Cheung KMC, et al; Growing Spine Study Group. Traditional growing rods versus magnetically controlled growing rods for the surgical treatment of early-onset scoliosis: a case-matched 2-year study. Spine Deform 2014;2(6):493–497
15. Glattes RC, Bridwell KH, Lenke LG, Kim YJ, Rinella A, Edwards C II. Proximal junctional kyphosis in adult spinal deformity following long instrumented posterior spinal fusion: incidence, outcomes, and risk factor analysis. Spine 2005;30(14):1643–1649
16. Shah SA, Karatas AF, Dhawale AA, et al; Growing Spine Study Group. The effect of serial growing rod lengthening on the sagittal profile and pelvic parameters in early-onset scoliosis. Spine 2014;39(22):E1311–E1317
17. Lee C, Myung KS, Skaggs DL. Proximal junctional kyphosis in distraction-based growing rods: Paper# 48. LWW; 2011:79–80
18. Thompson GH, Akbarnia BA, Campbell RM Jr. Growing rod techniques in early-onset scoliosis. J Pediatr Orthop 2007;27(3): 354–361
19. Stokes OM, O'Donovan EJ, Samartzis D, Bow CH, Luk KDK, Cheung KMC. Reducing radiation exposure in early-onset scoliosis surgery patients: novel use of ultrasonography to measure lengthening in magnetically-controlled growing rods. Spine J 2014; 14(10):2397–2404
20. Newton PO, Farnsworth CL, Upasani VV, Chambers RC, Varley E, Tsutsui S. Effects of intraoperative tensioning of an anterolateral spinal tether on spinal growth modulation in a porcine model. Spine 2011;36(2):109–117
21. Braun JT, Ogilvie JW, Akyuz E, Brodke DS, Bachus KN. Creation of an experimental idiopathic-type scoliosis in an immature goat model using a flexible posterior asymmetric tether. Spine 2006;31(13):1410–1414
22. Lonner BS, Ren Y, Yaszay B, et al. Evolution of surgery for adolescent idiopathic scoliosis over 20 years: have outcomes improved? Spine 2018;43(6):402–410
23. von Elm E, Altman DG, Egger M, Pocock SJ, Gøtzsche PC, Vandenbroucke JP; STROBE Initiative. The Strengthening the Reporting of Observational Studies in Epidemiology (STROBE) statement: guidelines for reporting observational studies. J Clin Epidemiol 2008; 61(4):344–349
24. Crawford CH III, Lenke LG. Growth modulation by means of anterior tethering resulting in progressive correction of juvenile idiopathic scoliosis: a case report. J Bone Joint Surg Am 2010;92(1):202–209
25. Samdani AF, Ames RJ, Kimball JS, et al. Anterior vertebral body tethering for idio_ pathic scoliosis: two-year results. Spine 2014; 39(20):1688–1693
26. Newton PO, Kluck DG, Saito W, Yaszay B, Bartley CE, Bastrom TP. Anterior spinal growth tethering for skeletally immature patients with scoliosis: a retrospective look two to four years postoperatively. J Bone Joint Surg Am 2018;100(19):1691–1697
27. Hoernschemeyer DG, Boeyer ME, Robertson ME, et al. Anterior vertebral body tethering for adolescent scoliosis with growth remaining: a retrospective review of 2 to 5-year postoperative results. J Bone Joint Surg Am 2020;102(13):1169–1176

28. Miyanji F, Pawelek J, Nasto LA, Rushton P, Simmonds A, Parent S. Safety and efficacy of anterior vertebral body tethering in the treatment of idiopathic scoliosis. Bone Joint J 2020;102-B(12):1703–1708
29. Stokes IAF, Spence H, Aronsson DD, Kilmer N. Mechanical modulation of vertebral body growth. Implications for scoliosis progression. Spine 1996;21(10):1162–1167
30. Stokes IAF, Aronsson DD, Spence H, Iatridis JC. Mechanical modulation of intervertebral disc thickness in growing rat tails. J Spinal Disord 1998;11(3):261–265
31. Samdani AF, Ames RJ, Kimball JS, et al. Anterior vertebral body tethering for immature adolescent idiopathic scoliosis: one-year results on the first 32 patients. Eur Spine J 2015;24(7):1533–1539
32. Baroncini A, Trobisch PD, Migliorini F. Learning curve for vertebral body tethering: analysis on 90 consecutive patients. Spine Deform 2021;9(1):141–147
33. Smith AD, Von Lackum WH, Wylie R. An operation for stapling vertebral bodies in congenital scoliosis. J Bone Joint Surg Am 1954;36(A:2):342–348
34. Betz RR, Kim J, D'Andrea LP, Mulcahey MJ, Balsara RK, Clements DH. An innovative technique of vertebral body stapling for the treatment of patients with adolescent idiopathic scoliosis: a feasibility, safety, and utility study. Spine 2003; 28(20, 20S): S255–S265
35. Betz RR, D'Andrea LP, Mulcahey MJ, Chafetz RS. Vertebral body stapling procedure for the treatment of scoliosis in the growing child. Clin Orthop Relat Res 2005;(434):55–60
36. Cuddihy L, Danielsson AJ, Cahill PJ, et al. Vertebral body stapling versus bracing for patients with high-risk moderate idiopathic scoliosis. BioMed Res Int 2015;2015: 438–452
37. Murray E, Tung R, Sherman A, Schwend RM. Continued vertebral body growth in patients with juvenile idiopathic scoliosis following vertebral body stapling. Spine Deform 2020;8(2):221–226

Index